Neurology & Psychiatry:

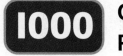 **Questions to Help You Pass the Boards**

Neurology & Psychiatry:

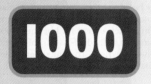 **Questions to Help You Pass the Boards**

Kumar Budur, MD (MS)

Board certified in Psychiatry and Sleep Medicine
Staff Physician
Departments of Psychiatry and Sleep Disorders Center
Assistant Professor in Medicine
Cleveland Clinic Lerner College of Medicine at Case Western
    Reserve University
Cleveland Clinic

Asim Roy, MD

Assistant Clinical Professor
Board Certified in Neurology and Sleep Medicine
Departments of Neurology and Sleep Medicine
University of Pittsburgh Medical Center

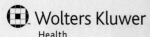 Wolters Kluwer | Lippincott Williams & Wilkins
Health

Philadelphia • Baltimore • New York • London
Buenos Aires • Hong Kong • Sydney • Tokyo

Acquisitions Editor: Frances Destefano
Managing Editor: Leanne McMillan
Marketing Manager: Brian Freiland
Production Editor: Beth Martz
Design Coordinator: Stephen Druding
Compositor: Maryland Composition/ASI

351 West Camden Street   530 Walnut Street
Baltimore, MD 21201   Philadelphia, PA 19106

Printed in China

9 8 7 6 5 4 3 2 1

Library of Congress Cataloging-in-Publication Data

Budur, Kumar.
  Neurology and psychiatry : 1,000 questions to help you pass the boards / Kumar Budur, Asim Roy.
    p. ; cm.
  Includes bibliographical references and index.
  ISBN 978-0-7817-9263-9
  1. Neurology—Examinations, questions, etc. 2. Psychiatry—Examinations, questions, etc. 3. Neurologists—Licenses—United States—Examinations—Study guides. I. Roy, Asim. II. Title.
  [DNLM: 1. Nervous System Diseases—Examination Questions. 2. Mental Disorders—Examination Questions. 3. Neurology—methods—Examination Questions. 4. Psychiatry—methods—Examination Questions. WL 18.2 B927n 2009]
  RC343.5.B83 2009
  616.80076—dc22

                                                                    2008051327

To my brother, Dhanunjaya

KB

To my wife Priya and my parents for
their support and encouragement

AR

Neurology & Psychiatry is written specifically to help neurologists prepare for the American Board of Psychiatry and Neurology Part I examination. This examination is based on the knowledge learned during residency and is based on questions from adult and pediatric neurology as well as psychiatry. Most neurologists who are taking Part I are either in fellowship or active clinical practice and therefore have limited time to study and prepare for the exam. We hope that this book will help Neurologists preparing for Part I of the boards. We also hope that this book will also benefit general neurologists, neurology residents, psychiatry residents, and medical students who are rotating through neurology and psychiatry. Most people can use this book as a self-assessment tool or concise review of high-yield topics.

Preparing for the boards is always an intimidating process to go through. However, all candidates who have completed residency training in neurology and have adequate knowledge should be able to pass the exam. We have attempted to cover all the important topics in a thorough, organized, and systematic way to help save valuable time and sincerely hope that we succeed in our efforts to make the board examination a bit less intimidating.

Kumar Budur, MD (MS)
Asim Roy, MD

Contents

Neurology & Psychiatry:

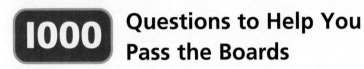 Questions to Help You
Pass the Boards

SECTION

I

Neurology

Anatomy and Physiology

QUESTIONS

1. The diencephalon consists of all of the following structures except:
   A. thalamus
   B. subthalamus
   C. pons
   D. putamen
   E. all of the above

2. Which subclavian artery would you inject with contrast to demonstrate both the carotid and vertebral circulation?
   A. Left subclavian
   B. Right subclavian
   C. Neither, you cannot see both the carotid and vertebral circulation.
   D. Either, you can see both the carotid and vertebral circulation with either subclavian artery.

3. An epidural hemorrhage results in a tear in what vessel?
   A. Bridging veins
   B. Middle meningeal artery
   C. Anterior choroidal artery
   D. None of the above
   E. All of the above

4. Occlusion of which area of the circle of Willis will result in total unilateral blindness?
   A. Ophthalmic artery
   B. Anterior choroidal artery
   C. Vertebral artery
   D. Anterior spinal artery

5. Hemisection of the spinal cord at the level of T1 actually produces contralateral loss of pain/temperature sensation at what level?
   A. T1
   B. T2
   C. T3
   D. C7

6. A 35-year-old male presents with bilateral paralysis, fasciculations, and muscle atrophy at and below T1 along with bilateral pain and temperature loss at the level of T2. What is the cause of his symptoms?
   A. Middle cerebral artery (MCA) stroke
   B. Carbon monoxide poisoning
   C. Syringomyelia
   D. Amyotrophic lateral sclerosis (ALS)
   E. None of the above

7. Common causes of carpal tunnel syndrome include all of the following except:
   A. rheumatoid arthritis
   B. diabetes mellitus
   C. acromegaly
   D. pregnancy
   E. all of the above are possible causes of carpal tunnel syndrome

8. Which one of the following carries the majority of the information from the outside into the cerebellum?
   A. Granule cells
   B. Basket cells
   C. Mossy fibers
   D. Dentate nucleus

9. Dejerine-Roussy syndrome can be associated with?
   A. Lesion in the oculomotor nerve
   B. Lesion in the left occipital lobe
   C. Lesion in the ventral posterior area of the thalamus
   D. Lesion in the lateral geniculate nucleus

10. Klüver-Bucy syndrome is associated with which disease?
    A. Pick's disease
    B. Guillain-Barré syndrome
    C. Grave's disease
    D. Lambert-Eaton syndrome
    E. None of the above

11. A 42-year-old male with a history of alcoholism presents to the hospital with confusion, diplopia (ophthalmoparesis), unsteady gait, and nystagmus. The most likely cause for these symptoms is thiamine deficiency. Where is the lesion?
    A. Edinger-Westphal nucleus
    B. Mamillary bodies
    C. Left parietal lobe
    D. Nucleus solitarius
    E. None of the above

12. Which of the following is true regarding a lesion of the right vestibular nuclei?
    A. The left paramedian pontine reticular formation (PPRF) is more active than the right PPRF.
    B. The fast phase of nystagmus is to the right.
    C. Stumbling to the left
    D. The left lateral vestibulospinal tract is more active than the right.
    E. Slow phase of nystagmus to the left

13. Which of the following statements is not true?
    A. Weakness is the least common sign of a cerebellar lesion.
    B. Golgi cells in the cerebellum lie in the granule cell layer and are excitatory.
    C. Basket cells in the cerebellum excite Purkinje cell firing.
    D. Fastigial nucleus receives input from Purkinje cells in the cerebellum.

14. Which of the following statements is TRUE?
    A. Nerve root C3 exits above vertebra C3.
    B. A C6 radiculopathy results in pain from the dorsal aspect of the thumb and index finger.
    C. A C7 radiculopathy results in pain in the middle finger.
    D. Spinal nerve C7 exits below vertebra C6.
    E. All are true statements.

15. A complete transection of the spinal cord at C2 results in a spastic bladder immediately after the injury (during spinal shock).
   A. True
   B. False

16. Which of the following statement(s) is true?
   A. The supplementary motor area (SMA) and premotor cortex (PM) are both in Brodmann's area 6.
   B. The SMA and PM are both involved in premotor planning.
   C. Primary motor cortex is involved in the execution of a movement.
   D. Pyramidal tract neurons fire before the muscles contract in an intended movement.
   E. All of the above are true.
   F. None of the above

17. Which of the following statements is false?
   A. The SMA becomes active when thinking of a complex motor task, even when the task is not actually performed.
   B. The neurons in the SMA and primary motor cortex fire prior to a given movement.
   C. Lesions in the SMA result in apraxias, whereas lesions in primary motor cortex result in contralateral paresis and upper motor neuron signs.
   D. Both the SMA and primary motor cortex code for the force of a movement.

18. A 60-year-old male presents with a stroke in the left occipital lobe, and a 72-year-old male presents with controlled glaucoma for 1 year. Which patient will have worse visual acuity?
   A. The stroke patient
   B. The glaucoma patient
   C. Neither
   D. Both

19. Which of the following structures is not paired correctly with all or part of its blood supply?
   A. Anterior limb of internal capsule—medial striates
   B. Dorsal part of the posterior limb of internal capsule—middle cerebral
   C. Visual cortex—posterior cerebral
   D. Broca's motor speech area—middle cerebral
   E. Hippocampus—anterior cerebral

20. A lesion in the frontal association cortex on the left would most likely result in:
    A. ipsilateral homonymous hemianopsia
    B. resting tremor
    C. Wernicke's aphasia
    D. Broca's aphasia
    E. diplopia

21. A lesion of the ventromedial nucleus of the hypothalamus (which lies in the tuberal level) has been shown (in experimental animals) to produce:
    A. diabetes insipidus
    B. increased appetite (hyperphagia) and rage
    C. loss of appetite
    D. memory loss and aphasia
    E. lack of prolactin production

22. Bilateral lesions of the ventral portion of the temporal lobes involving the hippocampal formation would most likely result in patients exhibiting which of the following signs and symptoms?
    A. Difficulty expressing their thoughts
    B. Trouble understanding speech and also trouble with verbal expression
    C. Loss of the sensation of pain, without loss of pain sensitivity or discrimination
    D. Long-term memory loss
    E. Short-term memory loss

23. The mammillary bodies:
    A. are damaged in Korsakoff's syndrome
    B. receive input from the fornix
    C. project to the medial dorsal nucleus of the thalamus
    D. are involved in temperature regulation
    E. A and B
    F. C and D

24. Which of the following statements is not true regarding the paraventricular nucleus of the hypothalamus?
    A. Cells are involved in regulating circadian rhythm.
    B. It is involved in the production of oxytocin.
    C. It is involved in regulating of water balance.
    D. Cells project to the posterior lobe of the pituitary gland.

25. Which of the following statements is correct?
    A. Patients with prosopagnosia do not recognize fingers.
    B. Reading disorders are called dysphagia.
    C. Broca's aphasia can be accompanied by hemiplegia.
    D. Anton's syndrome is a type of aphasia.

26. Which of the following statements is correct regarding apraxias?
    A. A lesion in ideomotor apraxia involves the temporal parietal junction.
    B. A patient with ideomotor apraxia will use the wrong object to perform the correct action.
    C. Apraxias are always associated with hemiparesis.
    D. A patient with an ideal apraxia is unable to use the correct motor sequence.
    E. A lesion in ideomotor apraxia involves the parietal lobe and SMA.

27. Which of the following statements is TRUE regarding the mesocorticolimbic dopamine system?
    A. It comes from the ventral tegmental area and innervates the limbic structures and visual cortex.
    B. It is part of reinforcement and reward.
    C. It arises from the substantia nigra and innervates the limbic and prefrontal cortical region.
    D. It arises from the raphe nucleus and innervates the limbic cortical region.

28. The human circadian pacemaker is located in the:
    A. reticular activating system
    B. thalamus
    C. suprachiasmatic nucleus
    D. pons

29. Which of the following statements is not true regarding serotonin?
    A. Cell bodies lie in the substantia nigra and innervate the cortex and limbic system.
    B. It is increased by monoamine oxidase inhibitors and tricyclics.
    C. It is likely decreased in impulsive individuals.
    D. It is kept in synaptic cleft longer by fluoxetine.
    E. It is produced in raphe nuclei.

30. The tuberomammillary nucleus is the only location in the brain that produces histamine.
    A. True
    B. False

31. The severe short-term (explicit) memory deficits characteristic of Alzheimer's disease would most likely be due to:
    A. plaques and tangles in the hippocampal regions
    B. neurofilaments and tau protein in basal ganglia
    C. degeneration of the ventral tegmental area
    D. loss of norepinephrine in the amygdala

32. A 65-year-old female presents with headache, fever, and occasional jaw claudication. What is the most likely cause?
    A. Left MCA stroke
    B. Tension headache
    C. Trigeminal neuralgia
    D. Temporal arteritis

33. Which cranial nerve is affected in the syndrome known as tic douloureux?
    A. CN II
    B. CN V
    C. CN VII
    D. CN X
    E. CN IV

34. Horner's syndrome is often associated with which one of the following?
    A. Cluster headache
    B. Multiple sclerosis
    C. Lyme disease
    D. Anton's syndrome

35. A 73-year-old female presents with symptoms consistent with amaurosis fugax. Which vessel is most likely involved?
    A. Vertebral artery
    B. PCA
    C. Ophthalmic artery
    D. Central retinal vein
    E. Lenticulostriate artery

36. A 93-year-old male presents with left leg weakness, irritability, and mood disturbance that occurred suddenly this morning. Which artery is most likely involved?
    A. Right anterior choroidal artery
    B. Left anterior cerebral artery
    C. Left middle cerebral artery (MCA)
    D. Right posterior cerebral artery
    E. None of the above

37. A 67-year-old right-handed male presents to the emergency department (ED) with decreased consciousness, ophthalmoplegia, pupillary constriction, and bilateral paralysis. Which artery or arteries would most likely be involved?
    A. Left posterior cerebral artery
    B. Basilar artery
    C. Bilateral anterior cerebral arteries
    D. Bilateral external carotid arteries
    E. All of the arteries above could cause these symptoms.

38. A 36-year-old female with a congenital berry aneurysm of the circle of Willis may also have one of the following?
    A. Ulcerative colitis
    B. Polycystic ovarian syndrome
    C. Turner's syndrome
    D. Polycystic kidney disease
    E. Abdominal aortic aneurysm

39. A 54-year-old male with a history of hypertension presents with sudden onset of hemiballistic movements of his right upper extremity. If these symptoms were due to a stroke, the most likely location and artery involved would be?
    A. Thalamus; MCA
    B. Subthalamic nucleus; posterior cerebral artery
    C. Genu of the internal capsule; anterior choroidal artery
    D. Caudate; MCA
    E. None of the above

40. A 28-year-old right-handed male presents to the ED with confusion and headache. A computed tomography (CT) scan of the head is performed and reveals hydrocephalus. This condition may be associated with an overproduction of cerebrospinal fluid (CSF), which would be associated with which structure?

    A. Meninges
    B. Choroid plexus
    C. Foramen of Luschka
    D. Foramen of Magendie

41. A 35-year-old male presents to the ED after a motor vehicle accident with decreased consciousness. On CT scan of his head, an epidural hemorrhage is noted. What is the most likely vessel involved?

    A. External carotid artery
    B. Middle meningeal artery
    C. Anterior choroidal artery
    D. Bridging vein

42. An 84-year-old male with a history of a right MCA territory stroke about 6 months ago presents to your office. The hallmark features on his examination could include all of the following except?

    A. Spastic paralysis
    B. Fasciculations
    C. Hyperreflexia
    D. No significant muscle atrophy

43. A 78-year-old female presents with a history of polio and has residual lower extremity weakness, atrophy, fasciculations, and hyporeflexia. Where did the polio virus cause the damage?

    A. Dorsal root ganglion
    B. Anterior horn cells
    C. C2 spinal root
    D. Lumbosacral plexus
    E. None of the above

44. An 18-year-old male presented to the ED after a recent MVA and hemi-section of his spinal cord at T2. At what level would he have pain and temperature loss?
    A. T1
    B. T2
    C. T4
    D. C7
    E. None of the above; pain and temperature would be preserved.

45. A 54-year-old male presented to the clinic with recent damage to his S2 and S3 nerve root. What is the most likely autonomic system that is involved?
    A. Sympathetic
    B. Parasympathetic
    C. Both are involved
    D. Neither are involved

46. Which pathway connects the hippocampus, hypothalamus, thalamus, and the cortex?
    A. Gatz pathway
    B. Papez circuit
    C. Mendel circuit
    D. Klüver-Bucy pathway

47. The parasympathetic system has what kind of effect on the adrenal medulla?
    A. It stimulates the secretion of adrenaline via cholinergic fibers.
    B. It stimulates the secretion of the rennin-angiotensin system.
    C. It has no significant effect.
    D. It increases aldosterone production.

48. The sympathetic system exerts its affects on the lungs by:
    A. constricting the bronchial tubes
    B. stimulating bronchial gland secretion
    C. increasing carbon dioxide production
    D. dilating the bronchial tubes

49. A 32-year-old female presents with episodes of high blood pressure, sudden fevers, and vomiting without an infectious etiology. She also states her eyes are dry, and she has decreased ability to form tears. She is very anxious and occasionally irritable. She states there may be someone in the family with similar complaints but is not sure. What is the most likely diagnosis?
    A. A variant of Guillain-Barré syndrome
    B. Charcot-Marie-Tooth disease type Va
    C. Riley-Day syndrome
    D. Korsakoff's syndrome
    E. None of the above

50. Congenital central hypoventilation syndrome (CCHS) is sometimes associated with what abnormality?
    A. Shoulder dystocia
    B. Absence of parasympathetic ganglion cells in the colon
    C. Diabetes insipidus
    D. Horner's syndrome

51. A 72-year-old male presents with weakness and decreased sensation in his left leg up to his hip as well as hyperreflexia. What is the most likely cause?
    A. Right anterior cerebral artery occlusion
    B. Left MCA occlusion
    C. Left posterior cerebral artery occlusion
    D. Right superior cerebellar artery occlusion
    E. None of the above

52. A 64-year-old female presents with bilateral upper and lower extremity muscle atrophy, fasciculations, and hyperreflexia. What is the most likely etiology?
    A. Guillain-Barré syndrome
    B. ALS
    C. Tertiary syphilis
    D. Brown- Séquard syndrome
    E. Syringomyelia

53. A 57-year-old male veteran presents with a history of severe pain in both lower extremities, decreased proprioception up to the hip, and a positive Romberg's sign. What is the most likely cause of his symptoms?
    A. Left thalamic infarct
    B. Polio
    C. Diabetic polyneuropathy
    D. Tertiary syphilis
    E. Cerebellar infarct

54. A 39-year-old female presents after an MVA with bilateral shoulder and arm numbness. She has decreased pain and temperature in the shoulder and arms, but light touch and proprioception is intact. What is likely the cause?
    A. Pernicious anemia
    B. Copper metabolism defect
    C. Cytomegalovirus (CMV) radiculitis
    D. Syringomyelia
    E. Brown-Séquard syndrome

55. A 23-year-old female presented with a rapid onset of weakness that started in her feet and moved up her body. She complained of having diarrhea about 2 weeks ago. Which one of the following is associated with this condition?
    A. Anti-GAD ab
    B. Anti-Hu ab
    C. *Campylobacter jejuni*
    D. Anti-Ma ab
    E. *Clostridium difficile*

56. A 72-year-old male presented with onset of pain, numbness, and tingling around both gluteal regions and atrophy. The patient also stated that he had become impotent. What is the likely location of his lesion?
    A. L1–L4
    B. S2–S4
    C. C3–C5
    D. Lumbosacral plexus
    E. None of the above

57. A 56-year-old female suddenly developed left severe neck pain, tongue deviation to the left, right-sided paralysis, loss of proprioception on the right side, and hyperreflexia. Pain and temperature were intact throughout. What is the likely location of the lesion?
    A. Left C5 nerve root
    B. Left medulla
    C. Right thalamus
    D. Left globus pallidus

58. A 45-year-old male with chronic alcohol use presented with a seizure. In the ED, he was given D5NaCl solution and lorazepam. A head CT scan was performed, which was negative for any acute pathology. The patient then progressed and started to have amnesia of his current visit but had retained all his previous memory. He also started making up answers to questions that were not true. What is the most likely location of his lesion and what is the cause?
    A. Occipital lobe; B_{12} deficiency
    B. Left temporal lobe; lorazepam
    C. Bilateral mamillary body; thiamine deficiency
    D. Reticular activating system; niacin deficiency
    E. None of the above

59. Which of the following groups is paired incorrectly?
    A. CN XII lesion; tongue deviates toward the side of the lesion
    B. CN V motor lesion; the jaw deviates away from the side of the lesion
    C. Cerebellar lesion; falls toward the side of the lesion
    D. CN X lesion; uvula deviates away from the side of the lesion
    E. CN XI lesion; head turns to the same side of the lesion

60. What path connects Wernicke's to Broca's area?
    A. Longitudinal fasciculus
    B. Arcuate fasciculus
    C. Cingulate gyrus
    D. Brodmann's area 44
    E. Splenium of the corpus callosum

61. A 63-year-old female presents to her ophthalmologist with complaints of being unable to see anything in her left upper quadrant. Where is the lesion located?
    A. Right optic tract
    B. Left lateral geniculate body
    C. Right calcarine fissure
    D. Right Meyer's loop
    E. Optic chiasm

62. Which artery occlusion would cause the classic "lacunar" syndromes?
    A. Anterior inferior cerebellar artery
    B. PCA
    C. Lenticulo-striate artery
    D. Vertebral artery
    E. None of the above

63. Which of the following is the most important risk factor for Alzheimer's disease?
    A. Age
    B. Down syndrome
    C. Family history
    D. Female gender
    E. None of the above

64. Which of the following is associated with "locked-in syndrome"?
    A. ALS
    B. Central pontine myelinolysis
    C. Vertebral artery dissection
    D. Bilateral carotid artery occlusion
    E. A and D
    F. A B, and C

65. Neologisms are part of which of the following?
    A. Motor aphasia
    B. Receptive aphasia
    C. Transcortical motor aphasia
    D. Lewy body dementia

66. A 34-year-old male presents with intermittent dizziness, nausea, vomiting, and hearing loss. The patient also complains of ear fullness and ringing in his ear. What is the most likely etiology?

    A. Trauma
    B. Syphilis
    C. Idiopathic
    D. All of the above
    E. None of the above

67. What is the most common cranial neuropathy associated with berry aneurysm?

    A. CN II
    B. CN III
    C. CN IV
    D. CN X

68. What is the major difference between a subdural hematoma and an epidural hematoma on CT scan?

    A. The subdural hematoma will look isodense.
    B. The epidural will have a lens-shaped convex hyperdensity.
    C. The subdural will have a crescent-shaped concave hypodensity.
    D. There is no difference shown by CT scan to distinguish the two.
    E. None of the above

69. An 87-year-old male presents to your clinic with resting tremor in both hands, stooped posture, and masked facies. What is the most likely cause of his symptoms?

    A. Serotonin depletion in the raphe nucleus
    B. Dopamine depletion in the substantia nigra
    C. Copper depletion in the reticular activating system
    D. B_{12} deficiency
    E. None of the above

70. A 56-year-old male presents with hearing loss, tinnitus, vertigo, and disequilibrium. Which of the following could be a potential cause?

    A. Excessive growth of astrocytes
    B. Excessive growth of Schwann cells
    C. Acetazolamide therapy
    D. Cavernous sinus thrombosis
    E. None of the above

71. A 34-year-old male presents with a long-standing history of abnormal movements, aggressive behavior, and memory difficulties. There is a strong family history of similar symptoms, and his father had committed suicide at age 41. The patient is extremely irritable and demonstrates antisocial behavior. What would be the most likely finding on magnetic resonance imaging (MRI)?

    A. Hydrocephalus
    B. Frontal lobe infarct
    C. Arnold-Chiari malformation
    D. Diffuse atrophy; more prominent in the caudate and putamen
    E. None of the above

72. A 74-year-old male with a history of cancer presents with new-onset seizures and focal deficits on his left side that have gradually worsened. His cancer had been in remission but has spread to his liver and bone. He had an MRI of his brain, which demonstrated multiple lesions consistent with metastatic disease. They were primarily located at the gray-white junction. What type of cancer does the patient most likely have?

    A. Squamous cell carcinoma
    B. Small cell carcinoma of the lung
    C. Meningioma
    D. Prostate carcinoma
    E. Leukemia

73. A 54-year-old male presents in a coma. He is found to have a severe subarachnoid bleed with left-sided uncal herniation. What is the most likely examination finding to confirm this?

    A. Right-sided paralysis
    B. Left-sided paralysis
    C. Left mydriatic pupil; this is nonreactive
    D. Right miotic pupil
    E. Tongue deviation to the right

74. A 74-year-old male presented with a history of resting tremor in his right hand, rigidity of his lower extremities, slow gait, and occasional falls. Which of the following could not have caused this man's symptoms?

    A. History of encephalitis
    B. Manganese ingestion
    C. Ethylene glycol
    D. History of anoxic brain injury
    E. Metoclopramide

75. A 67-year-old female presents with a 3-week history of headaches and low-grade fever. She states she has had scalp tenderness over her left eye and occasional jaw claudication. The reason she came into the hospital now is that she has lost vision in her left eye. Which vessel is the cause of her symptoms?

    A. Left ophthalmic artery
    B. Right carotid artery
    C. Left central retinal artery
    D. Left central retinal vein
    E. Left MCA

76. A 34-year-old male presents with rapid onset of diplopia, difficulty swallowing, and weakness that started in his arms and progressed downward. His pupils are dilated and non-reactive. You find out that he had recently eaten a can of soup that caused some diarrhea the day prior. What is the most likely cause of his symptoms?

    A. Difficulty for acetylcholine to be released
    B. Difficulty for acetylcholine to bind to the postsynaptic area
    C. Difficulty for norepinephrine reuptake
    D. Poor ATP release
    E. Defective glucose metabolism

77. A 69-year-old male presented with a 5-year history of progressive apathy, emotional lability, inappropriate behavior, and difficulty balancing his checkbook. He also stopped playing golf, which was his favorite hobby. An MRI demonstrated atrophy marked in the temporal region and frontal region. What is the pathologic hallmark for this disease?

    A. Argentophilic pick bodies
    B. Neurofibrillary tangles
    C. Spongiform changes to the gray matter
    D. Loss of dopamine cells in the substantia nigra
    E. Hippocampal atrophy bilaterally

78. A 82-year-old male with a long-standing history of dementia has been placed on an acetylcholinesterase inhibitor with some improvement of his symptoms. The area of the brain most likely involved is:

    A. caudate
    B. Raphe nucleus
    C. nucleus basalis of Meynert
    D. Brodmann's area 41
    E. Edinger-Westphal nucleus

79. A 49-year-old woman presents with sudden onset of left-sided facial weakness, hearing loss, and ear pain for 2 days. On examination, she has a vesicular rash on her left ear and sensorineural hearing loss on the left, as well as left face weakness. What is the most likely diagnosis?

A. Carcinomatous meningitis
B. Ramsay Hunt syndrome
C. HHV-6
D. HTLV-1
E. None of the above

80. A 27-year-old man with a history of HIV presents with 3 weeks of dysarthria and progressive left-sided weakness. He has been noncompliant with his antiretroviral medications. His last CD4 count was 72. An MRI brain scan demonstrated large confluent areas of T2 hyperintensities in the subcortical white matter bilaterally consistent with severe demyelination. Diffusion-weighted images were negative. An LP was performed and demonstrated normal opening pressure, normal cell count, glucose, and protein. CSF polymerase chain reaction (PCR) for John Cunningham (JC) virus was positive. What is the most likely location of this virus?

A. Astrocytes
B. Macrophages
C. Schwann cells
D. Oligodendrocytes
E. Basket cells
F. None of the above

81. A 60-year-old man with a history of untreated venereal disease complains of sudden lancinating pain in both legs. On examination, the patient has unequal pupils. The involved pupil does not react to light but constricts during accommodation. Sensory examination reveals decreased vibration and joint position sense. The patient exhibited a mild decrease in sensation to pinprick and temperature. Absent reflexes and a wide-based gait were demonstrated. Laboratory findings showed that his rapid plasma regain was positive and FTA-ABS was also positive. An LP demonstrated increased lymphocytes, elevated protein, and positive Venereal Disease Research Laboratory results (VDRL) in the CSF. The patient's eye findings are known as:

A. Marcus-Gunn pupil
B. Adie's pupil
C. Argyll-Robertson pupil
D. tonic pupil
E. There is no known name for his eye findings.

82. A 43-year-old right-handed woman presents with a 6-month history of numbness and tingling in her right hand (particularly in her first three digits). She denies any symptoms in her palm or her fourth or fifth digit. She types all day at a computer and states her symptoms are worse at night and when she wakes up in the morning. What is the most likely location of her problem?
    A. Anterior cruciate ligament
    B. Flexor retinaculum
    C. Antecubital fossa
    D. Right brachial plexus
    E. C6 root

83. A 75-year-old woman presents with an unsteady gait, generalized weakness, fatigue, and a burning sensation in her tongue. On examination, she is found to have bilateral weakness and decreased positional sense in her legs more than her arms. She has diminished reflexes and a positive Babinski reflex. She also has a positive Romberg's test. Which of the following conditions is associated with her problem?
    A. Atrophic gastritis
    B. Decreased ferritin
    C. Abnormal copper metabolism
    D. Niacin deficiency
    E. Elevated homocysteine

84. What is the most common cranial nerve palsy associated with subarachnoid hemorrhage?
    A. CN II
    B. CN IV
    C. CN VI
    D. CN III
    E. All cranial nerves can be equally involved.

85. A 34-year-old woman presents with an acute onset of vertigo, nausea, and vomiting. She also complains of pain and numbness on the right side of her face as well as difficulty with swallowing. On examination, she falls to the right and has decreased pain and a decrease in the left hand's skin temperature. She has nystagmus in all directions, which is worse when looking to the right. The patient also has ptosis on the right eyelid, and her right pupil is smaller in diameter than her left along with decreased sweating on the right side. What is the most likely involved artery?

    A. PCA
    B. MCA
    C. Anterior cerebral artery (ACA)
    D. Posterior inferior cerebellar artery (PICA)
    E. Anterior inferior cerebellar artery (AICA)

86. What is the characteristic lesion seen in the arteries in amyloid angiopathy?

    A. Silver stain amyloid
    B. Congo-red positive amyloid
    C. Apple-green birefringence under polarized light
    D. B and C
    E. A and C

87. What two structures make up the lentiform nucleus?

    A. Caudate and thalamus
    B. Globus pallidus and putamen
    C. Globus pallidus interna and externa
    D. Substantia nigra and putamen
    E. None of the above

88. What is the most common cause of basal ganglia calcifications?

    A. Fahr's disease
    B. Huntington's disease
    C. Wilson's disease
    D. Carbon dioxide poisoning
    E. None of the above

89. The parasympathetic fibers that control papillary constriction arise from?
    - A. CN III
    - B. CN IV
    - C. Superior cervical chain
    - D. Vagus nerve
    - E. None of the above

90. A 76-year-old man presents with sudden onset of monocular blindness in his left eye as well as difficulty seeing objects in his right lateral field. What is the most likely location of his lesion?
    - A. Right optic nerve
    - B. Left distal optic nerve
    - C. Optic chiasm
    - D. Left proximal optic nerve
    - E. Right temporal lobe

91. Which of the following cranial nerves is the smallest?
    - A. CN I
    - B. CN IV
    - C. CN XII
    - D. CN V

92. An 87-year-old male presents with a sudden onset of unresponsiveness. During examination, he is found to have absent corneal reflex. What are the most likely nerves involved?
    - A. CN II and III
    - B. CN IV and VI
    - C. CN V and VII
    - D. CN VII and III
    - E. None of the above

93. A 54-year-old female presents with left facial weakness (both upper and lower), a change in her taste sensation, and increased auditory sensitivity. What is the most likely cause of these symptoms?
    - A. Idiopathic
    - B. Herpes zoster
    - C. JC virus
    - D. A and B
    - E. B and C
    - F. None of the above

94. A 34-year-old female with refractory seizures was recently treated with a vagus nerve stimulator. The patient returns to the office with continued complaints of hoarseness in her voice. She denies any problems with swallowing. On examination, she does not have difficulty elevating her uvula or soft palate. What is the most likely nerve involved?
    A. Glossopharyngeal n.
    B. Recurrent laryngeal n.
    C. Accessory n.
    D. Hypoglossal n.
    E. Trochlear n.

95. A 45-year-old male presents with weakness. On examination, there is winging of his scapula. What is the most likely nerve involved?
    A. Pectoral n.
    B. Anterior thoracic n.
    C. Long thoracic n.
    D. Dorsal scapular n.
    E. Axillary n.

96. A 78-year-old female with left hand numbness is sent for electromyography/nerve conduction studies. She is noted to have a Martin-Gruber anastomosis. What nerves are involved?
    A. Ulnar n. and median n.
    B. Radial n. and brachial n.
    C. Axillary n. and ulnar n.
    D. None of the above

97. A 23-year-old man presents with severe pain in his left shoulder. He had a recent viral infection. His left arm is numb, weak, and has severe pain with movement. What is the most likely cause of his symptoms?
    A. Parsonage-Turner syndrome
    B. Erb-Duchenne syndrome
    C. Guillain-Barré syndrome
    D. Lambert-Eaton myasthenic syndrome

98. Muscle contraction is a complex phenomenon. The electrolyte mostly involved and stored in the sarcoplasmic reticulum is:
    A. sodium
    B. potassium
    C. calcium
    D. magnesium
    E. None of the above

99. The Golgi tendon organ is in a series in the muscle in contrast to muscle spindles that are in parallel. True or false?
    A. True
    B. False

100. In a lesion of CN XII, the way to differentiate an upper motor neuron (UMN) lesion versus a lower motor neuron (LMN) lesion is:
    A. The tongue deviates away from the lesion in the UMN.
    B. The tongue deviates toward the side of the lesion in the UMN.
    C. The tongue deviates away from the lesion in the LMN.
    D. It is impossible to tell without an MRI.

101. An 18-year-old male comes to the office with his caretaker. He has a history of perinatal damage to his basal ganglia resulting in glial scars that resembles "marbles." What is the name of this disorder?
    A. Striatonigral degeneration
    B. Status marmoratus
    C. Hallervorden-Spatz disease
    D. Status lacunaris
    E. None of the above

ANSWERS

1. **Answer: C.** The pons
2. **Answer: B.** Right subclavian
3. **Answer: B.** The middle meningeal artery, which lies outside the dura and forms a groove in the cranial bone. Epidural hemorrhage generally coincides with a skull fracture.
4. **Answer: A.** Ophthalmic artery

5. **Answer: C.** T3 and below. Fibers do not all cross over immediately. Most ascend one or two segments before they cross over. Also, the pain-temperature fibers in the spinothalamic tract are arranged so that the leg fibers are lateral to the arm fibers. Outside compression of the cord on the spinothalamic tract may affect the fibers of the lower extremities first.

6. **Answer: C.** Syringomyelia is a degenerative disease of the spinal cord (or brain stem) of unknown cause, which usually affects the pain and temperature fibers that are crossing at the level of involvement. It can vary in size, shape, and symmetry and can sometimes involve other parts of the cord (such as the anterior horn as in this case).

7. **Answer: E.** All are possible causes of carpal tunnel syndrome.

8. **Answer: C.** Mossy fibers make up 99% of the incoming fibers. They transmit impulses exclusively from the spinal cord and the vestibular and pontine nuclei by using granule cells as mediators; enter via all three peduncles. Aspartate is probably the main neurotransmitter.

9. **Answer: C.** Lesions in the ventroposterior (VP) area of the thalamus produce contralateral sensory loss to all modalities and can be associated with the thalamic pain syndrome in affected areas as anesthesia dolorosa.

10. **Answer: A.** Pick's disease. Any process that results in bilateral damage to the temporal lobes can cause this syndrome. The classic symptoms associated are hyperoral, increased appetite, hypersexual, and docile behavior.

11. **Answer: B.** Mamillary bodies. Wernicke's encephalopathy due to thiamine deficiency is often seen in alcoholics. The lesion is usually located in the mamillary bodies, dorsomedial nucleus of the thalamus, periaqueductal gray, and oculomotor nuclei.

12. **Answer: D.** The lateral vestibulospinal tract is an ipsilateral tract that runs down the entire length of the spinal cord. Therefore, the left vestibulospinal tract would be the primary functioning tract.

13. **Answer: C.** Granule cells are the only excitatory cells in the cerebellum, and the basket cells are inhibiting the Purkinje cells. Basket cells surround or wrap around the Purkinje cells.

14. **Answer: E.** All of the above are true statements.

15. **Answer: B.** False. Consider complete transection of the spinal cord to interrupt (UMN) input to the bladder. Initially, the bladder would be atonic and fill and retain the urine immediately following the injury. Later, spasticity follows the spinal shock.

16. **Answer: E.** All of the above are true statements.

17. **Answer: D.** Only the primary motor cortex codes for force. The SMA controls the "planning" of movements.

18. **Answer: C.** Neither. Both patients should have preserved acuity. Glaucoma does not affect acuity until very, very late in the course of the disease.

19. **Answer: E.** The hippocampus—anterior cerebral. Of note, the dorsal part of the posterior limb of the internal capsule receives input from the lateral striates, which come off the middle cerebral, and the ventral part comes from the anterior choroidal.

20. **Answer: D.** Broca's aphasia. Frontal association cortex is Brodmann's area 45, which is Broca's area, and lesions result in nonfluent or expressive aphasia.

21. **Answer: B.** Increased appetite

22. **Answer: E.** Short-term memory loss

23. **Answer: E.** Both A and B are correct.

24. **Answer: A.** The suprachiasmatic nucleus comprises the cells that regulate our circadian rhythm.

25. **Answer: C.** Broca's aphasia is a motor speech disorder and is also called *nonfluent aphasia*. Broca's speech area lies in the inferior frontal lobe, is near the motor area, and can be associated with a left MCA occlusion.

26. **Answer: E.** It involves the parietal lobe (motor cortex) and SMA. Patients with ideomotor apraxia lose the ability to perform motor actions in the correct sequence.

27. **Answer: B.** It is part of the reinforcement and reward mechanism. The mesocorticolimbic dopamine system arises from the ventral tegmental area, which lies dorsal to the substantia nigra.

28. **Answer: C.** The suprachiasmatic nucleus houses the circadian generator for humans.

29. **Answer: A.** The substantia nigra houses dopamine and GABA. The raphe nucleus is the primary serotonin producer in the brain.

30. **Answer: A.** True

31. **Answer: A.** Plaques and tangles in the hippocampus are the pathologic hallmark of Alzheimer's disease.

32. **Answer: D.** Temporal arteritis or giant cell arteritis is a chronic inflammatory disease of large blood vessels, and untreated patients are at risk for blindness.

33. **Answer: B.** CN V. It is also known as *trigeminal neuralgia* and is typically seen in older adults. Its etiology is not well understood, however, microvascular compression is thought to be one possible cause.

34. **Answer: A.** Cluster headaches are severe, brief, nonthrobbing unilateral headaches that recur. Horner's syndrome (ptosis, miosis, anhidrosis) and ipsilateral nasal congestion, rhinorrhea, and tearing are often associated with it. Treatment includes oxygen therapy, ergots, and triptans.

35. **Answer: C.** Ophthalmic artery. Occlusion of this artery temporarily would lead to brief, ipsilateral blindness.

36. **Answer: E.** The anterior cerebral artery would affect the contralateral leg, which in this case would have to be the right anterior cerebral artery. Behavioral changes are often seen as well.

37. **Answer: B.** Basilar artery occlusion would lead to these symptoms. Vertebrobasilar artery involvement is often fatal. Dysphagia and dysarthria may also be common symptoms.

38. **Answer: D.** Congenital berry aneurysms occurring around the circle of Willis are common and are sometimes associated with polycystic kidney disease and aortic coarctation. Typically, these aneurysms are asymptomatic until they bleed.

39. **Answer: B.** Occlusion of the posterior cerebral artery may lead to hemiballistic movement disorder, contralateral homonymous hemianopsia, sensory loss, and spontaneous thalamic pain.

40. **Answer: B.** The walls of each ventricle contain a specialized structure called the *choroid plexus*, which secretes the clear CSF.

41. **Answer: B.** The middle meningeal artery, which lies outside the dura (hence, epidural) and forms a groove in the cranial bone. Epidural bleeds generally coincide with skull fracture.

42. **Answer: B.** Fasciculations and fibrillations are a sign of a lower motor neuron deficit. All the rest are often seen with upper motor neuron lesions.

43. **Answer: B.** The anterior horn cells would be the location.

44. **Answer: C.** T4. Pain and temperature fibers do not all cross over immediately. Many ascend one or two segments before crossing over.

45. **Answer: B.** The parasympathetic area in the spinal cord is S2-S4. The sympathetic area in the spinal cord is T1-L2. The hypothalamus is the primary control center for the autonomic system.

46. **Answer: B.** The Papez circuit is believed to be involved in the emotional content of conscious thought process. There is some input from the olfactory system as well.

47. **Answer: C.** The parasympathetic system has no significant effect on the adrenal medulla.

48. **Answer: D.** It causes the dilations of the bronchial tubes.

49. **Answer: C.** Riley-Day syndrome or familial dysautonomia is a disease associated with degenerative changes in the central nervous system (CNS) and the peripheral autonomic system. Other symptoms could include impairment of taste or insensitivity to pain.

50. **Answer: B.** Absence of the parasympathetic ganglion cells in the colon is Hirschsprung's disease, which is often associated with CCHS. The phox2b gene is involved.

51. **Answer: A.** The right anterior cerebral artery occlusion would result in contralateral leg weakness and sensory finding.

52. **Answer: B.** ALS; usually the distal extremities are affected first.

53. **Answer: D.** Tertiary syphilis or tabes dorsalis. The upper extremities are often spared.

54. **Answer: D.** Syringomyelia; cervical levels are most commonly affected often with atrophy of the intrinsic/small muscles of the hands.

55. **Answer: C.** This is Guillain-Barré syndrome. *C. jejuni* is the bacterial illness most often associated with Guillain-Barré syndrome. About 60% of the patients with the axonal variant have diarrhea prior to onset.

56. **Answer: B.** S2-S4; this is cauda equina syndrome. Cauda equina syndrome has been defined as low back pain, bilateral sciatica (occasionally unilateral), saddle sensory disturbances, bladder and bowel dysfunction, and variable lower extremity motor and sensory loss.

57. **Answer: B.** The lesion is in the left medulla. The combination of symptoms could only be explained by a medullary lesion on the left of all the options available.

58. **Answer: C.** Bilateral mamillary body infarction or damage occurs in the setting of thiamine deficiency and providing a glucose load (D5NaCl). The patient has developed Wernicke-Korsakoff's encephalopathy.

59. **Answer: B.** A CN V motor lesion would result in the jaw deviating toward the side of the lesion. The rest of the options are correctly paired.

60. **Answer: B.** The arcuate fasciculus connects Wernicke's to Broca's area. Lesions in this area result in conduction aphasia—poor repetition with good comprehension and fluent speech.

61. **Answer: D.** Lesion in Meyer's loop result in contralateral upper quadrantic anopsia. This would be in the temporal lobe.

62. **Answer: C.** The lateral striate artery supplies the internal capsule, thalamus, caudate, putamen, and globus pallidus

63. **Answer: A.** Age is the most important risk factor for developing Alzheimer's dementia. The rest are also risk factors but not as great as age. Pathology includes neuritis plaques with amyloid deposition, neurofibrillary tangles, amyloid angiopathy, and neuronal loss.

64. **Answer: F.** Patients that are locked in are awake and alert but are unable to move anything but their eyes and eyelids. All of the choices listed are associated with this syndrome except bilateral carotid artery occlusion, which would cause the patient most likely not to be awake and alert.

65. **Answer: B.** Receptive aphasia or Wernicke's aphasia is a disorder of comprehension of language with intact production of words, yet it is "nonsensical." Neologism or made-up words and paraphrasic errors or word substitution is often part of this disorder.

66. **Answer: D.** All of the above. The patient has Ménière's disease, also known as *endolymphatic hydrops*. This is episodic peripheral vertigo that is due to enlargement of the endolymphatic compartment of the inner ear.

67. **Answer: B.** CN III is the most common cranial nerve involved with berry aneurysms. The anterior communicating artery is the most common location for the aneurysm. A rupture of this aneurysm results in subarachnoid hemorrhage.

68. **Answer: B.** The epidural will have a lens-shaped convex hyperdensity. Choice C would be correct, however, the question states hypodensity instead of hyperdensity. The other difference is that the epidural is bound by suture lines, whereas subdural can span the entire hemisphere but will not cross the midline.

69. **Answer: B.** The patient presents with signs and symptoms of Parkinson's disease, and it is caused by dopamine depletion in the substantia nigra. Life expectancy from diagnosis is 9 years.

70. **Answer: B.** The potential cause of this patient's symptoms could be an acoustic neuroma or schwannoma. The only treatment is surgical removal. If there are bilateral schwannomas, it is associated with the genetic disorder of neurofibromatosis type II (chromosome 22).

71. **Answer: D.** The patient most likely has Huntington's disease, and therefore the most common MRI finding is atrophy, which is usually more prominent in the caudate and putamen region. This is a rare, hyperkinetic, autosomal dominant disease involving multiple abnormal CAG (triple) repeats on chromosome 4p.

72. **Answer: B.** Lung cancer is one of the most common tumors to metastasize to the brain. The typical location is at the gray-white junction, and the tumors are typically found in multiple locations. The other common tumors are breast, kidney, GI tract tumors, and melanoma.

73. **Answer: C.** The typical clinical finding with a patient with uncal herniation is an ipsilateral "blown" pupil or a large dilated nonreactive pupil on the side of the herniation.

74. **Answer: C.** The patient has Parkinson's-type features. All of the above except ethylene glycol has been associated with Parkinsonism. Other issues that have been associated with Parkinsonism are carbon disulfide use, MPTP, trauma, and other neuroleptic drugs.

75. **Answer: C.** The patient has temporal arteritis, which is also known as *giant cell arteritis* and usually affects women more often. It is caused by subacute granulomatous inflammation of the large vessels, including the aorta, external carotid (especially the temporal branch), and vertebral arteries. The most serious complication is blindness, which is due to occlusion of the central retinal artery (branch of the internal carotid artery).

76. **Answer: A.** The patient has botulism. The toxin that is released binds irreversibly to the presynaptic terminals and prevents the release of acetylcholine at the neuromuscular junction. This disorder can be distinguished clinically from myasthenia gravis due to the involvement of the pupils.

77. **Answer: A.** The patient has frontotemporal dementia, previously known as Pick's disease. The MRI demonstrated atrophy in the frontal and temporal regions. Silver-staining Pick bodies would be seen on histology, which is the only way to confirm this disease.

78. **Answer: C.** The patient most likely has Alzheimer's dementia (the most common type of dementia). A deficiency in cholinergic transmission has been hypothesized as the mechanism of memory loss. The loss of cholinergic projections to the nucleus basalis of Meynert and the acetylcholine-synthesizing enzyme choline acetyltransferase is markedly depleted in the cortex and hippocampus.

79. **Answer: B.** The patient has Ramsay Hunt syndrome or herpes zoster oticus. It is caused by the reactivation of the herpes zoster virus and is often associated with radiation and immune compromise. When the virus involves the seventh and eighth nerve, it is called Ramsay Hunt.

80. **Answer: D.** The patient has progressive multifocal leukodystrophy, which is due to the reactivation of a papovavirus called JC virus. It is often present in healthy individuals. In immunocompromised patients, however, the virus can activate and gain access to the CNS via hematogenous spread and attacks oligodendrocytes leading to demyelination. Death usually occurs within 6 months.

81. **Answer: C.** The patient has tertiary syphilis (tabes dorsalis), which generally occurs 20 years after primary infection. The patient's eye finding is known as Argyll Robertson pupil. There are also signs of progressive degeneration of the posterior columns and dorsal root ganglia.

82. **Answer: B.** The patient has carpal tunnel syndrome, which is a mononeuropathy usually caused by compression of the median nerve at the anterior wrist, under the flexor retinaculum. It is characterized by numbness and paresthesias in the distribution of the median nerve.

83. **Answer: A.** The patient has vitamin B_{12} deficiency, which is most commonly caused by pernicious anemia. This is due to antibodies to intrinsic factor and the gastric parietal cell that produces intrinsic factor. Intrinsic factor is necessary to bind vitamin B_{12} and to allow ileal absorption. Other causes can include a vegan diet, poor absorption (multiple causes), increased requirements (tapeworms), or increased excretion. The neurologic manifestation is one of "combined" systems involving both central white matter and peripheral nerves (posterior column and corticospinal tracts).

84. **Answer: D.** The most common cranial neuropathy associated with subarachnoid hemorrhage is the third. The most common cause of spontaneous subarachnoid hemorrhage is a berry aneurysm.

85. **Answer: D.** The patient has Wallenberg syndrome (also called lateral medullary infarct or PICA syndrome). This is a brain stem infarct of the lateral medulla that usually results from vertebrobasilar insufficiency and compromise of the PICA.

86. **Answer: D.** Amyloid angiopathy demonstrates the characteristic lesion of Congo-red-positive, apple-green, birefringent amyloid in the media and adventitia of arteries. It can be associated with Alzheimer's disease but can occur in otherwise healthy elderly individuals. It may result in simultaneous intracerebral, subarachnoid, or lobar hemorrhages.

87. **Answer: B.** The putamen and globus pallidus form the lentiform nucleus. There is no functional overlap; this is just an anatomical term. They lie like lens-shaped structures wedged between the internal and external capsules.

88. **Answer: A.** Fahr's disease. None of the other diseases listed cause basal ganglia calcifications.

89. **Answer: A.** The inferior division of CN III carries the parasympathetic fibers via the ciliary ganglion and then the short ciliary nerves to the iris and ciliary body resulting in papillary constriction. Therefore, any external compression of the CN III results in papillary dilations (e.g., aneurysm, pituitary tumor).

90. **Answer: D.** The left optic nerve near the chiasm would be the only possible location that would cause ipsilateral monocular blindness as well as the temporal field of the contralateral side (affecting Willebrand's knee fibers).

91. **Answer: B.** The fourth cranial nerve is known as the smallest and contains approximately 2,500 axons. It is the only cranial nerve that exits the brain stem on the dorsal aspect and the only one that decussates (crosses) and the longest intracranial course.

92. **Answer: C.** The corneal reflex pathways consist of sensation on the cornea via CN V (first division), then to the principal sensory nucleus, and then to bilateral CN VII resulting in eyelid constriction.

93. **Answer: D.** The patient has Bell's palsy, which is usually idiopathic but can be caused by the herpes zoster virus (Ramsay Hunt syndrome). The typical treatment is prednisone with acyclovir. Abnormal reinnervation after these lesions may result in synkinetic movements and paradoxical gusto-lacrimal reflex also known as "crocodile tears."

94. **Answer: B.** The recurrent laryngeal nerve is a branch of the vagus nerve that when affected can cause hoarseness. Other possible etiologies of damage to this nerve are surgery in the neck, aortic aneurysm, or metastatic cancer with lymph nodes compressing the nerve.

95. **Answer: C.** The long thoracic nerve that contains cervical roots C5, C6, and C7 innervates the serratus anterior, and damage to this nerve results in "winging of the scapula."

96. **Answer: A.** Martin-Gruber anastomosis is a communicating branch from the median nerve to the ulnar nerve in the forearm. It supplies the adductor pollicis, abductor digiti minimi, and the first dorsal interosseous.

97. **Answer: A.** Parsonage-Turner syndrome or brachial plexus neuritis (neuralgic amyotrophy) is a postinfectious neuritis that causes localized pain, weakness, and atrophy of the affected muscles. The usual course is partial-to-complete resolution.

98. **Answer: C.** Calcium is stored in higher concentrations in the sarcoplasmic reticulum. The depolarization of the T-tubule activates voltage-gated channels within the sarcoplasmic reticulum, triggering the release of calcium.

99. **Answer: A.** True. The contraction of the muscle results in stretching of the Golgi tendon organ, which in turn stretches the Ib afferent ending. These depolarize, resulting in an action potential. The Golgi tendon organs are sensitive to muscle force rather than muscle length. The Golgi tendon organs are thought to serve a protective role, preventing dangerous levels of tension in the muscle.

100. **Answer: A.** Lesions to CN XII that are due to upper motor neuron cause the tongue to deviate away from the lesion versus lower motor neuron lesions that cause the tongue to deviate toward the side of the lesion. CN XII exits the skull via the hypoglossal foramen.

101. **Answer: B.** Status marmoratus. It results in involuntary movements, bizarre postures, and spasmodic outbursts of laughing or crying. The patient's intelligence can be normal.

Headache

QUESTIONS

1. What are the classic symptoms associated with migraine headaches?
   A. Anxiety
   B. Numbness
   C. Throbbing
   D. None of the above

2. A 23-year-old female presents with onset of headache on one side, which spreads to involve the whole side of her head. She describes it as pulsatile, and it stays on one side. The headache is usually self-limiting lasting 30 minutes to a few hours. What is the most likely diagnosis?
   A. Occipital migraine
   B. Cluster headache
   C. Classic migraine
   D. Tension headache
   E. None of the above

3. What is the most common headache type?
   A. Tension headache
   B. Classic headache
   C. Vasospastic migraine
   D. Low pressure headache

4. What is the ratio of men to women affected by cluster headaches?
   A. 1:1
   B. 2:1
   C. 5:1
   D. 3:2
   E. 1:4

5. What percentage of migraine sufferers are women?
   A. 10%
   B. 25%
   C. 50%
   D. 75%
   E. None of the above

6. Which of the following is not a type of vascular headache?
   A. Migraine
   B. Toxic
   C. Tension
   D. Cluster
   E. All of the above are vascular headaches.

7. A 34-year-old female presents with daily headache. She has been taking ibuprofen 800 mg three to four times a day. She also drinks four cups of coffee per day. She states she used to have headaches on the left side of her head but now the pain is diffuse and bilateral. What is the best treatment for this type of headache?
   A. Triptan
   B. Oxygen
   C. Stop ibuprofen
   D. Increase her caffeine intake
   E. Get more sleep

8. A 40-year-old male presents to the emergency department (ED) with a severe, stabbing, burning, and throbbing headache. He describes the pain as piercing and unbearable. He also describes a runny nose on the same side as his headache. This happened once about 6 months ago but went away naturally. He was given oxygen and a sumatriptan, which provided pain relief. What is the most likely neuropeptide involved?
   A. Acetylcholine
   B. Dopamine
   C. Histamine
   D. Aldosterone
   E. Melatonin

9. Which of the following is the most common aura associated with tension headaches?

    A. Zig-zag lines
    B. Blurry vision
    C. Taste change
    D. Strange smell
    E. None of the above

10. A 35-year-old female presents with chronic daily headache and depression. She reports severe tenderness on her scalp and neck. She also complains of pain with neck flexion. She denied any visual changes, and the rest of her neurologic examination was normal. She works in an office and sits in front of a computer all day. She does drink one cup of coffee per day but does not associate her headaches with this. She also states her son recently was evicted out of his apartment. She denies taking any over-the-counter medications for this pain. Which of the following is not a cause of her headache?

    A. Stress or anxiety
    B. Depression
    C. Poor posture
    D. Caffeine

11. In the patient above, what is the best first-line treatment?

    A. Exercise
    B. Adequate sleep
    C. Cognitive behavioral therapy
    D. Nonsteroidal anti-inflammatory drugs (NSAIDs)
    E. All of the above

12. A 45-year-old tall, rugged man presents with severe headaches that debilitate him once a year. He states that oxygen is the only treatment that helps. He is diagnosed with cluster headaches. What is the most likely mode of inheritance?

    A. Autosomal recessive
    B. X-linked dominant
    C. Sporadic
    D. Anticipation
    E. None of the above

13. Which of the following has recently been associated with increased attack frequency and severity of migraines?
    A. Hypertension
    B. Chronic renal insufficiency
    C. Obesity
    D. Diabetes
    E. None of the above

14. The development of cutaneous allodynia during a migraine attack is due to sensitization of?
    A. Basal ganglia
    B. Trigeminal nucleus
    C. Dorsal column
    D. Supplementary sensory area
    E. None of the above

15. Which of the following medication is not effective during allodynia during a migraine?
    A. Parental COX-1 inhibitor
    B. Parental COX-2 inhibitor
    C. Triptans
    D. All of the above are effective.

16. Which of the following combinations has recently been found to be more effective than monotherapy for the treatment of migraines?
    A. Triptan/opiate
    B. NSAID/triptan
    C. NSAID/opiate
    D. DHE/opiate

17. The new international classification of headache disorders classifies chronic migraine as:
    A. seven days of continuous migraine
    B. fifteen days or more for 3 or more months without medication overuse
    C. one month of medication overuse
    D. forty-five days of continuous migraine
    E. None of the above

18. Which group is affected by idiopathic intracranial hypertension?
    - **A.** Young teenage men
    - **B.** Postmenopausal women
    - **C.** Overweight women of childbearing age
    - **D.** Overweight men
    - **E.** All of the above

19. Which of the following is the most serious complication of idiopathic intracranial hypertension?
    - **A.** Brain death
    - **B.** Stroke
    - **C.** Visual loss
    - **D.** Headache
    - **E.** Nausea and vomiting

20. What approximate percentage of women have recurrence of idiopathic intracranial hypertension?
    - **A.** 10%
    - **B.** 35%
    - **C.** 75%
    - **D.** 100%
    - **E.** None of the above

21. A 19-year-old obese female with sixth nerve palsy presents to the ED, complaining of a severe headache. The most likely opening pressure on her LP would be?
    - **A.** >20 cm H_2O
    - **B.** 5 cm H_2O
    - **C.** 10–15 cm H_2O
    - **D.** <5 cm H_2O

22. In the above patient, what would be the best first line of treatment?
    - **A.** Optic nerve fenestration
    - **B.** Dietitian
    - **C.** Diuretics
    - **D.** A and C
    - **E.** B and C

23. A 23-year-old female with a recent diagnosis of idiopathic intracranial hypertension presents to the ED with worsening blurry vision. She has been on steroids, acetazolamide, and furosemide in the past without relief. Which surgical option is the most effective treatment?
    A. Optic nerve sheath fenestration
    B. Cerebrospinal fluid (CSF) diversion procedure
    C. Burr hole
    D. Lumbar fusion
    E. Laser surgery

24. What percentage of patients presenting to a neurologist with idiopathic intracranial hypertension have headaches?
    A. 5%
    B. 25%
    C. 75%
    D. 99%
    E. 50%

25. Which of the following has been associated with causing or worsening idiopathic intracranial hypertension?
    A. Tetracycline
    B. Acetazolamide
    C. Furosemide
    D. Lumbar puncture
    E. None of the above

26. Which of the following best represents episodic focal neurologic symptoms without headache or vomiting?
    A. Hemiplegic migraine
    B. Carotidynia
    C. Migraine equivalent
    D. Cluster headache
    E. None of the above

27. Which of the following fits the current theory of the cause of migraine?
    A. Vasodilatory mechanism
    B. Interleukin 1, 6, and 11 mediated
    C. Spreading depression
    D. Histamine mediated
    E. Acetylcholine mediated

28. Which of the following frequency of headaches would prophylaxis treatment indicate?
    A. Once a month
    B. Perimenstrual
    C. Once a week
    D. Stress related
    E. None of the above

29. What percentage of patients that complain of severe head pain after coughing, sneezing, or lifting have an Arnold-Chiari malformation?
    A. 100%
    B. 10%
    C. 25%
    D. 50%
    E. 75%

30. Which of the following chromosomes has been linked to hemiplegic migraine?
    A. 1
    B. 10
    C. 19
    D. 15
    E. None of the above

ANSWERS

1. **Answer: C.** Throbbing. Although throbbing is always emphasized as a typical feature of migraine, it does not have to be of this character to be a migraine.
2. **Answer: C.** Classic migraine. The description above fits only with the classic migraine.
3. **Answer: A.** According to the American Academy of Neurology, the most common headache type is tension headache.
4. **Answer: C.** Men are more affected by cluster headaches than women, and the ratio is 5 to 1.
5. **Answer: D.** According to the National Institute of Health, about 75% of migraine sufferers are women.
6. **Answer: C.** Tension headaches are caused by muscle contraction or tightening of the facial and neck muscles.

7. **Answer: C.** The type of headache she has is rebound headaches. It results due to over-medication for a previous headache. The National Headache Foundation states they are more common if the part of the drugs include caffeine. The "rebound" happens as the effects from the medication start to wear off. The person then continues to take more and more medication and perpetuates the cycle.

8. **Answer: C.** The patient has cluster headache. The National Headache Foundation states that histamine is the most likely culprit; however, antihistamines have not proven to be effective treatment.

9. **Answer: E.** Tension headaches are not associated with any preheadache syndrome (aura). Also, there has been no link to hormones, foods, or any strong hereditary association.

10. **Answer: D.** The patient has a tension headache, and caffeine is not a known trigger for this type of headache. The other possibilities are all probably contributing to the patient's headache.

11. **Answer: E.** There are various modalities to treat tension headaches.

12. **Answer: C.** Cluster headaches have consistently been found to be caused by a sporadic model of inheritance. There are cases of an autosomal dominant pattern within single families, which suggests there may be a genetic component.

13. **Answer: C.** A recent study has proposed obesity as a risk factor for the development of chronic daily headache. The results demonstrated that obesity is not a risk factor for having migraines, but it is a risk factor for increased frequency and severity of migraines in patients who already suffer.

14. **Answer: B.** The proposed mechanism that causes cutaneous allodynia, a painful response from nonpainful stimuli, is sensitization of the central trigeminovascular neurons. During a migraine, pain receptor stimulation on the dura activates the second sensory neurons in the trigeminal nucleus.

15. **Answer: C.** Triptans cannot abort migraines when there is ongoing allodynia.

16. **Answer: B.** Results from a recent study suggest that concurrently targeting the serotonin dysmodulation and inflammation in migraine improves outcomes over monotherapy. A short-acting triptan and a long-acting NSAID provide additional benefit.

17. **Answer: B.** The International Classification of Headache Disorders distinguishes subtypes of chronic daily headache, primarily chronic migraine, and medication overuse headache. Chronic migraine is a new entity defined by migraine headaches on 15 or more days per month for 3 or more months in the absence of medication overuse. If medication overuse is present, the diagnosis of medication overuse headache can be made as long as the headache developed or worsened with concomitant use of medications.

18. **Answer: C.** Idiopathic intracranial hypertension is a disorder of overweight younger women of childbearing age. The incidence in this population is 19 in 100,000.

19. **Answer: C.** The most serious complication is visual loss. This can occur early or late in the course of the disease and is usually insidious and may be asymptomatic. Weight gain is the primary associated factor with visual acuity change.

20. **Answer: B.** One study that reviewed this demonstrated a 38% recurrence rate at 5 years.

21. **Answer: A.** The patient most likely has idiopathic intracranial hypertension. Most people agree that an opening pressure of >20 cm H_2O with optic disc edema qualifies for the diagnosis.

22. **Answer: E.** The medical management of idiopathic intracranial hypertension is multifaceted, and weight control is the main treatment, however extremely difficult to task and use of diuretics. Acetazolamide appears to be the most effective. Corticosteroids are effective in lowering intracranial pressure; however, there are significant adverse effects (e.g., weight gain and diabetes).

23. **Answer: B.** Refractory idiopathic intracranial hypertension to medical management has two surgical options: optic nerve sheath fenestration and CSF diversion (i.e., lumboperitoneal shunt, ventriculoperitoneal shunt). Of the two, CSF shunting has been shown to be more effective. Optic nerve sheath fenestration has only shown a long-term success rate of 16%.

24. **Answer: D.** Headaches are recorded in 99% of patients presenting to a neurologist; there is a slightly lower percentage of patients with headaches that present to an ophthalmologist.

25. **Answer: A.** All of the above except tetracycline are associated with improving or treating idiopathic intracranial hypertension.

26. **Answer: C.** This is the definition of migraine equivalent. Often, ocular migraine is an example of this condition.

27. **Answer: C.** Cortical "spreading depression" of electrical activity is the current accepted theory in which there is a wave of excitation followed by a wave of complete inhibition of activity across the cortex.

28. **Answer: C.** Prophylaxis is recommended for attack frequency of more than two or three headaches per month. The probability of success is about 60% to 75%.

29. **Answer: C.** Transient, severe headache on coughing, bending, sneezing, or lifting would be considered a "cough" headache. Males are more affected than females. Most patients respond to indomethacin if no structural lesion is noted.

30. **Answer: C.** The familial form of hemiplegic migraine has been linked to chromosome 19 in an autosomal dominant fashion.

Sleep Medicine

QUESTIONS

1. What percentage of Americans suffer from insomnia (both acute and chronic)?
   A. 10%
   B. 40%
   C. 90%
   D. <1%
   E. None of the above

2. A 75-year-old man complains of difficulty falling asleep for the past 2 years. He was started on zolpidem by his primary care physician at that time and has been taking it since then. He states he is not sure if it is still helping and feels fatigued during the day. He goes to bed at the same time every night and lies in bed for hours thinking about things, watching the clock. The patient states he sleeps better at his sister's house. He denies any depression but does feel some anxiety about going to bed. He does watch TV in bed. About 2 years ago, he mentioned he had a significant amount of stress when his wife was sick, but she is much better now. What is the most likely diagnosis?
   A. Sleep apnea
   B. Circadian rhythm disorder
   C. Idiopathic insomnia
   D. Depression
   E. Psychophysiologic insomnia

3. A 22-year-old man comes to the office complaining of difficulty sleeping and daytime tiredness, which started right after college. His usual bedtime is 10:00 PM, but he cannot fall asleep until 1:00 or 2:00 AM, and then he wakes up for work around 6:00 AM. The patient states that on the weekends, he can stay in bed until 11:00 AM or noon, and he goes to bed around 2:00 AM. He does feel better on the weekends. He does not snore, is not obese, and had no problems as a child. The patient also denies any recent stressors. What is the best treatment for him?

   A. Light therapy
   B. Sedative hypnotic
   C. Antidepressant
   D. Stop working
   E. None of the above

4. Which of the following disorders is most commonly associated with chronic insomnia?

   A. Restless legs syndrome (RLS)
   B. Sleep apnea
   C. Narcolepsy
   D. Depression
   E. Obsessive compulsive disorder

5. A 35-year-old female presents to a sleep specialist for difficulty falling asleep and staying asleep over the course of 1 year. The patient also complains of daytime fatigue. She has been diagnosed with attention-deficit hyperactivity disorder (ADHD) in the past but has never been treated. The patient is diagnosed with primary insomnia. What is the best treatment for her?

   A. Stimulant
   B. Short-acting sedative hypnotic
   C. Cognitive behavioral therapy
   D. Antidepressant
   E. None of the above

6. Which of the following is not a behavioral therapy for insomnia?

   A. Relaxation therapy
   B. Stimulus control
   C. Biofeedback
   D. Sleep restriction therapy
   E. All of the above

7. Of all the treatments for insomnia, sedative hypnotics are commonly used. What length of time is generally recommended for this family of drugs?
   A. Six months
   B. Less than 1 month
   C. At least 1 year
   D. Nine months

8. A 67-year-old man presents with complaints of "acting out his dreams." He states they are very violent, and his wife has been injured on multiple occasions. He usually recalls the exact dream when his wife wakes him. There are no focal deficits on neurologic examination. He does have an uncle diagnosed with Parkinson's disease. What is the most likely location of this problem?
   A. Cortex
   B. Basal ganglia
   C. Pons
   D. Thalamus
   E. None of the above

9. In the above patient, what is the best line of treatment?
   A. Clonazepam
   B. Selective serotonin reuptake inhibitors (SSRIs)
   C. Gabapentin
   D. Carbidopa/levodopa
   E. There is no treatment.

10. What neurodegenerative disorder may rapid eye movement (REM) behavior disorder be associated with or be the prodrome of?
    A. Alzheimer's disease
    B. Huntington's chorea
    C. Mitochondrial myopathy
    D. Parkinson's disease
    E. All of the above

11. Which of the following is required to diagnose RLS?
    A. Polysomnogram
    B. History of iron deficiency
    C. Clinically meeting the four criteria
    D. Responsive to dopamine
    E. None of the above

12. Which of the following stages does not change significantly as we age?
    A. Stage I
    B. Stage II
    C. Delta sleep
    D. REM stage
    E. All of the above

13. A 16-year-old boy presents with complaints of difficulty sleeping during the school week. On the weekends, however, he is able to fall asleep around 2:00 AM and wakes around noon and feels refreshed. He is diagnosed with delayed sleep phase syndrome. What area of the brain controls this?
    A. Thalamus
    B. Parietal cortex
    C. Hypothalamus
    D. Pituitary gland
    E. Medulla

14. With decreased sleep, higher cognitive tasks are affected early and disproportionately. Which of the following is thought to be the reason?
    A. Increased acetylcholine levels
    B. Low melatonin levels
    C. Microsleep intrusion
    D. Visual neglect phenomenon
    E. A and D
    F. C and D

15. A 12-year-old boy presents with multiple episodes of somnambulism. He almost hurt himself in a recent episode, and therefore his parents came to seek help. When are these episodes likely occurring?
    A. Stage I sleep
    B. Wakefulness
    C. Delta sleep
    D. Stage II
    E. None of the above

16. A 54-year-old female with a history of anxiety presents with the sensation to move her legs at night. She is diagnosed with RLS. Which of the following treatments would not be appropriate?
    A. Fluoxetine
    B. Wellbutrin
    C. Clonazepam
    D. Ropinirole
    E. Carbidopa/levodopa

17. A 17-year-old female presents with excessive daytime sleepiness. She states she falls asleep in school and takes naps frequently that last 20 to 30 minutes and are refreshing. What else in her history could confirm the diagnosis of narcolepsy?
    A. Episodes of sleep paralysis
    B. Hypnagogic hallucinations
    C. Cataplexy
    D. All of the above

18. A 16-year-old boy is recently diagnosed with narcolepsy with cataplexy. Which of the following neuropeptides is thought to cause this disease?
    A. Increased dopamine
    B. Decreased acetylcholine
    C. Decreased hypocretin
    D. Increased interleukin-1
    E. None of the above

19. What percentage of narcoleptics have had to quit working due to their disease?
    A. <1%
    B. Almost 10%
    C. About 25%
    D. 100%
    E. None of the above

20. Which of the following are required on the polysomnogram to determine REM sleep?
    A. Rapid eye movements
    B. Mixed-frequency electroencephalogram (EEG)
    C. Atonia on electromyography (EMG)
    D. A and C
    E. All of the above

21. Which of the following is the most common sleep complaint?
    A. Sleep apnea
    B. Narcolepsy
    C. RLS
    D. Insomnia
    E. Sleepwalking

22. Which of the following has been closely associated with narcolepsy with cataplexy?
    A. Chromosome 4q
    B. HLA-DQB1*0602
    C. Chromosome 22
    D. X-linked
    E. None of the above

23. A 19-year-old male with a history of narcolepsy with cataplexy presents to your clinic. What is the most likely way to elicit his cataplexy?
    A. Making him jump
    B. Making him laugh
    C. Making him read
    D. Making him take a nap
    E. None of the above

24. A 23-year-old female with a long-standing history of narcolepsy with cataplexy presents to your office. She was recently placed on modafinil with significant improvement in her daytime sleepiness, however, she is still having frequent cataplectic attacks. Which of the following agents would help her?
    A. Methylphenidate
    B. Tricyclic antidepressant
    C. Benzodiazepine
    D. Clonidine

25. A 56-year-old female with chronic insomnia presents to the clinic. She is initiated on melatonin 3 mg about 4 hours before her target bedtime. Where in the brain is melatonin produced?
    A. Hypothalamus
    B. Pituitary gland
    C. Pineal gland
    D. Adrenal gland
    E. None of the above

ANSWERS

1. **Answer: B.** A survey conducted by the National Sleep Foundation in 2007 estimated 30% to 35% of the US population reported difficulty sleeping in the past year, and approximately 10% suffer from chronic insomnia. Although so many people suffer, only approximately 5% of the chronic insomniacs report it to their physician.

2. **Answer: E.** Psychophysiologic insomnia is a disorder of somatized tension and learned sleep-preventing associations resulting in a complaint of insomnia and daytime fatigue. It usually begins with a prolonged period of stress in a person who previously had no problems. The person tends to respond to this stress with increased tension and aggravation resulting in increased awakenings while in bed.

3. **Answer: A.** This patient has delayed sleep phase syndrome. Light therapy along with adjusting his schedule to a regular fixed schedule 7 days a week is the mainstay of his treatment. These steps will need to be done gradually, and chronotherapy is an option.

4. **Answer: D.** Depression is the most common disorder associated with insomnia. It is usually associated with early morning awakenings and inability to fall back asleep; some studies have shown that insomnia can lead to depression (especially if the insomnia has been present for more than 1 year).

5. **Answer: C.** Behavioral therapy is now considered the most appropriate treatment for patients with primary insomnia. If the patient had secondary insomnia, treating the underlying cause would be the primary focus. Behavioral therapy is based on the notion that the insomnia is associated with physiologic, cognitive, and emotional arousal as well as conditioned arousal in bed.

6. **Answer: E.** All of the above are types of behavioral therapy.

7. **Answer: B.** Most of the sedative hypnotics are not recommended for use for more than 2 to 3 weeks. Also, continued nightly use should not be recommended, and therapy should always be instituted with small doses and maintained at the smallest effective dose.

8. **Answer: C.** The patient has REM behavior disorder. Normally, generalized atonia of muscles occurs during REM. This atonia results from active inhibition of motor activity by the perilocus coeruleus (pons). In REM behavior disorder, the brain stem mechanisms generating the muscle atonia normally seen in REM sleep are interfered with, and therefore patients can "act out their dreams," which tend to be violent in nature.

9. **Answer: A.** Clonazepam has been shown to be very effective in the treatment of REM behavior disorder.

10. **Answer: D.** REM behavior disorder may be the prodrome to neurodegenerative diseases associated with synucleinopathies (e.g., Parkinson's disease, dementia with Lewy bodies, etc.).

11. **Answer: C.** The criteria for RLS consists of four basic elements: (1) a compelling urge to move the limbs, usually associated with paresthesias; (2) motor restlessness, such as pacing the floor, tossing and turning in bed, and rubbing the legs, etc.; (3) symptoms are worse or primarily occur only at rest with some degree of relief with movement; and (4) the symptoms are typically worse at night or in the evening.

12. **Answer: D.** REM sleep in general represents about 20% to 25% of total sleep time and does not significantly change as we age.

13. **Answer: C.** The patient has a circadian rhythm disorder that is controlled/modulated by the hypothalamus, specifically the suprachiasmatic nucleus. Light is the major influence on the suprachiasmatic nucleus also known as a "zeitgeber" or "time-giver."

14. **Answer: F.** Microsleep and visual neglect phenomenon have been proposed as reasons for decreased performance in sleep deprivation. Microsleep is defined as brief runs of slower EEG activity that intrudes during wakefulness (theta/delta activity). Visual neglect phenomenon is one of many sensory perceptual impairments that occur during sleep deprivation.

15. **Answer: C.** Sleepwalkers appear to have an abnormality in delta sleep (slow-wave sleep) regulation. Most parasomnias occur in a mixed state of transition from one sleep to the next (e.g., delta sleep to wakefulness).

16. **Answer: A.** SSRIs have been shown to worsen the symptoms of RLS. The other options have not been shown to worsen RLS and are actually often used in the treatment.

17. **Answer: C.** Although all of those features are helpful, if cataplexy is present, it confirms the diagnosis of narcolepsy, and a polysomnogram with multiple sleep latency test may not even be necessary.

18. **Answer: C.** Decreased hypocretin levels are thought to be the primary reason for narcolepsy. In one human study, hypocretin levels were undetectable in the cerebrospinal fluid in seven of nine patients.

19. **Answer: C.** In one study, about 24% of narcoleptic patients had to quit working, and 18% had been terminated by their employer.

20. **Answer: E.** REM, mixed-frequency EEG (almost like an awake pattern), and atonia on EMG are all part of REM sleep. Occasionally, sawtooth waves can be seen on EEG.

21. **Answer: D.** Insomnia is the most common sleep complaint, and more women than men suffer from insomnia.

22. **Answer: B.** Narcolepsy with cataplexy is closely associated with human leukocyte antigen (HLA)-DR2, specifically DQB1*0602. This HLA is not as closely associated with narcolepsy without cataplexy. In general, HLA typing is clinically helpful to exclude narcolepsy; it is less helpful to confirm the diagnosis because 20% to 30% of the general population is positive as well.

23. **Answer: B.** Cataplexy is an abrupt attack of muscle weakness and if severe can make someone fall. The most characteristic feature of cataplexy is that it is usually triggered by emotion (usually laughter or anger). It is seen in about 70% of patients with narcolepsy.

24. **Answer: B.** Cataplectic attacks are treated with tricyclic antidepressants (e.g., clomipramine) or SSRIs (e.g., fluoxetine).

25. **Answer: C.** Melatonin is a naturally occurring hormone secreted by the pineal gland. The concentration of melatonin is highest in the blood during normal sleep times and lowest during normal wakeful times.

Stupor and Coma

QUESTIONS

1. A 76-year-old male presents with the inability to maintain attention. He is easily distracted, fidgety, and occasionally mistakes the wires in the room for snakes. This has been going on for 2 days, but there are periods when he is completely alert. Which of the following describes this patient's disease?

    A. Frontotemporal dementia
    B. Dementia with Lewy bodies
    C. Delirium
    D. Transient global amnesia
    E. None of the above

2. Which of the following has not been associated with delirium?

    A. Cobalamin
    B. Niacin
    C. Thiamine
    D. Thyroxine
    E. All of the above are associated with delirium.

3. A 67-year-old woman presents with an acute confusional state. She is diagnosed with a stroke. Which of the following is most likely the location of the stroke?

    A. Basal forebrain
    B. Anterior inferior cerebellar artery territory infarct
    C. Left lateral geniculate
    D. Subthalamic nucleus

4. A 65-year-old man presents in an acute comatose state. Magnetic resonance imaging (MRI) is performed and shows a stroke affecting his ascending reticular activating system. Which of the following areas would correspond with this lesion?

   A. Right parietal lobe
   B. Left occipital lobe
   C. Cerebral peduncle
   D. Tegmentum of the upper pons
   E. Basal ganglia

5. A 40-year-old man presents to the intensive care unit in a comatose state. He is hyperventilating, on arterial blood gas, and there is a metabolic acidosis. Which of the following is probably not the cause of his coma?

   A. Diabetic ketoacidosis
   B. Acetaminophen overdose
   C. Ethylene glycol ingestion
   D. Excessive vomiting

6. A 35-year-old female who recently ran a marathon in the summer presents in a comatose state. Her core body temperature is 41°C. She is diagnosed with heat stroke. What are other possible causes for her hyperthermia?

   A. Wernicke's encephalopathy
   B. Adrenal failure
   C. Hypothyroidism
   D. Anticholinergic intoxication
   E. None of the above

7. An 87-year-old man is found unresponsive in his home. On presentation, he has ataxic breathing, fixed pinpoint pupils, absent vestibuloocular reflexes, and has no movement of his extremities. Which of the following is a possible etiology for his coma?

   A. Tumor compressing the lower pons
   B. Stroke to the midbrain
   C. Herpes encephalitis
   D. Bilateral thalamic infarcts
   E. None of the above

8. A 76-year-old man presents to the emergency department (ED) with Cheyne-Stokes respiration, which started acutely. On computed tomography (CT) scan of his head, bilateral parietal lobe infarcts are seen in the middle cerebral artery (MCA) distribution. Which of the following could also cause a similar breathing pattern?

   A. Right posterior cerebral artery infarct
   B. Alcohol intoxication
   C. Cardiomyopathy
   D. Opiate overdose
   E. None of the above

9. A 34-year-old female presents to the ED in a deep coma. Which of the following skin lesions would support that she had severe head trauma?

   A. Hypermelanosis
   B. Icterus
   C. Battle's sign
   D. Ecthyma gangrenosum
   E. None of the above

10. A 19-year-old female presents to the ED with severe head injury due to a recent motor vehicle accident. Her Glasgow coma scale is 4. Which of the following is not possible for her to be performing?

    A. Extension response to pain
    B. Incomprehensible sounds
    C. Eyes open in response to pain
    D. Inappropriate words
    E. None of the above

11. A 56-year-old female found unresponsive is brought to the ED. On examination, she is found to have decorticate posturing. Which of the following is consistent with this condition?

    A. Flexion at the elbow, plantar lower extremity extension
    B. Upper extremity extension, lower extremity extension
    C. Flexion at the wrist and fingers, lower extremity flexion
    D. All of the above
    E. None of the above

12. Which of the following is most likely the location of the lesion that may cause decerebrate posturing?

    A. Thalamus
    B. Caudate
    C. Red nucleus
    D. Cerebellar peduncle
    E. Medial longitudinal fasciculus

13. A 56-year-old male with a history of multiple psychiatric hospitalizations was recently admitted to the psychiatric ward with acute psychosis. He was given multiple doses of haloperidol. On the third day of admission, he developed a fever, increased bilateral muscle rigidity, and then went into a coma. Which of the following is the best next step?

    A. Place cooling blankets
    B. Start dantrolene
    C. Check creatine phosphokinase level
    D. Stop the neuroleptics
    E. None of the above

14. A 42-year-old female with a history of chronic alcohol abuse and hepatitis C presents with a decreased level of consciousness. She is found on examination to have a tremor in her extremities and elevated ammonia levels in her blood. Which of the following describes the type of tremor she most likely has?

    A. Transient increase in postural tone
    B. Transient decrease in postural tone
    C. Occasional twitches of her face
    D. A and C
    E. None of the above

15. A 32-year-old man with a history of berry aneurysm that was partially coiled 1 week ago presents in a coma and is completely unresponsive. What physical finding would be pathognomonic for a subarachnoid hemorrhage?

    A. Elevated blood pressure
    B. Loss of the vestibule-ocular reflex
    C. Pinpoint pupils
    D. Roth spots
    E. Subhyaloid hemorrhage

16. A 65-year-old man presents after a stroke in the brain stem, and on examination, you find that his pupillary light reflex is impaired and he has an oculomotor palsy. Which of the following could also have caused this?
    A. Syphilis
    B. Low vitamin B_{12}
    C. Herniation of medial temporal structures from an expanding supratentorial mass
    D. Thiamine deficiency
    E. None of the above

17. A 36-year-old male presents with pinpoint pupils bilaterally and feels drowsy and nauseated. His sister comes in later and states that he took an overdose of oxycodone. Which of the following could also cause his pupillary changes?
    A. Lesion in the pontine tegmentum
    B. Bilateral retinal artery occlusion
    C. Pilocarpine drops
    D. Left carotid artery dissection
    E. All of the above

18. A 76-year-old male presents to the ED with left-sided hemiparesis (worse in the leg than arm) and eye deviation to the left. He has some nystagmus to the left as well and is unresponsive. Which of the following is possible?
    A. Large left frontal lobe lesion
    B. Seizure
    C. Right occipital lobe infarct
    D. Tumor in the brain stem
    E. None of the above

19. A 19-year-old man presents in a coma after a major motorcycle accident. His cervical spine is cleared of any fracture. You attempt the oculocephalic maneuver. If the patient has a positive doll's eye reflex, which of the following would be seen?
    A. The eyes do not turn with the head but in the opposite direction
    B. The eyes turn with the head in the same direction
    C. The left eye turns with the head while the right eye does not turn
    D. Both eyes move upward
    E. None of the above

20. Which of the following is required for caloric testing of the doll's eye reflex?
    A. One milliliter of ice cold water
    B. Three liters of lukewarm water
    C. Fifty milliliters of ice cold water
    D. Thirty milliliters of lukewarm water
    E. None of the above

21. Which of the following results would be seen in a patient in a psychogenic coma after a cold caloric test?
    A. Sustained deviation of both eyes toward the ear being stimulated
    B. Eye deviation toward the stimulated ear with nystagmus
    C. Sustained eye deviation away from the stimulated ear
    D. Temporary eye deviation upward
    E. None of the above

22. A 65-year-old female presents to the toxicology service with an acute overdose of lorazepam and is comatose on examination. On cold caloric testing, there is no response. She has good papillary reflexes. Which of the following could also present these examination findings?
    A. Lyme disease
    B. Ethylene glycol
    C. Lead toxicity
    D. Botulism
    E. Wernicke's encephalopathy

23. A 45-year-old man with an acute myocardial infarction presents after cardiac arrest and was resuscitated for 45 minutes. He is currently comatose, and the family would like to know his prognosis. Which of the following examination findings at 24 hours would help support that the outcome would be poor?
    A. Absent ankle reflexes
    B. Absent bilateral corneal reflexes
    C. Roving eye movements
    D. Withdraws to noxious stimuli but no localization
    E. Pupils pinpoint but reactive

24. Which of the following occurs first in uncal herniation syndromes?
    A. Ipsilateral hemiplegia
    B. Third cranial nerve palsy
    C. Decerebrate posturing
    D. Ataxic breathing
    E. None of the above

25. A 64-year-old female presents to the ED with severe head trauma. Which of the following is not part of Cushing's triad?
    A. Increased intracranial pressure
    B. Papilledema
    C. Hypertension
    D. Bradycardia
    E. All of the above

26. A 36-year-old female presents in a metabolic coma. Most metabolic comas present with symmetrical neurologic deficits. Which of the following is often associated with lateralizing motor findings in metabolic coma?
    A. Uremia
    B. Elevated ammonia
    C. Hypoglycemia
    D. Hypothyroidism
    E. None of the above

27. Which of the following does not strongly suggest a metabolic coma?
    A. Tremor
    B. Multifocal myoclonus
    C. Asterixis
    D. Hemiparesis
    E. All of the above

28. A 21-year-old female presents with cocaine overdose. Which of the following will be seen on pupil examination?
    A. Miosis
    B. Mydriasis
    C. Pinpoint pupils
    D. Anisocoria
    E. None of the above

29. A 35-year-old female presents with a drug toxicity of unknown type. Her brother tells you she is on amitriptyline and has a history of cocaine abuse. Which of the following would help you be able to tell that she ingested the amitriptyline?
    A. Hyperthermia
    B. Tachycardia
    C. Dry flushed skin
    D. Pupils
    E. Diaphoresis

30. A 76-year-old male presents with an acute embolism to the top of the basilar artery and shows classic signs of locked-in syndrome. All of the following can mimic a patient in chronically locked-in syndrome except:
    A. severe upper cervical spinal cord lesion
    B. end-stage Parkinsonism
    C. Herpes encephalitis
    D. amyotrophic lateral sclerosis
    E. None of the above. They all can present like someone locked in.

31. A 46-year-old female is initially diagnosed with an acute psychotic episode. She has a CT scan of her head, which demonstrates there is a lesion. She is able to follow with her eyes but cannot initiate any other movement. She does not follow any other commands. Her reflexes and tone are intact. What is the most likely diagnosis?
    A. Pontine infarct
    B. Syphilis
    C. Premotor area infarct
    D. Frontotemporal dementia
    E. None of the above

32. Which of the following is a distinguishing characteristic that differentiates catatonia from a comatose state?
    A. Fixed eye movements
    B. Seizures
    C. Ability to maintain tone
    D. Withdrawal to pain
    E. None of the above

33. Which of the following is NOT used in comatose patients that have been suspected of drug ingestion?
    A. Naloxone
    B. Mannitol
    C. Flumazenil
    D. Activated charcoal
    E. None of the above

34. A 19-year-old female presents in a comatose state. On examination, she is noted to have papilledema. She also presents with a fever, and her family states there was another student at her college diagnosed with bacterial meningitis. Which of the following is the next best step?
    A. Electroencephalogram (EEG)
    B. Lumbar puncture
    C. CT scan of head
    D. Blood cultures
    E. None of the above

35. Which of the following is an acute encephalopathy?
    A. Frontotemporal dementia
    B. Anton's syndrome
    C. Korsakoff syndrome
    D. Wernicke's encephalopathy
    E. None of the above

36. A 36-year-old male with a history of chronic alcohol abuse presents with ophthalmoplegia, confusion, and gait ataxia. Which of the following has not been associated with this condition?
    A. Anorexia nervosa
    B. Prolonged parental nutrition
    C. HIV
    D. Megaloblastic mania
    E. All of the above are associated.

37. What percentage of patients with Wernicke's encephalopathy has been associated with an atrophic mamillary body?
    A. 10%
    B. 50%
    C. 80%
    D. 100%
    E. None of the above

38. A 65-year-old man presents with a history of malabsorption due to a colon resection many years ago for colon cancer. He exhibits confusion, lateral rectus palsy, nystagmus, and an unsteady gait. The patient is diagnosed with thiamine deficiency. Which of the following symptoms of Wernicke's encephalopathy occasionally precedes the other symptoms?

A. Nystagmus
B. Lateral rectus palsy
C. Ataxia
D. Encephalopathy
E. None of the above

39. Toxic metabolic encephalopathies are extremely common. Which of the following patients in the intensive care unit are at the greatest susceptibility to develop this encephalopathy?

A. A 50-year-old male with multiple medical problems
B. An 18-year-old male intubated for 4 weeks
C. A 75-year-old male with history of mild dementia
D. A 45-year-old male with no past medical history
E. None of the above

40. A 34-year-old female with a history of depression presents to the intensive care unit with an overdose of acetaminophen. What percentage of patients with acute hepatic encephalopathy have cerebral edema?

A. <1%
B. 25%
C. 50%
D. 80%
E. 99%

41. A 32-year-old male marathon runner presents with impaired mental status and develops nausea and malaise. He also developed headaches and then became lethargic. The patient is diagnosed with hyponatremia. Which of the following sodium levels corresponds to when he developed nausea and malaise?

A. 145 mEq/L
B. 135 mEq/L
C. 120 mEq/L
D. 155 mEq/L
E. None of the above

42. A 67-year-old male has been in the intensive care unit in a comatose state and is diagnosed with brain death. Which of the following is a prerequisite before anyone can even contemplate the diagnosis?
    A. The cause of the brain death should be known.
    B. Exclusion of any complicating medical condition that may confound clinical assessment (i.e., no severe electrolyte imbalance)
    C. No drug intoxication or poisoning that may impair the clinical assessment
    D. The core body temperature is greater than or equal to 32°C.
    E. All of the above are prerequisites.

43. Which of the following would exclude brain death?
    A. Absent gag reflex
    B. Absent corneal reflex
    C. Coma
    D. Triple flexion response with foot stimulation
    E. None of the above

44. Which of the following meets the criteria for a positive apnea test in brain death?
    A. Absent respiratory response with a $PaCO_2 > 45$ mm Hg
    B. Absent respiratory response to $PaCO_2 > 60$ mm Hg
    C. Breathing below the ventilator
    D. Ten-second or longer stoppage of breathing
    E. None of the above

45. What is the number of hours in between examinations and physicians required for brain death in the United States?
    A. 72;3
    B. 6;2
    C. 96;1
    D. 1;2
    E. None of the above

46. Which of the following is the traditional "gold standard" test for brain death?
    A. Transcranial Doppler
    B. Carotid ultrasound
    C. Cerebral angiography
    D. CT angiography
    E. None of the above

47. A 56-year-old male presents to the emergency department (ED) after severe head trauma. After two physicians examine him, and after a positive apnea test, the patient is confirmed brain dead. Which of the following has been misdiagnosed with brain death?

   A. Locked-in syndrome
   B. Hypothermia
   C. Drug intoxication
   D. Guillain-Barré syndrome
   E. All of the above

48. A 60-year-old man presents to the emergency department (ED) after cardiac arrest. It was reported that cardiopulmonary resuscitation (CPR) was performed for approximately 25 minutes. What is the likelihood that the patient will survive after 6 weeks?

   A. 44%
   B. 30%
   C. 13%
   D. <1%
   E. None of the above

49. Which of the following improves neurologic outcome after cardiac arrest?

   A. Administer mannitol
   B. Hypothermia
   C. Craniectomy
   D. Magnesium infusion
   E. Thiamine IV

50. Which of the following is required in brain death criteria in the United States?

   A. EEG
   B. MRI
   C. Transcranial Doppler
   D. Lumbar puncture
   E. None of the above

ANSWERS

   1. Answer: C. Delirium is distinguished from dementia, which is a nonacute progressive process and is not associated with psychomotor, autonomic, and level of consciousness alterations that characterize delirium.

2. **Answer: E.** All of the above have been associated with causing or being associated with delirium.

3. **Answer: A.** Basal forebrain strokes have been implicated in confusion/delirium. Other locations that have been associated with delirium are caudate nucleus, thalamic lesions (that include the Papez circuit), and the hippocampus.

4. **Answer: D.** The ascending reticular activating system is a group of neurons that originate in the tegmentum of the upper pons and midbrain. They project their axons to the diencephalons and then on to the cortex. These neurons are thought to be integral in maintaining alertness.

5. **Answer: D.** All of the above except excessive vomiting could cause hyperventilation with a metabolic acidosis. Excessive vomiting would cause a metabolic alkalosis with hypoventilation, and usually, there should be no impairment of consciousness; if present, suspect psychogenic coma or some other etiology.

6. **Answer: D.** Besides heat stroke, anticholinergic intoxication could cause a hyperthermic coma as well as infection. All the other etiologies listed could cause hypothermic coma.

7. **Answer: A.** Based on the clinical picture, the most likely location for ataxic breathing and fixed pinpoint pupils is a lesion to the lower pons or upper medulla.

8. **Answer: C.** Cheyne-Stokes respiration (a crescendo-decrescendo pattern of breathing with apneic episodes) may occur with impaired cardiac output, bilateral cerebral dysfunction, and also in the elderly during sleep.

9. **Answer: C.** Bruises can often indicate head trauma, especially periorbital ecchymosis, also known as "raccoon eyes" and Battle's sign, which is bruising over the mastoid. All of the above are skin lesions but are do not indicate head trauma.

10. **Answer: D.** Inappropriate words gives her a score of 3 with best verbal response and therefore a minimum score of 5. The scale ranges between 3 and 15. A Glasgow coma scale score of 3 means no eye opening, no verbal response, or no motor response. The scale is used more as a prognostic indicator than used in the diagnosis of coma.

11. **Answer: A.** Decorticate posturing consists of upper extremity adduction and flexion at the elbow, wrists, and fingers along with lower extremity extension. Decerebrate posturing consists of upper extremity extension, adduction, and pronation along with lower extremity extension.

12. **Answer: C.** A lesion below or at the red nucleus has been traditionally associated with decerebrate posturing, therefore allowing the vestibulospinal tract to dominate.

13. **Answer: D.** All of the above are good options and are part of the management of neuroleptic malignant syndrome. However, stopping the neuroleptics is the first and foremost step in the management.

14. **Answer: B.** The patient most likely has hepatic encephalopathy, which is a type of metabolic coma. With elevated ammonia levels, the type of tremor she most likely has is asterixis, which is defined as transient loss of postural tone and therefore occasionally falling transiently when the tone is decreased.

15. **Answer: E.** A subhyaloid hemorrhage is pathognomonic for subarachnoid hemorrhage in a comatose patient. Although all the others can be present except Roth spots (which are often seen with bacterial endocarditis, leukemia, vasculitis, and diabetic retinopathy), none are diagnostic in a comatose patient for a subarachnoid hemorrhage.

16. **Answer: C.** Disruption of the papillary light reflex in a comatose patient (excluding medication effect) typically implies downward herniation of medial temporal structures due to an expanding supratentorial mass or a brain stem lesion. Usually, the third cranial nerve or the nuclei in the midbrain have been injured.

17. **Answer: A.** Lesions in the pontine tegmentum, which selectively interfere with sympathetic outflow, can produce pinpoint pupils (sometimes known as pontine pupils). Opiate overdose is also a common cause.

18. **Answer: B.** Persistent eye deviation especially to the same side as the hemiparesis in an unresponsive patient is possibly due to a seizure. The lesion most likely is in the right frontal lobe (contralateral to the hemiparesis).

19. **Answer: A.** If the oculocephalic reflex is present or positive (or positive doll's eye reflex), the eyes do not turn with the head but move in the opposite direction, as if the person is trying to maintain a visual fix on a single point (for example, one tile on the ceiling).

20. **Answer: C.** Caloric testing requires the head to be in a 30-degree position from horizontal and at least 50 mL of ice cold water. You must first verify there is no obstruction in the ear as well as no perforated eardrum. You should also wait 5 minutes before testing the opposite ear.

21. **Answer: B.** A cold caloric test done on an awake person (psychogenic coma) would result in deviation in the eye toward the stimulated ear but also severe vertigo, nystagmus, nausea, and probably vomiting.

22. **Answer: E.** Wernicke's encephalopathy selectively interferes with the vestibule-ocular reflex and spares other brain stem functions or reflexes.

23. **Answer: B.** Absent corneal reflexes 24 hours after a cardiac arrest has been associated with poor prognosis in many instances (not 100%). This is assuming no sedation has been used.

24. **Answer: B.** Third cranial nerve palsy is very first sign of uncal herniation syndromes. The other options occur later (however, they can occur very rapidly).

25. **Answer: B.** Although papilledema is a sign of increased intracranial pressure, it is traditionally not part of Cushing's triad.

26. **Answer: C.** Most metabolic comas typically present in a symmetrical fashion; however, with hypo- and hyperglycemia, they are often associated with lateralizing signs.

27. **Answer: D.** As mentioned in the previous question, metabolic comas typically present in a symmetrical pattern. Tremor, myoclonus, and asterixis (if seen) are very suggestive of a metabolic coma.

28. **Answer: B.** With sympathomimetic toxicity, the patient's pupils are enlarged. Cocaine is an example of a sympathomimetic and therefore would result in her pupils being dilated.

29. **Answer: C.** The major difference between sympathomimetic and anticholinergic toxicity would be the diaphoresis (seen in sympathomimetics) and dry flushed skin (seen in anticholinergics). The other options are similar in both overdose situations.

30. **Answer: C.** Locked-in syndrome results from a lesion at the base of the pons, most typically due to occlusion at the top of the basilar artery. The person still retains consciousness, but paralysis of all muscles except the eyelids and vertical eye movements are still intact. All of the above except herpes encephalitis could present similar to a locked-in syndrome.

31. **Answer: C.** The patient has akinetic mutism. This is caused by a lesion in the prefrontal or premotor area, which is the area that is involved in initiating movements.

32. **Answer: C.** Catatonia is usually differentiated from coma usually by the person's ability to maintain a posture (e.g., sitting or standing). All of the other options cannot definitively differentiate the two.

33. **Answer: B.** Mannitol is often used when increased intracranial pressure is suspected. The others are all options when overdose or ingestion is thought to be involved.

34. **Answer: C.** The presence of papilledema suggests structural etiology of the comatose and therefore possible impending herniation. A spinal tap would be helpful and necessary once a CT scan of the head is performed. Any signs of increased intracranial pressure or structural lesion would contradict the lumbar puncture, which could lead to herniation.

35. **Answer: D.** Wernicke-Korsakoff syndrome is related to thiamine deficiency. There are two parts to the syndrome: Wernicke's encephalopathy is an acute syndrome, whereas Korsakoff's amnestic syndrome is a chronic condition. None of the other options are acute encephalopathies.

36. **Answer: D.** The patient has Wernicke's encephalopathy, which occurs typically in the setting of thiamine deficiency with chronic alcoholism. It has also been seen in the setting of poor nutrition (e.g., malabsorption, poor dietary or increased metabolic requirement). Megaloblastic mania has been associated with vitamin B_{12} deficiency.

37. **Answer: C.** Atrophy of the mamillary bodies is a highly specific finding in Wernicke's encephalopathy as well as Korsakoff's syndrome and is present in up to 80% of cases.

38. **Answer: C.** The symptoms of Wernicke's encephalopathy typically present more or less at the same time. Occasionally, however, ataxia precedes other symptoms by a few days or even weeks.

39. **Answer: C.** Toxic metabolic encephalopathy is common among patients who are admitted to the intensive care unit. Older patients and those with underlying dementia are at greatest risk. About 31% of patients older than 65 years of age develop delirium in the intensive care unit.

40. **Answer: D.** Cerebral edema is found in 80% of patients with acute hepatic encephalopathy and is caused by cytotoxic edema and breakdown of the blood-brain barrier leading to increased permeability.

41. **Answer: C.** Nausea and malaise are the earliest signs of hyponatremia and usually are seen with plasma sodium concentration below 125 to 130 mEq/L. Seizures, coma, and respiratory arrest can be seen when plasma sodium concentration falls below 115 to 120 mEq/L.

42. **Answer: E.** All four of the above are prerequisites needed to start evaluating patients for brain death.

43. **Answer: E.** All of the above would not exclude brain death. Movements originating from the spinal cord or peripheral nerve may occur in brain death. Approximately 33% to 75% of patients may have these reflex movements related to tactile stimuli or they may occur spontaneously.

44. **Answer: B.** A positive apnea test is when there is no respiratory response to a $PaCO_2 > 60$ mm Hg or a 20-mm Hg increase from baseline.

45. **Answer: B.** In the United States, two physicians and an observation time of 6 hours is the minimum requirement to diagnose brain death, and ancillary tests are optional.

46. **Answer: C.** Cerebral angiography (four-vessel) is the traditional test among cerebral blood flow test for brain death. This test is very invasive, risky, and also requires moving the patient. This test in brain death demonstrates absent blood flow around the carotid bifurcation (it can also occur at the circle of Willis). There are false-negative results in the setting of profound hypotension.

47. **Answer: E.** The options listed may produce a neurologic examination that can mimic brain death; however, they should not be mistaken if the proper brain death criteria are applied.

48. **Answer: D.** The duration of CPR correlates with outcome. No patients that require more than 15 minutes of CPR survived more than 6 weeks. Out-of-hospital cardiac arrest has shown approximately 44% of patients that receive CPR survive initially, 30% survived 24 hours, 13% were alive at 1 month, and 6% were alive at 6 months.

49. **Answer: B.** The induction of hypothermia (32°C to 34°C) for 24 hours after cardiac arrest improves neurological outcome of patients successfully resuscitated after cardiac arrest, even when the patient remains comatose after resuscitation.

50. **Answer: E.** The apnea test and examination by two physicians separated by 6 hours is the only requirement for brain death in the United States. Ancillary tests are not mandatory but are sometimes recommended.

Behavioral Neurology and Dementia

QUESTIONS

1. What percentage of people in the United States older than 80 have Alzheimer's dementia (AD)?

   A. 5%
   B. 25%
   C. 40%
   D. 75%
   E. None of the above

2. Which of the following areas is most involved in AD?

   A. Occipital lobe
   B. Basal ganglia
   C. Pons
   D. Medial temporal lobe
   E. None of the above

3. Which of the following is not seen in AD?

   A. Granulovacuolar degeneration
   B. Neuropil threads
   C. Neuronal loss and synaptic degeneration
   D. Neurofibrillary tangles
   E. All of the above

4. Which of the following structures is most affected by neurofibrillary tangles?

   A. Entorhinal cortex
   B. Caudate
   C. Layer III of the parietal lobe
   D. Cerebral peduncle
   E. None of the above

5. A 76-year-old male with a history of dementia presents to your office. He seems to be doing well, and his caretaker confirms this. Which of the following most likely will cause this patient's death?

   A. Myocardial infarction
   B. Stroke
   C. Motor vehicle accident
   D. Pneumonia
   E. All of the above

6. What percentage of AD is familial?

   A. 10%
   B. 35%
   C. 75%
   D. 100%
   E. None of the above

7. Which of the following is the most common presenting symptom in AD?

   A. Focal weakness
   B. Gait disturbance
   C. Urinary incontinence
   D. Language difficulty
   E. Memory problems

8. Which of the following needs to be excluded to diagnose AD?

   A. Syphilis
   B. Hypothyroidism
   C. Stroke
   D. Cobalamin deficiency
   E. All of the above

9. Which of the following is associated with a variant of AD?

   A. Urinary incontinence
   B. Spastic paraparesis
   C. Right facial droop
   D. Ataxia
   E. None of the above

10. A 76-year-old male is sent to your clinic for evaluation of AD. You have ruled other possible causes and diagnose him with AD. Which of the following is associated with this condition?
    A. Presenilin IV
    B. Chromosome 2
    C. Amyloid precursor protein
    D. Alpha-amyloid peptide
    E. None of the above

11. Which of the following chromosomes has been associated with the amyloid precursor protein?
    A. Chromosome 14
    B. Chromosome 1
    C. Chromosome 21
    D. X-linked
    E. None of the above

12. Which of the following statements is true regarding AD?
    A. No intervention has been shown to prevent AD or slow its progression.
    B. N-methyl-D-aspartate (NMDA) antagonists are extremely effective.
    C. Cholinesterase inhibitors are third-line agents for the treatment of AD.
    D. Psychotropic medications should always be avoided in AD patients.
    E. None of the above

13. An 87-year-old female with severe AD presents with extreme anger and rage. Which of the following medications has been approved by the FDA for the treatment of behavioral changes in AD?
    A. Haloperidol
    B. Risperidone
    C. Gabapentin
    D. Quetiapine
    E. None of the above

14. Which of the following should be part of the routine work-up for dementia?

    A. Complete blood count
    B. Cobalamin
    C. Liver enzyme
    D. Cortisol
    E. Thyroid-stimulating hormone blood test
    F. All of the above

15. A 65-year-old male presents with a long-standing history of dementia. He is seen by a specialist and is recommended to have further testing to help confirm AD. Which of the following tests could be ordered?

    A. Serum ferritin
    B. Cerebrospinal fluid (CSF)-tau levels
    C. CSF hypocretin-1
    D. Serum amyloid
    E. None of the above

16. A 90-year-old female presents with a history of AD for 10 years. She has steadily progressed over the past 10 years requiring all her ADLs and language deficit. Which of the following anatomical locations would be most depleted or damaged in this patient?

    A. Nucleus solitarius
    B. Basal nucleus of Meynert
    C. Reticular nucleus of the thalamus
    D. Medial geniculate nucleus
    E. None of the above

17. NMDA antagonists are often used to treat AD. In which of the following scenarios would this drug be favored over cholinesterase inhibitors?

    A. Parkinson's disease
    B. Late-stage AD
    C. Hepatic encephalopathy
    D. Huntington's disease
    E. B and D
    F. C and D

18. A 63-year-old female with a recent diagnosis of AD presents to the clinic. Her husband states she has become very depressed lately. She is initiated on an antidepressant. Which of the following is the percentage of patients with AD that have depression as well?
    A. 5%
    B. 31%
    C. 70%
    D. 99%
    E. None of the above

19. A 71-year-old man presents with his son for the treatment of AD. His son states that he has been placed on memantine, and they have seen good results. Which of the following could also be done as an adjunct to help his father?
    A. Increase the memantine
    B. Provide the patient with brainteaser puzzles
    C. Add cholinesterase inhibitor
    D. Use diphenhydramine to help his father sleep
    E. None of the above

20. Which of the following is the main difference between AD in Down syndrome and AD in the general population?
    A. Patients with Down syndrome do not have amyloid deposits.
    B. In Down syndrome patients, dementia occurs at an earlier age.
    C. Down syndrome patients have Lewy body deposition as well.
    D. All of the above
    E. None of the above

21. Which of the following is part of a theory regarding why Down syndrome patients develop AD?
    A. They often graduate college.
    B. Trisomy 2
    C. Someone else in the family has AD.
    D. Cognitive reserve hypothesis
    E. None of the above

22. A 35-year-old male with Down syndrome is starting to develop memory difficulty. He wants to know how long he may live. What would you tell him?
    A. About 1 year
    B. At least 10 years
    C. More than 50 years
    D. Less than 6 months
    E. None of the above

23. A 21-year-old man with Down syndrome presents with increasing aggression. He is also noted to be very stubborn and refuses to do his chores. His parents are extremely frustrated. His neurologic examination is unchanged, and he denies any headaches or visual changes. His parents state there is nothing else wrong. Which of the following is the most likely cause of this patient's symptoms?
    A. Lack of sleep
    B. Exaggeration of a previous long-standing trait
    C. Stroke
    D. Behavioral changes are not usually seen in Down syndrome, and therefore looking for a structural lesion is crucial.
    E. None of the above

24. A 45-year-old female with Down syndrome presents with advanced-stage dementia. Which of the following would most likely demonstrate her current condition?
    A. Decreased muscle tone
    B. Vegetative state
    C. Some mild language difficulty
    D. Able to perform some ADLs
    E. None of the above

25. For patients with AD with or without Down syndrome, which of the following is the most important risk factor for AD?
    A. Presence of trisomy 21
    B. Age
    C. Family history of AD
    D. Small head circumference
    E. History of multiple concussion

26. Which of the following has been associated with decreased risk of AD?

    A. Stroke
    B. Low IQ
    C. Mediterranean diet
    D. Sedentary lifestyle
    E. None of the above

27. Which of the following is associated with aphasia?

    A. Left middle cerebral artery (MCA) territory stroke involving Broca's area
    B. Developmental disorders of language
    C. Stuttering
    D. Schizophrenia-associated language difficulty
    E. All of the above

28. What percentage of left-handed people have language control in their left hemisphere?

    A. <1%
    B. 15%
    C. 60%
    D. 100%
    E. None of the above

29. A 56-year-old man presents with difficulty expressing himself and right-handed weakness. What percentage of patients develop aphasia due to stroke?

    A. 5%
    B. 20%
    C. 75%
    D. 99%
    E. None of the above

30. Which of the following statements regarding gender and aphasia is true?

    A. Women develop aphasia more than men.
    B. Men are equal to women in developing aphasia.
    C. Men develop Wernicke's aphasia more than women do.
    D. Women develop aphasia less than men.
    E. None of the above

31. Which of the following is considered part of aphasic syndromes?
    A. Global
    B. Conduction
    C. Aphemia
    D. Anomic
    E. All of the above

32. In the previous question, which choice is considered the most common and most widely understood and accepted?
    A. Global
    B. Conduction
    C. Aphemia
    D. Anomic
    E. None of the above

33. A 77-year-old male presents with acute onset of confusion. He is later found to have aphasia. Which of the following are good language tests to help elucidate his aphasia?
    A. Boston Diagnostic Aphasia Examination
    B. Token test
    C. Action Naming Test
    D. Western Aphasia Battery
    E. All of the above
    F. None of the above

34. Which of the following is not a common bedside test for aphasia?
    A. Naming
    B. Repetition
    C. Comprehension
    D. Pursuit
    E. All of the above

35. A 65-year-old female who presented with a recent stroke to her left temporal-parietal region is being evaluated. She is asked to name as many animals as she can think of in 1 minute. Which of the following area is being assessed during this test?
    A. Occipital lobe
    B. Frontal lobe
    C. Right parietal lobe
    D. Brain stem
    E. None of the above

36. A 56-year-old male is being evaluated for acute aphasia. He has severe difficulty with repetition. What is the most likely location of his deficit?
    A. Left mesial temporal region
    B. Right thalamus
    C. Perisylvian region
    D. Nonperisylvian region
    E. None of the above

37. A 46-year-old female with atrial fibrillation presents with a right hemispheric stroke. She has difficulty attending to her left and misses reading the left side of the book. Which of the following accurately describes her?
    A. Neglect apraxia
    B. Neglect dyslexia
    C. Aphemia
    D. Agraphia without acalculia
    E. None of the above

38. A 72-year-old man presents with nonfluent aphasia. Which of the following would help support the location of the lesion?
    A. Left hemiparesis
    B. Buccofacial apraxia
    C. Urinary incontinence
    D. Acalculia
    E. None of the above

39. With Broca's aphasia, where is the most likely location of the lesion?
    A. Posterior temporal horn
    B. Cingulate gyrus
    C. Inferior frontal gyrus operculum
    D. Posterior parietal lobe
    E. None of the above

40. A 56-year-old female with recent left MCA distribution infarct is diagnosed with Wernicke's aphasia. Primarily, she is found to have word substitution difficulty but has other deficits as well, consistent with the lesion. Which of the following is true?
    A. Comprehension of language is intact.
    B. Naming is impaired but repetition is intact.
    C. Neologism may be present.
    D. Grammar is not as preserved as it is in Broca's aphasia.
    E. None of the above

41. Patients with Wernicke's are not always aware of their deficits. They are often mistaken to be confused and sometimes even psychotic. Which of the following is true?

    A. The lesion usually involves the posterior one third of the superior temporal gyrus.
    B. Wernicke's aphasia is often due to a stroke involving the left anterior cerebral artery.
    C. The amount of recovery from Wernicke's aphasia is independent of age.
    D. Superior quadrantanopsia is not a helpful sign in Wernicke's aphasia.

42. Lesions of the occipital gyrus or fusiform gyrus would result in what deficit?

    A. Difficulty in naming inanimate objects
    B. Impaired verb naming
    C. Impaired ability to name living things
    D. A and B
    E. None of the above

43. A 54-year-old female presents with an acute aphasia. She is found to have conduction aphasia. Which of the following is a hallmark feature?

    A. Repetition impairment
    B. Nonfluent aphasia
    C. Right hemiparesis
    D. Right hearing deficit
    E. None of the above

44. In the patient above, which of the following locations would correlate with her language deficit?

    A. Right posterior temporal lobe
    B. Left amygdala
    C. Left supramarginal gyrus
    D. Right posterior frontal lobe
    E. None of the above

45. In the patient in question 43, which of the following signs would also help confirm the diagnosis?
   A. Acalculia
   B. Contralateral superior quadrantanopsia
   C. Contralateral limb apraxia
   D. A and C
   E. B and C

46. A patient presents with global aphasia. Which of the following is spared in this setting?
   A. Spontaneous speech
   B. Naming
   C. Repetition
   D. Reading
   E. None of the above

47. An 80-year-old male with a history of diabetes presents with global aphasia. The rest of his examination is normal. There are no signs of hemiparesis. Which of the following could explain this finding?
   A. Cerebellar lesion
   B. Thalamic lesion
   C. Caudate lesion
   D. Pontine lesion
   E. None of the above

48. A 63-year-old female with atrial fibrillation presents with a stroke. Magnetic resonance imaging demonstrates a lesion in both superior temporal gyri. Which of the following would be associated with this?
   A. Wernicke's aphasia
   B. Broca's aphasia
   C. Pure word deafness
   D. Conduction aphasia
   E. None of the above

49. Which of the following differentiates auditory nonverbal agnosia from pure word deafness?
    A. Auditory nonverbal agnosia involves failure to recognize familiar sounds.
    B. Pure word deafness has language deficits.
    C. Pure word deafness has no sparing of pure-tone hearing.
    D. Auditory nonverbal agnosia involves both language and nonlinguistic sounds.
    E. None of the above

50. Which of the following is associated with transcortical motor aphasia?
    A. Repetition is impaired.
    B. Mutism may be present initially.
    C. Initiation of speech is intact.
    D. There is no difference between transcortical motor aphasia and Broca's aphasia.
    E. None of the above

51. A 78-year-old male presents with an acute stroke. Which of the following locations would explain why the patient has lost the ability to perform skilled movements but has full motor strength?
    A. Supplementary motor cortex
    B. Left inferior parietal lobe
    C. Corpus callosum
    D. All of the above
    E. None of the above

52. A 55-year-old female presents with ideomotor apraxia on examination. Which of the following would be an example of a bedside test for this problem?
    A. Tandem walk
    B. Showing how to hammer a nail into the wall
    C. Asking to repeat three words
    D. Asking the patient for different ideas about her symptoms
    E. None of the above

53. A 45-year-old male presents to the emergency department (ED). On examination, he is found to have difficulty performing tasks with his mouth. He cannot demonstrate how to blow out a candle or how to kiss. Which of the following could cause this?
    A. Lesion in the left inferior frontal region
    B. Chronic alcohol use
    C. History of gastric bypass surgery
    D. Hypoglycemia
    E. None of the above

54. Which of the following is part of Gerstmann's syndrome?
    A. Confusion of handedness
    B. Alexia with agraphia
    C. Inability to count numbers
    D. All of the above
    E. None of the above

55. An 89-year-old male presents with progressive difficulty with ADLs. His memory is intact, however, he demonstrates unilateral apraxia. Which of the following is possible?
    A. Vertebral dissection
    B. Corticobasal degeneration
    C. Reye's syndrome
    D. Anton's syndrome
    E. None of the above

56. Dementia with Lewy bodies accounts for what percentage of dementias?
    A. 15%
    B. 1%
    C. 50%
    D. 99%
    E. None of the above

57. Which of the following helps differentiate AD from dementia with Lewy bodies?
    A. Patients with AD have visual hallucinations.
    B. Patients who have dementia with Lewy body have Parkinsonian features.
    C. Patients with AD have intact rapid eye movement behavior disorder.
    D. Patients with AD have more visuospatial impairment.
    E. None of the above

58. A 65-year-old male presents with progressive dementia. While in the examination room, he goes from being alert, coherent, and oriented to a period of confusion and becomes unresponsive to questions but wide awake and then back. Which of the following is consistent with the patient's symptoms?

    A. Dementia with Lewy bodies
    B. AD
    C. Parkinson's dementia
    D. Frontotemporal dementia
    E. Vascular dementia

59. Which of the following statements regarding dementia with Lewy bodies is true?

    A. Myoclonus never occurs.
    B. Resting tremor occurs less frequently than in Parkinson's disease.
    C. Gait is rarely an issue.
    D. The etiology of this dementia is known.
    E. None of the above

60. An 80-year-old female with severe dementia, hallucinations, and Parkinson's features is found to be very agitated, and her hallucinations are becoming worse. Which of the following would be the next best step?

    A. Initiate antipsychotics.
    B. Initiate a psychiatry consult.
    C. Initiate acetylcholinesterase inhibitors.
    D. Administer neuropsychological testing.
    E. None of the above

61. A 78-year-old male who has dementia with Lewy bodies has severe agitation while being hospitalized. Donepezil was ineffective. Which of the following medications would be the treatment of choice?

    A. Quetiapine
    B. Haloperidol
    C. Metoclopramide
    D. Lorazepam
    E. None of the above

62. Which of the following may be the cause of depression in patients who have dementia with Lewy bodies?

   A. Damage to the locus ceruleus
   B. Axonal degeneration of the vagus nerve
   C. Psychological response to their impairment
   D. Depression is rarely seen in this type of dementia.
   E. A and C
   F. B and D

63. A 56-year-old male with a history of motor neuron disease presents with a gradual change in his personality per his wife. He was recently at a social gathering and suddenly became very disinhibited and took off all his clothes and started making inappropriate jokes. Which of the following is consistent?

   A. The patient is acutely psychotic and should be evaluated by a psychiatrist.
   B. This behavior is due to pyramidal cell loss in the frontal and temporal lobes.
   C. This behavior is due to Lewy bodies in the basal ganglia.
   D. This behavior is the patient's normal personality.
   E. None of the above

64. Which of the following tests is an adequate bedside test for frontal lobe dysfunction?

   A. Montreal Cognitive Assessment
   B. Mini-Mental State Examination
   C. Antisaccade task
   D. A and C
   E. B and C

65. A 56-year-old male with a history of traumatic brain injury presents to the clinic. He is found to have abnormal digit span forward and backward testing. Which of the following would meet criteria for abnormal digit span?

   A. 4/4
   B. 7/2
   C. 5/3
   D. 6/1
   E. None of the above

66. A 78-year-old male with a long-standing history of dementia has had urinary incontinence. Which of the following areas could be the cause of the incontinence?
    A. Posterior superior frontal gyri
    B. Amygdala
    C. Left posterior temporal lobe
    D. Lateral medullary lesion
    E. None of the above

67. A 59-year-old male with a history of atrial fibrillation presents with an acute stroke. He is found to have abulia as well as some personality changes. There is a period of time that he is agitated and confused, but then he progresses to abulia. Which of the following is correct?
    A. This is psychogenic and not organic.
    B. Occlusion of the artery of Heubner
    C. Bilateral parietal lobe infarcts
    D. Hypertensive bleed in the left thalamus
    E. None of the above

68. A 45-year-old male presents with a gradual decline of cognitive function. He is found to have anosmia, loss of inhibition, memory difficulty, and occasional visual changes. Which of the following could explain his symptoms?
    A. Basilar migraine
    B. Olfactory groove meningioma
    C. Early-onset AD
    D. Frontotemporal dementia
    E. None of the above

69. Which of the following are frontal release signs?
    A. Glabellar
    B. Snout
    C. Grasp
    D. Palmomental
    E. All of the above

70. A 61-year-old male with progressive problems presents to the neurologist. He is found to have normal pressure hydrocephalus. Which of the following is not part of the classic syndrome of normal pressure hydrocephalus?

    A. Incontinence
    B. Dementia
    C. Gait apraxia
    D. Headache
    E. All of the above are part of normal pressure hydrocephalus.

71. An 80-year-old male is found to have communicating hydrocephalus on computed tomography (CT) scan of his head. He has progressive difficulty with gait and memory. Which of the following is the most likely cause?

    A. Overproduction of CSF
    B. History of intraventricular hemorrhage
    C. Venous drainage insufficiency
    D. Aqueductal stenosis
    E. None of the above

72. A 55-year-old male presents with obstructive hydrocephalus. He is evaluated and treated by the neurosurgeon with a ventriculoperitoneal shunt. Which of the following represents the amount of CSF he produces in 1 hour?

    A. 10 mL
    B. 1 mL
    C. 20 mL
    D. 100 mL
    E. None of the above

73. A 40-year-old male with a recent diagnosis of minimal cognitive impairment is in your clinic. He is worried that he may develop AD. Which one of the following choices represents his annual risk of developing AD?

    A. 1% per year
    B. 15% per year
    C. 50% per year
    D. 90% per year
    E. None of the above

74. A 32-year-old female who has a history of migraines with aura presents to the ED with left-sided weakness and facial droop. She is found to have had an acute stroke with multiple areas of gliosis in the subcortical white matter predominately in the frontal lobe as well as in the basal ganglia. She is noted to have some mild dementia. Which of the following would help confirm her diagnosis?
    A. Homocysteine levels
    B. Thyroid status
    C. Notch3 gene mutation
    D. CT angiogram
    E. None of the above

75. A 45-year-old male presents with a history of chronic renal failure for 20 years. He has been on dialysis for that period of time. On examination, he is found to have dysarthria, myoclonus, dementia, and some apraxia. Which of the following is the cause of the encephalopathy?
    A. Medication
    B. Elevated ammonia levels
    C. Aluminum toxicity
    D. Increased protein 14-3-3
    E. None of the above

ANSWERS

1. **Answer: C.** The lifetime risk for Alzheimer's disease is approximately 1:4. It is estimated that more than 14% to 15% of people older than 65 have AD, and this figure increases to 40% in the over-80 age group.

2. **Answer: D.** Patients with AD have atrophy of the association areas, particularly the medial aspect of the temporal lobe.

3. **Answer: E.** All of the above choices are associated with AD. In addition, senile plaques are also seen. The neurofibrillary tangles and senile plaques are often thought of as the hallmark of the disease but are not pathognomonic.

4. **Answer: A.** Neurofibrillary tangles are initially and most densely distributed in the medial aspect of the temporal lobe and mostly affect the entorhinal cortex and the hippocampus.

5. **Answer: D.** The most common and primary cause of death in AD patients is concurrent illnesses (e.g., pneumonia), especially in patients who have had AD for many years and are debilitated by the disease.

6. **Answer: A.** Alzheimer's disease is typically sporadic (about 90%). Early-onset AD occurs in the familial form and has about 10% or less prevalence. This can occur as early as the patient's third decade in life.

7. **Answer: E.** Memory loss is the most common presenting symptom. After memory loss, the patient often develops anomia and aphasia. Impairment of executive function and visuospatial skills follows as well.

8. **Answer: E.** All of the above are necessary to be ruled out before anyone is labeled with AD.

9. **Answer: B.** Spastic paraparesis and right parietal lobe syndrome along with the other features of AD are associated with the visual variant of AD. This presentation of AD is extremely unusual.

10. **Answer: C.** Mutations that alter the way amyloid precursor protein is processed is thought to be the mechanism for AD. The amyloid precursor protein leads to aggregation of the 40 to 43 amino acid residues also known as beta-amyloid peptide. This peptide is thought to have neurotoxic effects.

11. **Answer: C.** The amyloid precursor protein is associated with chromosome 21.

12. **Answer: A.** Up until now, there has been no convincing treatment that can prevent or even delay the onset or slow the progression of AD.

13. **Answer: E.** Currently, the FDA has not approved any agent for the treatment of AD behavioral manifestations.

14. **Answer: F.** All of the above as well as RPR are often part of the routine screening for dementia workup. Current recommendations from the AAN recommend cobalamin and thyroid function as screening tests; all other tests are left to the physician's discretion.

15. **Answer: B.** The tau protein test is advocated by some experts. It can be measured in the CSF to help diagnose AD. This protein is seen in neurofibrillary tangles and amyloid protein. This test, however, is not a reliable test or mandatory.

16. **Answer: B.** AD is thought of as a disease process that is caused by depletion of acetylcholine in the cerebral cortex. The subcortical cholinergic neurons are thought to be primarily depleted in AD. The basal nucleus of Meynert and the medial septal nuclei in the hippocampus are the main cholinergic neurons that send projections to the cortex.

17. **Answer: E.** NMDA antagonists are approved for the advanced stages of AD that cholinesterase inhibitors are not approved for (however, cholinesterase inhibitors do help improve cognitive function in late-stage AD). Also, NMDA antagonists may also be helpful in treating Huntington's disease,

dementia associated with AIDS, and vascular dementia (cholinesterase inhibitors may be helpful in this situation as well).

18. **Answer: B.** More than 30% of patients with AD develop depression. Often, the depression may precede the diagnosis of AD. Treatment of the depression often improves both the cognitive and noncognitive performance.

19. **Answer: B.** Both physical and mental activity should be recommended to patients with AD. Often, crossword puzzles and brainteasers are recommended to mentally challenge patients. These puzzles, however, should not be too challenging, which would end in frustration and less motivation for the patient to continue.

20. **Answer: B.** Patients with Down syndrome have clinically and neuropathologically indistinguishable characteristics from patients with AD.

21. **Answer: D.** All patients with AD have been found to have limited education or diminished baseline cognitive abilities and are at a higher risk for AD. In Down syndrome, patients are often mentally retarded and have poor baseline cognition.

22. **Answer: B.** Once patients with Down syndrome develop AD, they often have a sharp decline in survival after age 45. The mean age at the time of clinical diagnosis of AD in Down syndrome is around age 51.

23. **Answer: B.** Behavioral changes are usually the early signs of dementia in Down syndrome. These changes are usually subtle early on, and the family or individuals that are close to him or her would recognize them. These changes are typically considered an exaggeration of long-standing behavioral traits.

24. **Answer: B.** Down syndrome patients with advanced-stage dementia as well as non-Down syndrome patients are usually in a comatose/vegetative state and usually require 100% assistance and interact minimally with the environment.

25. **Answer: B.** Age is the most important risk factor of those listed above. The others are all risk factors but are not as important.

26. **Answer: C.** A Mediterranean diet as well as an active lifestyle have been associated with decreased risk of AD.

27. **Answer: A.** Aphasia is an acquired disorder of language caused by a lesion or damage to the brain. All of the others are not true aphasia.

28. **Answer: C.** Approximately 60% of left-handed people are language dominant on the left side. About 96% to 99% of right-handed people are language dominant on the left. Of the 40% of the left-handed people, 50% are mixed language and the 50% are right-hemisphere dominant.

29. **Answer: B.** Stroke is the most common cause of aphasia, and about 20% of stroke patients develop aphasia.

30. **Answer: D.** There are few studies that evaluate gender differences regarding aphasia. Some studies suggest, however, that women develop aphasia less often than men, and it is thought that women may have more bilateral language function. It has also been suggested that women develop Wernicke's aphasia more than men.

31. **Answer: E.** All of the above as well as many others are part of aphasic syndromes or language syndromes. The classics are Broca's and Wernicke's, conduction, and global aphasia. Anomic, transcortical sensory, transcortical motor, and mixed transcortical aphasias, however, are also included. Some of the more specific language deficits are aphemia, alexia with and without agraphia, and pure word deafness.

32. **Answer: B.** Conduction along with Wernicke's, and Broca's aphasia are considered to be the most common and widely accepted.

33. **Answer: E.** All of the above are classic language tests often used by neuropsychologists and speech therapists to help evaluate aphasia as well as to plan therapy and predict recovery.

34. **Answer: D.** Pursuit is not a test for language but rather is used to evaluate eye movements. All of the others are common bedside tests. Reading, writing, and assessing spontaneous speech are also part of the bedside evaluation.

35. **Answer: B.** She is performing the Boston Diagnostic Aphasia Examination. It is considered to evaluate frontal lobe function and not language directly; however, the evaluation does include the patient's ability to speak spontaneously. Fewer than 8 words in 1 minute is considered abnormal.

36. **Answer: C.** Deficit with repetition is the hallmark of lesions in the perisylvian area. These are known as *perisylvian aphasias* and consist of all the classic aphasias near the sylvian fissure. Broca's, Wernicke's, conduction, and global aphasia are all included.

37. **Answer: B.** Neglect dyslexia is due to right hemispheric lesions and results in decreased attention to the contralateral side including words or sentences.

38. **Answer: B.** Patients with Broca's aphasia often have buccofacial or limb apraxia along with contralateral (right) hemiparesis. Buccofacial apraxia is the inability to blow a kiss or blow out a candle although there is no facial weakness.

39. **Answer: C.** Broca's aphasia is localized to the dorsolateral frontal cortex, specifically, the posterior two thirds of the inferior frontal gyrus operculum. Some patients have had lesions in the anterior parietal lobe, lateral

striate, and periventricular white matter. Some argue that Broca's aphasia could not occur without the subcortical white matter tract involvement.

40. **Answer: C.** Wernicke's aphasia is a fluent aphasia. The patients often use nonexistent words (neologism). They also often have paraphasic errors with sound (phonemic paraphasia) or word substation (semantic paraphasias). Grammar is better preserved than in patients with Broca's aphasia.

41. **Answer: A.** The lesion location can be variable but typically involves the posterior one third of the superior temporal gyrus.

42. **Answer: C.** Lesions in this location are more likely to cause deficits in naming living things or highly imageable words. Lesions in the frontal lobe often result in impaired verb naming, and lesions in the temporal lobe lead to difficulty naming inanimate objects.

43. **Answer: A.** Repetition impairment is the hallmark feature of conduction aphasias. Language output is fluent, but occasionally, the patient may make phonemic errors.

44. **Answer: C.** The supramarginal gyrus is the most often implicated location for conduction aphasia, although there is probable involvement of the subcortical connections in the arcuate fasciculus.

45. **Answer: E.** Associated signs with conduction aphasia would include the superior quadrantanopsia and limb apraxia depending on location.

46. **Answer: E.** All aspects of speech and language are affected in global aphasia. It is typically caused by a large left MCA or left carotid artery occlusion. This rarely occurs without hemiplegia.

47. **Answer: B.** Thalamic lesions can cause a global aphasia without hemiparesis.

48. **Answer: C.** Pure word deafness results in the inability to comprehend spoken language, but patients are not deaf; therefore, verbal output as well as reading ability typically are intact. This occurs most commonly due to damage at the Heschl gyrus bilaterally.

49. **Answer: A.** Auditory nonverbal agnosia causes deficits in recognizing familiar sounds such as a dog barking or a telephone ringing.

50. **Answer: B.** All the other statements are not true. Often, mutism is present initially and then gradually improves. Sometimes, the patient speaks only one word at a time or may speak in a soft voice.

51. **Answer: D.** All of the above locations have been implicated in causing apraxia, which is described in the question. Apraxia is a syndrome that reflects motor dysfunction in the absence of weakness. The patient loses the ability to perform skilled movements.

52. **Answer: B.** Ideomotor apraxia is demonstrated at the bedside by testing the patient's ability to pantomime tool use (e.g., brushing one's teeth).

53. **Answer: A.** The patient has buccofacial apraxia, which is usually localized to Brodmann's area 44 (also called *Broca's area*). Often, these patients present with Broca's aphasia as well.

54. **Answer: D.** All of the above.

55. **Answer: B.** Unilateral apraxia is often the presenting sign of corticobasal degeneration. It precedes any memory difficulty. The other name for this entity is Rebeitz syndrome. Patients often can have a useless limb (on the affected side) or exhibit bizarre behaviors with the affected limb.

56. **Answer: A.** About 10% to 20% of all dementias are dementias with Lewy bodies. Up to 40% of patients with AD have concomitant Lewy bodies.

57. **Answer: B.** Dementia patients with Lewy bodies have visual hallucinations, daytime sleepiness, and Parkinsonian features.

58. **Answer: A.** Dementia patients with Lewy bodies often have these fluctuating mental status examination scores, which is a relatively specific feature of this dementia.

59. **Answer: B.** Dementia patients with Lewy bodies have less resting tremor than patients with Parkinson's disease and often cannot meet the full criteria of Parkinson's. The rest of the statements are not true.

60. **Answer: C.** Acetylcholinesterase inhibitors are the drugs of choice for the treatment of agitation and hallucinations. These patients also do better on neuropsychological testing after starting treatment.

61. **Answer: A.** Most patients that do not respond to acetylcholinesterase inhibitors are typically tried on an atypical antipsychotic. Standard antipsychotics should be avoided in these patients because of neuroleptic sensitivity.

62. **Answer: E.** Damage to the dorsal raphe nucleus and locus ceruleus has been hypothesized as the cause of dementia. Also, there is probably a psychological response to their realization of their impairment.

63. **Answer: B.** Patients with motor neuron disease can go on to develop frontotemporal dementia (sometimes, the cognitive changes can occur prior to the motor neuron disease). This is due to pyramidal cell damage in the frontal and temporal lobes and degeneration of motor neurons in the hypoglossal nucleus and spinal motor neurons.

64. **Answer: D.** The Montreal cognitive assessment and the frontal assessment battery are good bedside tests to assess frontal lobe function. Other sensitive tests are the Go/No-Go task, antisaccade task, Trail-Making Test and the Thurstone Test.

65. **Answer: C.** A normal digit span is six to seven digits forward and four to five backward. Abnormal digit span is the most common deficit in patients with traumatic head injury.

66. **Answer: A.** Lesions in the posterior superior frontal gyri and anterior parts of the cingulated gyrus can lead to incontinence of urine and stool. This type of incontinence is usually unannounced, and patients are usually shocked or surprised that it has even happened.

67. **Answer: B.** Occlusion of the artery of Heubner would lead to infarction of the head of the caudate and could result in the above scenario. None of the other answers could explain the clinical scenario.

68. **Answer: B.** Olfactory groove meningioma would give the classic description of the patient above. None of the other answers clinically would correlate with the constellation of symptoms.

69. **Answer: E.** All of the above are considered frontal release signs.

70. **Answer: D.** Headache is typically not seen in patients with normal pressure hydrocephalus. The others are part of the classic Hakim triad.

71. **Answer: B.** Communication hydrocephalus occurs when there is no obstruction in the ventricular system and subarachnoid space. The most common cause is defective absorption of CSF. The least likely cause is overproduction of CSF.

72. **Answer: C.** CSF is made approximately 15 to 25 mL per hour. The total volume of CSF in an adult is approximately 120 mL.

73. **Answer: B.** Amnestic minimal cognitive impairment is said to progress to AD at an annual rate of 10% to 15%. A study conducted at the Mayo clinic demonstrated at 6 years the likelihood of developing AD was 80%.

74. **Answer: C.** The patient has CADASIL (cerebral autosomal dominant arteriopathy with subcortical infarcts and leukoencephalopathy). This is the most common form of hereditary stroke disorders. The Notch3 gene mutation is the confirmatory test to determine this disorder. Homocysteine levels can be elevated but do not confirm the diagnosis.

75. **Answer: C.** The patient has dialysis encephalopathy, which is usually caused by aluminum toxicity. Most patients who develop the dementia have approximately 6 months to live. This encephalopathy is part of a multisystem disease that also includes bone disease, proximal myopathy, and anemia.

Pediatric Neurology

QUESTIONS

1. A 5-year-old boy presents to the clinic with a history of epilepsy, cognitive regression, and progressive blindness. A skin biopsy is done and demonstrates intracellular accumulation that is yellow-green in color and is fluorescent. How did the boy get this disease?
   - **A.** It is X-linked.
   - **B.** It is autosomal dominant.
   - **C.** It is autosomal recessive.
   - **D.** He has Trisomy 21.
   - **E.** None of the above

2. A 9-year-old boy presents to the clinic with a history of staring spells about 20 times per day over the past 2 months. There is no family history of seizure. An electroencephalography is performed and demonstrates a 3-Hz spike and wave during hyperventilation. Which of the following is the best next step?
   - **A.** Order a magnetic resonance imaging brain scan.
   - **B.** Initiate phenytoin.
   - **C.** Initiate ethosuximide.
   - **D.** Report the family to social services.
   - **E.** There is nothing to do.

3. A 4-year-old girl presents with ataxia and skin lesions. She is diagnosed with ataxia-telangiectasia. What should the parents look out for?
   - **A.** Leukemia
   - **B.** Renal cell carcinoma
   - **C.** Death before age 20
   - **D.** Pontine atrophy
   - **E.** None of the above

4. A mother brings her 1-week-old daughter to your clinic and states her daughter's face is "crooked." As you evaluate the infant, you do not see any abnormalities, but she then starts crying and develops a right-sided facial droop. What is the best next step?

   A. Lumbar puncture
   B. Vitamin B_{12}
   C. Echocardiogram
   D. Bone scan
   E. None of the above

5. Patients with craniofacial syndrome have an abnormality on what chromosome?

   A. 1
   B. 12
   C. 16
   D. 22
   E. 2

6. Which of the following is not a cardinal feature of neuronal ceroid lipofuscinosis?

   A. Motor regression
   B. Progressive blindness
   C. Epilepsy
   D. Ataxia
   E. None of the above

7. A 12-year-old boy is found to have a Chiari malformation type II. Which of the following does he also have?

   A. Arachnoid cyst
   B. Intracranial hypotension
   C. Lumbar meningomyelocele
   D. Hypoplastic cerebellum
   E. All of the above

8. During gestation, at what week does gyri formation occur?

   A. 6
   B. 14
   C. 24
   D. 36
   E. None of the above

9. A father brings his son in for a check-up. The child is able to wave hello, plays peekaboo, and can crawl and sit without support. He has been developing appropriately. What age must he at least be?

    A. 8 weeks
    B. 8 months
    C. 12 months
    D. 24 months
    E. None of the above

10. A term infant is found hypotonic and moderately weak at birth. Her mother has a history of myasthenia gravis. What percentage of infants born to mothers with myasthenia gravis will develop neonatal myasthenia?

    A. 1%
    B. 15%
    C. 50%
    D. 99%
    E. None of the above

11. In the infant in the previous question, what is the next best step?

    A. Administer treatment with oral medication.
    B. Supportive care
    C. Plasma exchange
    D. Intravenous steroids
    E. None of the above

12. A neonate presents with a seizure. On lab testing, he is found to have low blood glucose. Which of the following would not be the cause of the lab abnormality?

    A. Glycogen storage disease
    B. Fructose 1,6 diphosphatase deficiency
    C. Maple syrup urine disease
    D. Citrullinemia
    E. None of the above

13. A neonate is born comatose and with lower cranial nerve damage. The most likely etiology is neonatal asphyxia. Which of the following would help support this diagnosis?
    A. Enterocolitis
    B. Normal hepatic enzymes
    C. No evidence of irregular rhythm
    D. Usually no meconium is passed
    E. None of the above

14. Which of the following are causes of persistent hypoglycemia in a neonate?
    A. Maternal diabetes
    B. Prematurity
    C. Asphyxia
    D. Aminoaciduria
    E. Intrauterine malnutrition

15. A 1-month-old infant is found to have hypocalcemia. On further examination, she is found to have facial abnormality and absent or low T cells. Which of the following chromosomes are linked with her abnormality?
    A. 1
    B. 12
    C. 19
    D. 22
    E. None of the above

16. Which one of the following statements about primitive reflexes is true?
    A. Hand grasp reflex is present around 3 months and usually disappears around 4 months of age.
    B. Hand grasp reflex typically appears by 34 weeks and disappears around 6 months of age.
    C. The Moro reflex appears around 9 months and usually persists.
    D. The parachute reflex appears around 9 months of age and disappears by age 2 years.
    E. None of the above

17. A 6-year-old child presents with staring spells. She is diagnosed with absence seizures. Which of the following could be used as monotherapy?

    A. Tiagabine
    B. Gabapentin
    C. Lamotrigine
    D. Dilantin
    E. None of the above

18. A 3-year-old boy presents with worsening irritability, weight loss, and fever. There is a palpable abdominal mass on examination. Imaging shows a large mass arising from the adrenal gland. Which of the following paraneoplastic disorders is most classically associated with this type of tumor?

    A. Myasthenia gravis
    B. Stiff-person syndrome
    C. Myotonic dystrophy
    D. Myoclonic encephalopathy of infants
    E. None of the above

19. What is the most common type of focal epilepsy in children?

    A. West syndrome
    B. Landau-Kleffner syndrome
    C. Benign epilepsy with centrotemporal spikes (BECTS)
    D. Benign occipital epilepsy
    E. None of the above

20. A 13-year-old female presents with a history of choreoathetosis, dysarthric speech, grimacing, and awkward gait, which have been slowly progressing since early childhood. She has telangiectasias on her eye examination. Which of the following chromosomes is associated with this disorder?

    A. 11
    B. 20
    C. 4
    D. 9
    E. None of the above

21. Which of the following is often associated with Landau-Kleffner syndrome?
    A. Absence seizures
    B. Rheumatoid arthritis
    C. Electrical status epilepticus of sleep
    D. It is most often associated with an underlying tumor.
    E. None of the above

22. A 9-year-old boy presents with episodes of dystonia. He is diagnosed with dopamine-responsive dystonia. Which of the following is true?
    A. It occurs more often in boys than girls.
    B. It has a circadian pattern.
    C. The patient has no signs of gait abnormalities.
    D. It has no association with focal dystonias.
    E. None of the above

23. Which of the following is not part of the triad that comprises the clinical elements of Lesch-Nyhan syndrome?
    A. Uremia
    B. Neurologic impairment
    C. Uricemia
    D. Behavioral problems
    E. None of the above

24. A 5-year-old boy with swallowing difficulties is found to have a medulloblastoma. Which of the following is true?
    A. This is a type of glioma.
    B. It is primarily found in the posterior fossa.
    C. It is typically a hereditary disorder.
    D. Hydrocephalus rarely complicates the situation.
    E. None of the above

25. A 14-year-old female is diagnosed with neurofibromatosis type 1 (NF1). Which of the following is associated with NF1?
    A. Optic nerve glioma
    B. Inguinal freckles
    C. Café-au-lait spots
    D. Pseudoarthrosis
    E. All of the above
    F. None of the above

26. A 15-year-old boy presents to the office with complaints of frequent twitching of his right eye. He is diagnosed with motor tics. Which of the following is true?

    A. Symptom onset should be younger than age 18.
    B. Females are more often affected than males.
    C. The symptoms usually resolve by the third decade.
    D. Tics are not suppressible.
    E. None of the above

27. Which of the following is a core feature of pervasive developmental disorder?

    A. Impaired social skills
    B. Impaired verbal communication
    C. Impaired nonverbal communication
    D. Perseveration
    E. All of the above
    F. None of the above

28. A very small newborn is found to have a periventricular-intraventricular hemorrhage, which was noted to be located at the germinal plate with some ventricular involvement. What grade would the hemorrhage be classified as?

    A. I
    B. II
    C. III
    D. IV
    E. V

29. Which of the following is/are possible causes for hypoxic-ischemic encephalopathy at birth?

    A. Placental abruption
    B. Uterine rupture
    C. Umbilical cord infarction
    D. A and C
    E. All of the above

30. What is the predominant bacterial infection associated with neonatal meningitis?

    A. Group A streptococcus
    B. Herpes simplex virus
    C. Mycoplasma
    D. Group B streptococcus
    E. N. meningitis

31. What is the mortality rate associated with neonatal seizures?

    A. 5%
    B. 20%
    C. 50%
    D. 80%
    E. None of the above

ANSWERS

1. **Answer: C.** This is an autosomal recessive disorder. The patient has neuronal ceroid lipofuscinoses.

2. **Answer: C.** The patient has absence seizures of childhood. The first-line agent for monotherapy is ethosuximide. This is a generalized epilepsy.

3. **Answer: C.** Patients with ataxia-telangiectasia have an increased risk of death by age 20. Also, these patients are at increased risk of cerebellar degeneration, B-cell lymphoma, and hypertrichosis.

4. **Answer: C.** The patient has craniofacial syndrome, which is often accompanied by cardiac abnormalities.

5. **Answer: D.** These patients have a deletion at 22q11.

6. **Answer: D.** Ataxia is not part of neuronal ceroid lipofuscinosis. Along with the others, cognitive regression and intracellular accumulation of auto-fluorescent material are cardinal features.

7. **Answer: C.** There are four types of Chiari malformations. Type II patients typically have the lumbar meningomyelocele. Syringomyelia, syringobulbia, and hydrocephalus are often seen in the first three types of Chiari malformations. The classification of Chiari type IV is not typically used anymore. Patients present with cerebellar hypoplasia and no protrusion of the tonsils through the foramen magnum.

8. **Answer: B.** It begins during week 14 and usually continues until week 32.

9. **Answer: B.** At 8 months of age, these are the appropriate milestones that should be occurring. At 12 months, he should be walking.

10. **Answer: B.** About 15% of infants born to mothers with myasthenia gravis develop neonatal myasthenia.

11. **Answer: B.** Neonatal myasthenia is typically self-limiting, and symptoms usually resolve without any specific treatment or intervention.

12. **Answer: D.** Citrullinemia would lead to elevated blood ammonia. The rest are all possible causes of low blood glucose.

13. **Answer: A.** Enterocolitis, along with lactic acidosis, elevated hepatic enzymes, renal failure, and fatal myocardial damage are usually present in patients with severe HIE.

14. **Answer: D.** Aminoaciduria along with congenital hypopituitarism, defects in carbohydrate metabolism, hyperinsulinemia, and organic acidurias are other possible causes for persistent hypoglycemia. The rest of the options are all possible causes for transient/transitional hypoglycemia.

15. **Answer: D.** The infant has DiGeorge syndrome, and it is associated with an abnormality on chromosome 22.

16. **Answer: B.** The hand grasp reflex appears around 34 weeks and then is no longer present by 6 months.

17. **Answer: C.** A patient absence seizure is usually treated with ethosuximide. If motor symptoms are present, valproate is often used. Lamotrigine has been shown to be effective as monotherapy.

18. **Answer: D.** The boy has neuroblastoma. It is characterized by acute or subacute onset of ataxia and opsoclonus/myoclonus ("dancing eyes and tremors").

19. **Answer: C.** BECTS is benign childhood epilepsy with centrotemporal spikes (also known as *benign Rolandic epilepsy*) and is the most common focal epilepsy.

20. **Answer: A.** The patient has ataxia-telangiectasia, and it is associated with a defect on chromosome 11.

21. **Answer: C.** Landau-Kleffner syndrome is also known as *acquired epileptic aphasia* and is often thought of as a spectrum of epilepsy with electrical status epilepticus during sleep (ESES). Acquired epileptic aphasia (AEA) typically develops in healthy children who acutely or progressively lose receptive and expressive language ability coincident with the appearance of paroxysmal EEG changes. It is rarely associated with an underlying cause.

22. **Answer: B.** Dopamine-responsive dystonia usually presents in the first decade of life and typically affects girls more than boys. It is characterized by diurnal fluctuations, exquisite responsiveness to levodopa, and mild Parkinsonian features. Gait disturbance is the most common presenting symptom, and these patients are often mistaken for having cerebral palsy.

23. **Answer: A.** Uremia is not part of Lesch-Nyhan syndrome. The others are all characteristics of this syndrome. The classic behavioral problems are self-mutilation—type behavior. This is a genetic disorder caused by a defect on the X chromosome. Neurologically, patients are typically cognitively impaired.

24. **Answer: B.** Medulloblastoma is a type of primitive neuroectodermal tumor. It is primarily found in the cerebellum or posterior fossa. Most cases are sporadic, and hydrocephalus is the most common complication.

25. **Answer: E.** There are seven clinical criteria. All of those listed are part of the seven; in addition, a first-degree relative with involvement, two or more hamartomas (Lisch nodules), and two or more typical neurofibromas or one plexiform neurofibroma are also criteria.

26. **Answer: B.** The age of onset should be younger than 18; some criteria use age 21. Boys are often affected more, and the symptoms usually persist throughout a person's entire life but may fluctuate in severity. The tics are suppressible, but after prolonged suppression, a rebound effect often occurs.

27. **Answer: E.** Pervasive developmental disorders have variable symptoms, but the core features are impaired sociability, verbal, nonverbal communication, and decreased interests and activities. Some patients have stereotypical movements and self-injury.

28. **Answer: B.** Blood that is confined only to the germinal plate would be grade I. Once the blood extends into the ventricle, it is grade II. Grade II with increased intraventricular component and grade IV has blood in the brain parenchyma itself. There is no grade V.

29. **Answer: E.** HIE occurs in all the above scenarios and can occur despite optimal obstetric management. The incidence is two to four per 1,000 births.

30. **Answer: D.** Bacterial meningitis in neonates is usually seen with sepsis, and the predominate organism in the United States is group B streptococcus and gram-negative bacteria.

31. **Answer: B.** A mortality rate of at least 17% to 20% is seen with neonates with seizures, and almost one third of patients have serious morbidity.

Neurophysiology

QUESTIONS

1. A patient is found to be in a coma, and an electroencephalogram (EEG) is performed. Which of the following on the EEG would support the finding that this patient was in hepatic encephalopathy?

   A. POST
   B. Alpha rhythm
   C. Triphasic waves (TWs)
   D. 3-Hz spike and wave
   E. None of the above

2. Which of the following would be consistent with a brain tumor located in the left parietal lobe?

   A. Spike and wave discharges on the right hemisphere
   B. Delta wave in the left hemisphere
   C. POST
   D. Posterior dominant rhythm of 9 Hz
   E. None of the above

3. A 32-year-old female is diagnosed with optic neuritis. A visual evoked potential is tested. Which of the following is true?

   A. Retrochiasmatic lesions would be best detected with this test.
   B. Prolonged P-100 would be consistent with the diagnosis.
   C. Temporal axons of the optic nerve cross anterior to the optic chiasm.
   D. Carbamazepine usually shortens the latency of this test.
   E. None of the above

4. A 67-year-old male with early-onset dementia on no medication has an EEG. Which of the following would most likely be seen?

   A. Alpha frequency of 8 Hz
   B. Occasional temporal sharp waves
   C. No reactivity
   D. TWs
   E. None of the above

5. A 56-year-old male with an episode of confusion is found to have transient global amnesia. Which of the following would be consistent with this diagnosis on EEG?

   A. Normal
   B. Slow background rhythm
   C. 4-Hz spike and wave with photic stimulation
   D. Occasional occipital sharps
   E. None of the above

6. Which of the following diseases may be consistent with TWs?

   A. Multi-infarct dementia
   B. Creutzfeldt-Jakob disease
   C. Parkinson's disease
   D. Progressive supranuclear palsy
   E. None of the above

7. Which of the following would be seen in a patient in stage I sleep (drowsy)?

   A. Sleep spindles
   B. Rapid eye movements
   C. Slow roving eye movements
   D. Periodic leg movements
   E. None of the above

8. Which of the following are considered to be idiopathic generalized epilepsies?

   A. West syndrome
   B. Juvenile myoclonic epilepsy
   C. Autosomal dominant frontal lobe epilepsy
   D. Lennox-Gastaut syndrome
   E. None of the above

9. Which of the following are not considered EEG artifacts?
    A. Eye movements
    B. Glossokinetic
    C. Sweat
    D. Respiration
    E. None of the above
    F. All of the above

10. A 45-year-old male with acute head trauma is encephalopathic. An EEG is performed and shows some amplitude asymmetry from one side to the other. Which of the following is a likely etiology?
    A. Electrode malfunction
    B. Underlying hematoma
    C. History of seizures
    D. Mesial temporal sclerosis
    E. None of the above

11. A 56-year-old male with a recent stroke is undergoing transcranial magnetic stimulation in a research study to see if he can regain function. Which of the following would not be a contraindication?
    A. Pacemaker
    B. Recent head trauma
    C. History of epilepsy
    D. Metallic foreign body
    E. None of the above; they all are contraindications.

12. A 32-year-old female with a recent history of optic neuritis undergoes visual evoked potentials. Which of the following statements is true regarding the visual evoked potentials?
    A. Amplitude will be decreased
    B. Prolongation of the P-100
    C. Amplitude will be increased
    D. Shortened P-100
    E. None of the above

13. A 23-year-old male presents after severe head trauma due to a motor vehicle accident. He is found to be comatose, and an EEG is performed. Which of the following would favor a better prognosis?

    A. Widespread continuous spindles
    B. Minimal reactivity
    C. Spindle coma with reactivity
    D. Excessive alpha with no reactivity
    E. None of the above

14. Which of the following is the most common artifact seen on EEG?

    A. Muscle
    B. Sharp waves
    C. Alpha rhythm
    D. Sweat
    E. Photic

15. Which of the following is often seen during rapid eye movement (REM) sleep?

    A. K-complex
    B. Spindles
    C. POSTs
    D. Sawtooth waves
    E. None of the above

16. Which of the following frequencies would be consistent with spindle activity on EEG?

    A. 4 Hz
    B. 14 Hz
    C. 20 Hz
    D. 50 Hz
    E. None of the above

17. Which of the following aspects of stage II sleep is true?

    A. Rapid eye movements are seen.
    B. Lowest electromyography (EMG) tone
    C. Vertex sharp waves are required for this stage.
    D. Loud noises can cause K-complex.
    E. None of the above

18. A 12-year-old boy is found to be sleep walking and sleep talking regularly. His last sleep-walking episode led him to leave the house, but he did not injure himself. Which of the following is true?
    A. This occurred out of slow-wave sleep.
    B. This sounds like REM behavior disorder.
    C. Nightmares are the usual cause of sleep walking.
    D. The boy must be awake and should seek psychological evaluation.
    E. None of the above

19. A 56-year-old male is comatose after cardiac arrest. An EEG is performed using strict guidelines, and he is deemed to have electrocerebral inactivity. The intensive care team has told the family that he is brain dead. Which of the following statements is true?
    A. His core body temperature must be less than 32°C.
    B. He must be on sedation for his comfort.
    C. The patient must have passed the apnea test.
    D. He has no brain activity greater than 2 uV.
    E. None of the above

20. Which of the following are somatosensory evoked potentials (SSEPs) used in neurological patients?
    A. Prognosis in comatose patients
    B. Evaluation for epileptic activity
    C. Evaluating corticospinal tract abnormalities
    D. Spinal cord abnormalities are not evaluated using this modality.
    E. None of the above

21. The N20 is a critical value in the testing of SSEPs. In a patient with anoxic brain injury who has absent N20s bilaterally, which of the following would be true?
    A. This is a poor prognosis.
    B. All patients with absent N20s always have bad outcomes.
    C. EEG is more sensitive in abnormalities in the spinal cord.
    D. A and B
    E. None of the above

22. Which of the following are determinants of mortality and morbidity in status epilepticus?
    A. Etiology
    B. Family history
    C. Age
    D. A and C
    E. None of the above

23. In which of the following would a brain stem auditory evoked response be useful?
    A. Left parietal stroke
    B. Demyelinating disease
    C. Acoustic neuroma
    D. B and C
    E. All of the above

24. In a patient with AIDS dementia, which of the following is true?
    A. Magnetic resonance imaging (MRI) readings of the brain are usually normal.
    B. EEG abnormalities precede memory difficulties.
    C. Computed tomography (CT) scan of the head usually shows atrophy.
    D. Antiretroviral medications have no improvement in AIDS dementia.
    E. All of the above

25. What percentage of patients with focal slowing on EEG will have an abnormal MRI or CT scan of the head?
    A. 1%
    B. 10%
    C. 33%
    D. 70%
    E. 100%

26. REM sleep seen during a routine daytime EEG can be due to which of the following?
    A. Narcolepsy
    B. Sleep deprivation
    C. ETOH withdrawal
    D. Withdrawal from a selective serotonin reuptake inhibitor (SSRI)
    E. All of the above
    F. A and B

27. Which of the following are features on an EEG of a patient with rolandic epilepsy?
    A. Focal spikes in the parietal region
    B. Focal central-midtemporal sharp waves
    C. Slow background rhythm
    D. Focal intermittent delta
    E. None of the above

28. Which of the following is true of juvenile myoclonic epilepsy?
    A. Lifetime AED usage
    B. 3-Hz spike and wave with hyperventilation on EEG
    C. Photic stimulation has no effect on these patients.
    D. Responds well to ethosuximide
    E. None of the above

29. What percentage of patients with herpes encephalitis have focal EEG changes?
    A. 10%
    B. 20%
    C. 50%
    D. 80%
    E. 99%

30. Which of the following represents brachial plexus integrity during a somatosensory evoked potential?
    A. N13 wave
    B. Erb point potential
    C. P14
    D. N18
    E. N20

31. Which of the following waves is delayed on visual evoked potential in patients with optic neuritis?
    A. N20
    B. P-100
    C. Wave I
    D. Wave I to III interpeak
    E. None of the above

32. Which of the following is part of the principles of evoked potential recording?

    A. A large electrical signal is recorded at the cortex.
    B. A small electrical signal is recorded at the scalp.
    C. A small stimulus is given in the spinal cord.
    D. Delayed responses arise from axonal damage.
    E. None of the above

ANSWERS

1. **Answer: C.** TWs are a distinctive but nonspecific EEG pattern originally described in a stuporous patient. The pattern is most often associated with renal failure, hepatic encephalopathy, and anoxic brain injury.

2. **Answer: B.** Focal delta activity is the classic electrographic sign of a local disturbance in cerebral function. If continuous delta, typically, a structural lesion is present. If no structural lesion is seen on CT scan or MRI of the head, it may be seen in the setting of trauma or postictal state after a seizure.

3. **Answer: B.** Prolonged P-100 is diagnostic of an abnormality in the optic nerve anterior to the chiasm. The retrochiasmatic portion of the optic nerve is not well tested with visual evoked potentials. The temporal portion of the optic nerve never crosses.

4. **Answer: A.** The early signs of dementia on EEG are reflected with slowing of the alpha frequency. The lower end of normal for alpha frequency is approximately 8.5 Hz. Medications can slow this down and therefore need to be excluded. The other answers are seen in disorders rather than just dementia.

5. **Answer: A.** Patients with transient global amnesia typically have normal EEG readings. Multiple different types of EEG readings, however, have been described such as bitemporal delta or bioccipital theta.

6. **Answer: B.** The EEG shows a fairly typical repetitive pattern of BiPEDs (periodic epileptiform discharges) such as TWs, approximately 1 to 1.5 seconds apart. These are usually present during wakefulness and disappear during sleep. Periodic synchronous discharges are the hallmark of the disease.

7. **Answer: C.** Slow roving eye movements are typically seen during the drowsy state. Sleep spindles are part of stage II sleep. Rapid eye movements as stated are part of REM sleep. Periodic leg movements can be seen in any stage of sleep.

8. **Answer: B.** Idiopathic generalized epilepsies are genetic epilepsies that are not symptomatic or cryptogenic. Juvenile myoclonic epilepsy and absence are two of the more common generalized idiopathic epilepsies. The others listed are symptomatic (West syndrome, Lennox-Gastaut syndrome) or localized (autosomal dominant frontal lobe epilepsy).

9. **Answer: F.** All of the above are common EEG artifacts.

10. **Answer: B.** Any destructive lesion can clearly attenuate the amplitude of normal rhythms. The other options would not likely be causes of amplitude differences comparing hemispheres.

11. **Answer: E.** All of the above are contraindications. History of epilepsy, however, is a relative contraindication.

12. **Answer: B.** Prolongation of the waveform on visual evoked potential would help support the diagnosis of optic neuritis. This is a demyelinating process, and therefore, there will be delay in transmission.

13. **Answer: C.** Patients with reactivity typically favor a better prognosis. The other answers all bode worse prognosis. Lack of reactivity is a negative prognostic indicator.

14. **Answer: A.** Muscle or EMG artifact is the most common artifact seen on EEG.

15. **Answer: D.** Along with low EMG tone and rapid eye movements, sawtooth waves are often seen. However, sawtooth waves are not diagnostic or required for staging someone's sleep in REM sleep.

16. **Answer: B.** Typically, spindle activity is between 12 to 16 Hz (mostly 14 Hz).

17. **Answer: D.** The K-complex is part of stage II sleep and can be induced by "knocking" on the door, or any noise can cause the K-complex to appear. They can be associated with blood pressure variation.

18. **Answer: A.** The patient has non-REM parasomnias, which typically occur during slow-wave sleep. Confusional arousals and night terrors also occur during this state of sleep.

19. **Answer: D.** Electrocerebral inactivity is defined by no electrical activity greater than 2 uV. There are strict guidelines for diagnosing brain death by EEG.

20. **Answer: A.** SSEPs are used for clinical diagnosis in patients with neurologic disease for prognostication in comatose patients and for intraoperative monitoring during surgeries that place parts of the somatosensory pathways at risk. The dorsal column is the main pathway that SSEPs evaluate.

21. **Answer: A.** N20 is a useful value in the setting of comatose patients with traumatic brain injury. If a patient has a metabolic derangement or infection and has absent N20 value bilaterally, however, the prognosis is better.

22. **Answer: D.** Etiology, age, duration, and type of status epilepticus are all determinants of mortality and morbidity in status epilepticus.

23. **Answer: B.** Brain stem auditory evoked response is primarily useful in the setting of multiple sclerosis or acoustic neuroma, but it has limitations.

24. **Answer: C.** EEG abnormalities usually present after abnormalities on CT scan and on clinical examinations. Patients show neurological improvement shortly after initiation of intravenous and then oral zidovudine, which produces absolute EEG normalization.

25. **Answer: D.** Focal slowing seen on EEG correlates with a lesion on MRI or CT scan in 70% of cases.

26. **Answer: E.** REM can be seen during a daytime EEG with all of the above situations. SSRIs are REM suppressants, and therefore, withdrawal would cause a REM rebound.

27. **Answer: B.** Patients with benign rolandic epilepsy have focal central-midtemporal sharp waves and a normal background rhythm.

28. **Answer: A.** Patients with juvenile myoclonic epilepsy are dependent on AED for their entire life but are usually very responsive to medications. Photic stimulation often precipitates seizures, and the usual frequency on EEG is 4- to 8-Hz spike and polyspike wave discharges. They usually have a normal background.

29. **Answer: D.** Patients with herpes encephalitis have focal EEG changes in more than 80% of cases. Abnormal EEG changes are usually seen 2 to 30 days after symptom onset.

30. **Answer: B.** All of the above are components of the somatosensory evoked potential; Erb point potential is the first wave and reflects brachial plexus integrity.

31. **Answer: B.** The P-100 is delayed in patients with acute optic neuritis, and the delay is permanent. About 70% of patients with MS will have abnormal P-100 even without a history of optic neuritis. The N20 wave is seen in somatosensory evoked potentials, waves I and III are seen in brain stem auditory evoked potentials.

32. **Answer: B.** The principle of evoked potentials is a small electrical signal recorded at the scalp, and delay in response is due to demyelination. Attenuation or loss of the signal is caused by axonal damage.

CHAPTER

8

Neurochemistry

QUESTIONS

1. Which of the following lowers the seizure threshold?
   A. Carbamazepine
   B. Lamotrigine
   C. Phenytoin
   D. Wellbutrin
   E. None of the above

2. Which one of the following is an irreversible reaction or very slowly reversible reaction of antipsychotic medications?
   A. Resting tremor
   B. Dystonia
   C. Tardive dyskinesia
   D. Sedation
   E. None of the above

3. If comparing tricyclic antidepressants to selective serotonin reuptake inhibitors (SSRIs), which of the following statements is true?
   A. Patients on SSRIs usually have dry mouth.
   B. Tricyclic antidepressants have dopaminergic effects.
   C. SSRIs elevate norepinephrine levels.
   D. Tricyclic antidepressants cause sedation.
   E. None of the above

4. What is the pathway that is involved with Parkinson's disease side effects of antidopaminergic agents?
   A. Spinothalamic
   B. Mesocortical
   C. Mesolimbic
   D. Nigral striatal pathway
   E. None of the above

5. Which of the following inhibits prolactin?

   A. Adrenocorticotropic hormone (ACTH)
   B. Corticotropin-releasing hormone (CRH)
   C. Thyrotropin-releasing hormone (TRH)
   D. Dopamine
   E. Orexin

6. A 24-year-old male with a history of seizures presents in status epilepticus. Which of the following agents would be considered first-line therapy?

   A. Valproate
   B. Lorazepam
   C. Clonazepam
   D. Ethosuximide
   E. None of the above

7. Which of the following antiepileptic drugs has similar properties as tricyclic antidepressants?

   A. Topiramate
   B. Lamotrigine
   C. Carbamazepine
   D. Clonazepam
   E. None of the above

8. A 13-year-old boy with a history of seizure disorders presents with aplastic anemia. Which one of the following medications could he be on?

   A. Lamotrigine
   B. Diazepam
   C. Felbamate
   D. Gabapentin
   E. None of the above

9. An 87-year-old male with a history of Parkinson's disease has been on dopamine agents for the past year. Which one of the following has more peripheral effects than central effects?

   A. Bromocriptine
   B. Pergolide
   C. Carbidopa
   D. Trihexyphenidyl
   E. Levodopa

10. Which of the following has antiemetic effects via serotonin receptor blockade?
    A. Prochlorperazine
    B. Promethazine
    C. Metoclopramide
    D. Scopolamine
    E. Ondansetron

11. Which of the following agents has the least amount of sedation as a side effect?
    A. Doxepin
    B. Amitriptyline
    C. Protriptyline
    D. Amoxapine
    E. Clomipramine

12. A 56-year-old male with early-onset Parkinson's disease is evaluated and placed on medication. Which one of the following irreversibly inhibits monoamine oxidase type B?
    A. Phenelzine
    B. Paroxetine
    C. Maprotiline
    D. Bupropion
    E. Selegiline

13. A 45-year-old male with a history of severe depression is started on phenelzine. Which one of the following would not be recommended?
    A. Sertraline
    B. Isocarboxazid
    C. Alprazolam
    D. Bupropion
    E. Gabapentin

14. A 34-year-old female with a seizure disorder is started on valproic acid. Which one of the following also has a similar mechanism that results in inducing its own metabolism?
    A. Gabapentin
    B. Ethosuximide
    C. Phenytoin
    D. Lamotrigine
    E. None of the above

15. A 45-year-old male with a long-standing history of generalized seizures is noncompliant with his medications. Which one of the following agents has the longest half-life?

    A. Primidone
    B. Phenobarbital
    C. Gabapentin
    D. Phenytoin
    E. Topiramate

16. A 40-year-old male with a history of migraines uses sumatriptan when he has a migraine. Which one of the following receptors is where the medication works?

    A. D3
    B. Muscarinic acetylcholine
    C. Inhibits the reuptake of gamma-aminobutyric acid (GABA)
    D. 5HT1
    E. Mu receptors in the spinal cord

17. 5-HT imbalance has not been associated with which one of the following conditions?

    A. Depression
    B. Narcolepsy
    C. Attention deficit disorder
    D. Headaches
    E. All of the above

18. A 22-year-old male presents with a long-standing history of seizures. He is given diazepam for a recent seizure. Which of the following is a true statement?

    A. GABA receptors regulate the Cl- ion channel.
    B. Diazepam has not been shown to be effective in the treatment of seizures.
    C. Diazepam also binds to dopamine receptors.
    D. GABA receptors are on a 16-subunit complex.
    E. None of the above

19. Which of the following agents are considered opiate receptor agonists or associated with opiates?
    A. Endorphins
    B. Dynorphins
    C. Enkephalins
    D. Pro-opiomelanocortin
    E. All of the above

20. Which one of the following is associated with glutamate?
    A. Trihexyphenidyl
    B. Pergolide
    C. Riluzole
    D. Pimozide
    E. None of the above

21. Which one of the following tricyclic antidepressants has the longest half-life?
    A. Imipramine
    B. Phenelzine
    C. Protriptyline
    D. Maprotiline
    E. None of the above

22. A 38-year-old female with a history of schizophrenia presents in a coma, with a fever and rigidity. She is diagnosed with neuroleptic malignant syndrome. Which one of the following agents could have caused this?
    A. Chlorpromazine
    B. Theophylline
    C. Theobromine
    D. Pemoline
    E. None of the above

23. Which one of the following agent's elimination is enhanced by smoking?
    A. Methylphenidate
    B. Caffeine
    C. Maprotiline
    D. Fluvoxamine
    E. None of the above

24. A 21-year-old male presents with an amphetamine overdose. Which one of the following would be recommended in the treatment of the overdose?

    A. Acidifying the urine
    B. Chlorpromazine
    C. Clonidine
    D. Guanfacine
    E. All of the above
    F. None of the above

25. An 84-year-old male with Parkinson's disease presents to the clinic. Which one of the following could be used as an adjunct to his L-dopa?

    A. Trihexyphenidyl
    B. Benztropine
    C. Procyclidine
    D. Biperiden
    E. All of the above
    F. None of the above

26. A 40-year-old male presents with alcohol withdrawal. Which one of the following agents has the longest half-life?

    A. Midazolam
    B. Temazepam
    C. Chlordiazepoxide
    D. Alprazolam
    E. None of the above

ANSWERS

1. **Answer: D.** Wellbutrin lowers the seizure threshold. The other medications are all used to raise the seizure threshold.
2. **Answer: C.** Tardive dyskinesia is typically irreversible or has a slowly reversible reaction of antidopaminergic agents even when the drug is discontinued.
3. **Answer: D.** Tricyclic antidepressants cause sedation especially early in the treatment.
4. **Answer: D.** Parkinsonism is associated with a defect in the nigral-striatal pathway.
5. **Answer: D.** Dopamine has prolactin inhibitory properties. The others have other endocrinological effects, and orexin affects appetite.

6. **Answer: B.** Continuous seizures with awakening is status epilepticus. There is potential for brain damage. Intravenous lorazepam, diazepam, and phenytoin are recommended for the treatment.

7. **Answer: C.** Carbamazepine's chemical structure is similar to that of tricyclic antidepressants. It also has an antidiuretic effect. This drug is effective in all seizure types except absence.

8. **Answer: C.** Felbamate and carbamazepine have a potential serious side effect of aplastic anemia. It is highly recommended to follow blood counts when on these agents.

9. **Answer: C.** Carbidopa diminishes decarboxylation of L-dopa in the peripheral tissues and therefore increases the effectiveness of L-dopa in the brain and reduces the required dose by 75%.

10. **Answer: E.** Ondansetron blocks serotonin receptors and not dopamine receptors like the others. It is particularly helpful in treating chemotherapy-induced nausea.

11. **Answer: C.** Protriptyline has the least sedating effects of all the tricyclic antidepressants.

12. **Answer: E.** Selegiline is a MAO inhibitor that irreversibly binds monoamine oxidase type B. Phenelzine is also a MAO inhibitor, but it is reversible.

13. **Answer: A.** Sertraline and other SSRIs can lead to a life-threatening reaction when given in combination with MAO inhibitors especially in the first 2 weeks.

14. **Answer: D.** Lamotrigine is similar to valproic acid in that it induces its own metabolism.

15. **Answer: B.** Phenobarbital has a half-life of more than 50 hours. It also has a slow onset of action and is metabolized by the P450 system in the liver.

16. **Answer: D.** Sumatriptan is a vascular 5HT1 receptor agonist that leads to vasoconstriction.

17. **Answer: B.** Narcolepsy has not been clearly associated with serotonin. It is thought to be related to low hypocretin/orexin levels.

18. **Answer: A.** GABA receptors reside on two subunits of a four-subunit receptor complex that surrounds and regulates a chloride ion channel.

19. **Answer: E.** All of the above are opiate receptor agonists except pro-opiomelanocortin, which is the precursor molecule that the others are cleaved into.

20. **Answer: C.** Riluzole protects neurons (specifically anterior horn cells) from glutamate toxicity in animals and minimally slows progression of ALS.

21. **Answer: C.** Protriptyline has a half-life of 80 hours and is the longest of all the tricyclic antidepressants.

22. **Answer: A.** Neuroleptic malignant syndrome is seen with antidopaminergic agents, and chlorpromazine is the only antidopaminergic agent listed. The others listed are psychomotor stimulants.

23. **Answer: B.** Caffeine's elimination is enhanced by smoking. A typical cup of soda or tea has approximately 50 mg of caffeine.

24. **Answer: E.** Patients with amphetamine overdose are treated by acidifying the urine and giving chlorpromazine (an antipsychotic) as well as an alpha-receptor blocker to lower blood pressure is the typical regimen.

25. **Answer: E.** All of the above have anticholinergic properties that can lessen the acetylcholine-dopamine imbalance in Parkinson's disease. These agents are typically less effective than L-dopa for tremor and other symptoms.

26. **Answer: C.** Chlordiazepoxide has the longest duration of action and is often used in the setting of alcohol withdrawal.

Neuromuscular

QUESTIONS

1. A 42-year-old male presents to his neurologist complaining of right arm weakness that has progressed over the past 2 years. He states he occasionally feels some tingling in that same arm. The examination shows atrophy and fasciculations of his arm and weakness. His reflexes are normal, and his sensory examination is normal. What would be the findings on his electrodiagnostic studies, and what would be the treatment of choice?

   A. Decrease amplitude of the sensory nerve action potential amplitudes (SNAPs); intravenous immunoglobulin (IVIG)
   B. Conduction block; methylprednisolone
   C. Fifty percent reduction in compound muscle action potential (CMAP) amplitude and area; IVIG
   D. Normal sensory studies; cyclophosphamide
   E. Absent H-reflex; steroids

2. What antibody is found in myasthenia gravis patients with negative AchR antibodies?

   A. Anti-GAD antibody
   B. MuSK antibody
   C. Anti-Hu antibody
   D. Anti-GQ1b antibody

3. A 24-year-old male diagnosed with HIV was found to have increased myalgia in the proximal leg regions bilaterally. He has been taking antiretrovirals for 2 years. A muscle biopsy was performed, and ragged red fibers were seen. It was recommended that the patient discontinue one of his antiretrovirals. What else may be suggested to help improve the proximal leg weakness?

   A. Visit a physical therapist to improve his strength in the lower extremities.
   B. Stopping the antiretroviral medication will make no difference and should be restarted.
   C. Adding corticosteroids has been shown to improve the weakness in some patients.
   D. Nothing else can be done, and there has been evidence that his disease process will accelerate.

4. All of these neuromuscular disorders are often preceded by gastrointestinal (GI) symptoms EXCEPT:

   A. intermittent porphyria
   B. botulinism
   C. lead poisoning
   D. arsenic intoxication
   E. rabies

5. Duplication of the PMP22 gene on chromosome 17p11 results in:

   A. hereditary sensory and autonomic neuropathy (HSAN) type V
   B. hereditary neuropathy with liability to pressure palsies (HNPP)
   C. Charcot-Marie-Tooth disease type 1A (CMT 1A)
   D. Charcot-Marie-Tooth disease type 1B (CMT 1B)

6. Which of the following toxins causes hair loss, arthralgias, GI symptoms, and an axonal sensorimotor neuropathy (predominately sensory)?

   A. Mercury
   B. Lead
   C. Thallium
   D. Ethylene glycol
   E. None of the above

7. All of these are typical of amyloid neuropathy, EXCEPT:
   A. autosomal dominant inheritance
   B. occurs frequently below the age of 40
   C. motor findings are usually minimal
   D. course is slow and steady
   E. forty percent of patients have M-protein in their serum protein elec-
   trophoresis (SPEP)

8. The mechanism of action of nitric oxide damage to the spinal cord is:
   A. calcium channel blockade
   B. direct toxicity to the spinothalamic tracts
   C. prolonged opening of sodium channels
   D. cobalamin inactivation
   E. None of the above

9. All of the following are related to CMT type IV, EXCEPT:
   A. autosomal dominant inheritance
   B. accumulation of phytanic acid
   C. retinitis pigmentosa
   D. high consanguinity rate

10. Which of the following are inherited forms of autonomic neuropathy?
    A. Amyloidosis
    B. Shy-Drager syndrome
    C. Chagas' disease
    D. Bassen-Kornzweig syndrome
    E. Diabetes

11. A 45-year-old male presents with complaints in his fourth and fifth digit
    on his right hand having numbness and tingling. He has also noticed his
    fifth digit gets caught in his pants when he tries to put his hand in his
    pant pocket. Which of the following is the possible site of pathology for
    this patient?
    A. Medial epicondyle area
    B. Carpal tunnel
    C. Femoral groove
    D. C1 root
    E. None of the above

12. The lateral cutaneous femoral nerve has motor function of which of the following muscles?
    A. Serratus anterior
    B. Adductor magnus
    C. Sartorius
    D. Rectus femoris
    E. None of the above

13. A 23-year-old male with a recent history of an upper respiratory illness presents with progressive weakness. He is diagnosed with Guillain-Barré syndrome. Which of the following supports the diagnosis?
    A. Areflexia
    B. Progressive weakness
    C. Relative symmetry
    D. Absence of fever
    E. All of the above

14. A 56-year-old male presents with distal weakness, tongue fasciculations, and atrophy in two limbs. He is diagnosed with amyotrophic lateral sclerosis (ALS). What is the percentage of ALS that is familial in nature?
    A. 1%
    B. 10%
    C. 75%
    D. 90%
    E. None of the above

15. Which of the following is the most common heredity neuropathy?
    A. Hereditary motor sensory neuropathy type 1
    B. Guillain-Barré syndrome
    C. Lambert-Eaton myasthenic syndrome (LEMS)
    D. Postural tachycardia syndrome (POTS) disease
    E. Diabetes

16. A 35-year-old female with muscle cramps and weakness is found to have polymyositis. Which of the following muscles will not be involved?
    A. Cardiac muscle
    B. Distal hand muscles
    C. Proximal leg muscles
    D. Ocular muscles
    E. None of the above

17. A 60-year-old male with numbness and tingling in his feet presents to your clinic. He has had diabetes for 10 years. Which of the following is the most common manifestation of diabetic neuropathy?
    A. Small fiber neuropathy
    B. Distal symmetric polyneuropathy
    C. Diabetic autonomic neuropathy
    D. Diabetic neuropathic cachexia
    E. None of the above

18. A 20-year-old female presents with acute weakness and is found to be in tetany with carpopedal spasm. Which one of the following could be a cause of her symptoms?
    A. Hyperthyroidism
    B. Hypopituitarism
    C. Hyperparathyroidism
    D. Hypoparathyroidism
    E. Polymyalgia rheumatica

19. A 30-year-old female presents with onset of hemifacial spasms. There is no family history, and her symptoms have progressively worsened. Which one of the following is true?
    A. This is most commonly idiopathic, and nothing further needs to be done.
    B. It is unusual at her age and may be a sign of multiple sclerosis.
    C. Hemimasticatory spasm is not analogous to hemifacial spasms.
    D. Fatigue or reading usually improves the symptoms.
    E. All of the above are true.

20. Which of the following is not true or associated with inclusion body myositis (IBM)?
    A. Proximal and distal muscles are often involved.
    B. Cardiac disease is common.
    C. Dysphagia is common.
    D. The disease is typically symmetrical.
    E. None of the above is associated with IBM.

21. Kennedy's disease is associated with which of the following?

    A. Lower motor neurons
    B. Upper motor neurons
    C. Eye musculature
    D. Sporadic
    E. A and B

22. A 65-year-old male with a long history of smoking presents with weakness. An electromyography/nerve conduction study (EMG/NCS) is performed, and the patient is found to have LEMS. Which one of the following is associated with LEMS?

    A. Anti-Hu antibody
    B. Voltage-gated calcium channel antibody
    C. Anti-Jo
    D. *Campylobacter jejuni* infection
    E. Anti-GQ1B antibody

23. A 21-year-old female with myasthenia gravis is on immunosuppressant agents. Which one of the following would place her in class V rating?

    A. Oropharyngeal muscle involvement
    B. Limb or axial muscle involvement
    C. Intubation
    D. Feeding tube
    E. None of the above

24. A 15-year-old male with periodic paralysis would have which one of the following channel defects?

    A. Sodium
    B. Calcium
    C. Potassium
    D. A and C
    E. All of the above

25. A patient presents with increasing muscle rigidity and stiffness. She is found to have stiff syndrome. Which of the following is an associated antibody with this disorder?

    A. Anti-GQ1b antibody
    B. Anti-GAD antibody
    C. Anti-Hu antibody
    D. HLA-DQB106
    E. None of the above

ANSWERS

1. **Answer: C.** Multifocal motor neuropathy (MMN) is a rare disorder and is more common in males with a ratio of 2:1. The presenting features are painless, asymmetrical weakness, atrophy, and fasciculations in the arms usually restricted to one or two nerves. Findings on sensory examination are normal, and reflexes are out of proportion to the weakness of the involved muscles. The electrodiagnostic findings are usually conduction block (typically a 50% reduction in CMAP amplitude and area), segmental demyelination, and normal sensory studies.

2. **Answer: B.** Approximately 30% of AchR-seronegative patients with myasthenia gravis have the MuSK antibody. These patients are phenotypically different in that they have severe ophthalmoparesis, bulbar, facial, and posterior neck symptoms. The other antibodies are related to other neurologic disorders, anti-GAD with stiff-man syndrome, Ant-Hu with paraneoplastic disease, and anti-GQ1b with Guillain-Barré syndrome.

3. **Answer: C.** Patients with HIV taking zidovudine (AZT) have been found to develop an inflammatory myopathy with mitochondrial involvement. There are no good controlled studies to date that have proven AZT directly causes this. Some patients have shown improvement with the addition of corticosteroids. This treatment produces increased risk of opportunistic infections, however, and there has been no evidence that there is acceleration of the HIV disease.

4. **Answer: E.** Rabies involves the medullary respiratory centers that usually produce disproportionate respiratory weakness and usually have no GI prodrome. The rest of the diseases or toxins listed are preceded either by hours to weeks with nausea, vomiting, and abdominal pain.

5. **Answer: B.** Eighty-five percent of patients with HNPP have shown a deletion of the PMP22 gene on chromosome 17p11. The duplication of the same gene results in CMT type 1A. HSAN type V is Strümpell's disease, which is CMT plus spastic paraparesis, and CMT type 1B is a mutation in the P0 gene on chromosome 1q22–23.

6. **Answer: C.** Thallium has been shown to produce all of the symptoms listed. Lead toxicity predominately causes motor weakness; mercury poisoning may cause mood change along with gingivitis, and ethylene glycol causes renal failure, metabolic acidosis, and a severe axonal neuropathy with cranial mononeuropathy.

7. **Answer: B.** Amyloidosis rarely occurs below the age of 40, has primarily sensory and autonomic findings, 40% of the patients have M-protein on

their SPEP, the course is slow and steady and is inherited in an autosomal dominant fashion.

8. **Answer: D.** The mechanism of action is via inactivation of cobalamin, resulting in myeloneuropathy.

9. **Answer: A.** Patients with CMT type IV, also known as Refsum's disease, have autosomal recessive inheritance. It is caused by an accumulation of phytanic acid in many systems, results in night blindness, and is associated with a high consanguinity rate.

10. **Answer: B.** Of the diseases listed, only Shy-Drager syndrome and Bassen-Kornzweig syndrome (abetalipoproteinemia) are inherited. Shy-Drager syndrome causes an autonomic neuropathy. Abetalipoproteinemia primarily affects large fiber sensory modalities.

11. **Answer: A.** The patient has an ulnar neuropathy, and therefore the medial epicondyle area is the most common sight of compression. The carpal tunnel leading to median neuropathy is the most common compression neuropathy.

12. **Answer: E.** The lateral cutaneous femoral nerve is a pure sensory nerve that controls sensation of the lateral aspect of the proximal leg. It is often known as *meralgia paresthetica* when it is damaged, typically with focal entrapment by the inguinal ligament.

13. **Answer: E.** Diagnostic criteria for Guillain-Barré syndrome include the presence of progressive weakness and areflexia, relative symmetry, mild sensory involvement, cranial nerve involvement, at least partial recovery, autonomic dysfunction, and absence of fever. Cerebrospinal fluid features that strongly support the diagnosis are an increase in protein beyond the first week (albuminocytologic dissociation) in the setting low cell count (<10).

14. **Answer: B.** About 10% of ALS patients have the familial form, and it is transmitted in an autosomal dominant fashion. Therefore, the majority of ALS cases are sporadic in nature.

15. **Answer: A.** HMSN type 1 is the most common form of hereditary neuropathy. Severely and uniformly slowed nerve conduction velocities (NCVs) and secondary axonal changes are the hallmarks of the disease.

16. **Answer: D.** Ocular muscles are not involved even in severe cases. Facial muscles are rarely involved and if so, usually in severe cases.

17. **Answer: B.** Distal symmetric polyneuropathy is the most common manifestation of diabetic neuropathy. Chronic symmetrical symptoms affect peripheral nerves in a length-dependent pattern (the longest nerves are affected first). The dominant feature is sensory abnormalities.

18. **Answer: D.** Hypoparathyroidism results in tetany with or without carpopedal spasm. Muscle pain, cramps, and spasms are present in up to 50% of patients. Muscle weakness is usually mild.

19. **Answer: B.** Hemifacial spasms typically when idiopathic occurs in the fifth or sixth decade. When patients are under the age of 40, it often precedes a neurologic disorder such as demyelinating diseases.

20. **Answer: D.** IBM typically presents in an asymmetrical pattern and not a symmetrical pattern like polymyositis or dermatomyositis. The rest of the other answers are true and are associated with IBM.

21. **Answer: A.** Kennedy's disease is an inherited disorder characterized by degeneration of both motor and sensory neurons. It involves loss of lower motor neurons supplying the limb and bulbar musculature. Extraocular muscles are spared, possibly because of reduced numbers of androgen receptors in these muscles.

22. **Answer: B.** VGCC antibodies have been reported in 75% to 100% of patients with LEMS who have SCLC and in 50% to 90% of patients with LEMS without underlying cancer. They are also found in fewer than 5% of patients with MG, in up to 25% of patients with lung cancer without LEMS, and in some patients who do not have LEMS but have high levels of circulating immunoglobulins (e.g., systemic lupus erythematosus, rheumatoid arthritis).

23. **Answer: C.** Intubation by definition places a patient in class V with myasthenia gravis.

24. **Answer: E.** Hypokalemic or hyperkalemic periodic paralysis has been associated with all three channel defects.

25. **Answer: B.** There are three associated antibodies with stiff person syndrome. Anti-GAD is the most common associated antibody. The other two are amphiphysin antibody (paraneoplastic) and gephyrin antibody in one case report.

Infectious Disease

QUESTIONS

1. A 25-year-old female presents to the clinic with neck stiffness, fever, and headache. She is found to have aseptic meningitis. Which one of the following is most likely the cause?

   A. Lyme disease
   B. Sarcoidosis
   C. Coxsackievirus
   D. Adenovirus
   E. None of the above

2. A 45-year-old female with a history of AIDS develops encephalopathy. Which one of the following is the most common cause for encephalopathy in AIDS patients?

   A. Toxoplasmosis
   B. Herpes
   C. Medication side effects
   D. *Staphylococcus aureus*
   E. None of the above

3. A 29-year-old male with a history of AIDS is diagnosed with progressive multifocal leukoencephalopathy (PML). Which of the following is true?

   A. PML damages white matter of the brain including U-fibers.
   B. PML is diagnosed only by brain biopsy.
   C. Polymerase chain reaction (PCR) for the John Cunningham (JC) virus shows high specificity.
   D. Highly active antiretroviral therapy (HAART) has not shown benefit for AIDS patients.
   E. None of the above

4. A 45-year-old male who recently traveled to South Korea is found to have a headache, encephalopathy, and an acute infection with brucellosis. Which of the following is another possible neurologic complication?

   A. Bell's palsy
   B. Trigeminal neuralgia
   C. Exophthalmos
   D. Sensorineural hearing loss
   E. None of the above

5. Which of the following is the most common virus associated with neonatal herpes encephalitis?

   A. Human herpesvirus-6 (HHV-6)
   B. Herpes simplex virus-1 (HSV-1)
   C. Human immunodeficiency virus (HIV)
   D. Human T-cell lymphotropic virus (HTLV-1)
   E. Herpes simplex virus-2 (HSV-2)

6. Patients treated for herpes encephalitis often have neurologic sequelae. Which one of the following is the most common sequelae?

   A. Hemiparesis
   B. Developmental delay
   C. Seizures
   D. Stroke
   E. Hematoma

7. Prior to effective immunizations, which one of the following was one of the most common causes of bacterial meningitis but is currently seen much less often and rarely occurs in children over age 5?

   A. *Neisseria meningitidis*
   B. *Streptococcus pneumoniae*
   C. *Escherichia coli*
   D. *Listeria monocytogenes*
   E. *Haemophilus influenzae*

8. A 34-year-old male complaining of muscle pain is found to have pyomyositis. What is the most likely location of his abscess?

   A. Psoas
   B. Quadriceps
   C. Biceps
   D. Triceps
   E. All of the above

9. Which one of the following is the most common neurologic manifestation of acute Lyme disease?

    A. Cranial neuropathy
    B. Meningitis
    C. Cerebritis
    D. Radiculopathy
    E. Myositis

10. A 54-year-old male from Connecticut presents with a rash and history of tick bite. What percentage of patients with Lyme disease have erythema migrans at the site of the tick bite?

    A. 5%
    B. 25%
    C. 50%
    D. 90%
    E. None of the above

11. A patient presents with acute meningitis. She is found to have meningococcal meningitis. Which of the following is true?

    A. The patient is most likely 60 years old.
    B. Smoking does not increase the risk of disease.
    C. The patient must be in high school.
    D. Irritability is unlikely in the patient.
    E. None of the above

12. Which of the following is associated with Waterhouse-Friderichsen syndrome?

    A. Disseminated intravascular coagulation (DIC)
    B. Large petechial hemorrhage
    C. Fever
    D. Septic shock
    E. All of the above

13. A 34-year-old Hispanic male presents with new-onset seizures. He is found to have neurocysticercosis. Which of the following is the most likely etiology?

    A. HIV
    B. HSV
    C. *Taenia solium*
    D. Coccidiomycosis
    E. None of the above

14. Which of the following is the only reliable way of confirming the diagnosis of neurocysticercosis?
    A. Computed tomography (CT) scan of the head with and without contract
    B. Magnetic resonance imaging (MRI) of the brain with and without gadolinium
    C. Plain X-ray of the skull
    D. Whole body bone scan
    E. None of the above

15. A 45-year-old male presents with an acute stroke. He is found to have endocarditis. Which one of the following is the most likely organism?
    A. *Enterococcus* species
    B. *Streptococcus* viridans
    C. HSV type II
    D. *Pseudomonas*
    E. None of the above

16. Which of the following is the most common neurologic examination finding in neurosyphilis?
    A. Optic atrophy
    B. Charcot's joint
    C. Romberg's sign
    D. Hyporeflexia
    E. None of the above

17. A 56-year-old male with progressive dementia is found to have sporadic prion disease. What is the most likely cause, and what is the mean duration of mortality?
    A. Sporadic fatal insomnia; 6 months
    B. Scrapie; 12 months
    C. Sporadic Creutzfeldt-Jakob disease (CJD); 8 months
    D. Familial fatal insomnia; 12 months
    E. None of the above

18. A 34-year-old female presents with acute onset of vertigo, tinnitus, and facial paresis. She is diagnosed with Ramsay Hunt syndrome. Which of the following is associated with this disease?
    A. HIV
    B. Coxsackie virus
    C. *Borrelia*
    D. HSV III
    E. Arbovirus

19. A 55-year-old male with a history of IV drug abuse presents with fever, back pain, incontinence, and is found to have an epidural abscess. Which of the following is true regarding epidural abscess?
    A. Fever is present in 10% of cases.
    B. Fever is present in 33% of cases.
    C. Fever is present in 75% of cases.
    D. Fever is present in all cases.
    E. None of the above

20. A 35-year-old male presents with bacterial meningitis. Which of the following tests has a prognostic value in bacterial meningitis?
    A. Cerebrospinal fluid (CSF) leukocyte count
    B. Serum protein
    C. CSF glucose
    D. CSF lactate dehydrogenase
    E. CSF protein

21. Which of the following is the most common cause of subdural empyema?
    A. Pulmonary spread
    B. Trauma
    C. Postsurgical
    D. Paranasal sinusitis
    E. None of the above

22. What often causes tropical ataxic neuropathy?
    A. Malnutrition
    B. Virus
    C. Trauma
    D. Diabetes
    E. Genetic disorder

23. Which of the following is the strongest risk factor for *Mycobacterium tuberculosis* to progress into active tuberculosis (TB)?
    A. Smoking
    B. HIV coinfection
    C. Hx of lymphoma
    D. Chronic obstructive pulmonary disease (COPD)
    E. None of the above

24. A 23-year-old male with sudden onset of fever, personality change, and confusion is found to have HSV encephalitis. What is the mortality rate of this disease if it is untreated?
    A. 1%
    B. 20%
    C. 70%
    D. 100%
    E. None of the above

25. Which of the following is part of the clinical triad associated with CNS Whipple's disease?
    A. Dementia
    B. Vertical ophthalmoplegia
    C. Myoclonus
    D. A and C
    E. B and C
    F. All of the above

ANSWERS

1. **Answer: C.** Coxsackie viruses and echoviruses (types of enteroviruses) account for about half of the cases of aseptic meningitis. The others can cause aseptic meningitis but are not as common.

2. **Answer: A.** Toxoplasmosis along with PML and HIV encephalopathy are the three most common causes for encephalopathy in AIDS patients.

3. **Answer: C.** PCR for the JC virus has high specificity for diagnosing the disease and therefore can usually replace the need for brain biopsy.

4. **Answer: D.** Sensorineural hearing loss is the second most common focal neurologic side effect of brucellosis after encephalopathy. Most symptoms of brucellosis are nonfocal or non-specific symptoms such as headache, fever, and malaise.

5. **Answer: E.** HSV-1 is the more common cause of adult encephalitis. HSV-2 is the more common cause of newborn encephalitis, which is associated with maternal genital infections.

6. **Answer: C.** Seizures are the most common neurologic sequelae; approximately 44% of patients go on to develop epilepsy. It is associated with developmental delay in approximately 25% of patients. Despite adequate therapy, patients still have poor long-term neurologic outcome.

7. **Answer: E.** *Haemophilus influenzae* type b (Hib) has been identified as one of the three most common causes of bacterial meningitis. The others are *Neisseria meningitidis* and *Streptococcus pneumoniae*. These three bacteria have accounted, before the development of effective immunizations, for more than 80% of all cases of meningitis in industrialized nations. Prior to effective immunizations, Hib has been the most important cause of meningitis in children younger than 5 years of age. Since immunization, the frequency has reduced significantly.

8. **Answer: B.** The quadriceps is the most common location of pyomyositis. The psoas is the second most common location.

9. **Answer: A.** Cranial neuropathies are the most common neurologic presentation. The others are associated but are not as common. Approximately 5% to 10% of untreated patients with Lyme disease have signs of cranial neuropathies, and up to 60% of patients with early Lyme disease develop cranial neuritis. It usually begins 3 weeks after infection. Seventh nerve palsy is by far the most common. Bilateral facial palsy can be seen in 35% of patients.

10. **Answer: D.** About 90% of patients develop the classic expanding rash at the site of the tick bite. Erythema migrans starts as a flat to slightly raised erythematous lesion at the site of the tick bite within days to weeks. Over days, the lesion spreads to a diameter of approximately 5 to 6 inches. The center of the bite may clear, giving this lesion its typical bull's-eye appearance or target lesion.

11. **Answer: C.** Meningococcal meningitis most commonly affects individuals between 3 years of age and adolescence. It rarely occurs in individuals older than 50 years. Irritability is the most common presenting sign. The bacteria are transmitted via direct contact or respiratory transmission.

12. **Answer: E.** All of the above are associated with Waterhouse-Friderichsen syndrome. This syndrome is associated meningococcal infection and develops in 10% to 20% of children that are infected.

13. **Answer: C.** Neurocysticercosis is the most common parasitic disease of the nervous system and is the main cause of acquired epilepsy in developing countries. It results from accidentally ingesting of *Taenia solium* eggs (i.e., pork tapeworm).

14. **Answer: E.** The only truly reliable standard for diagnosis is pathologic confirmation through biopsy or autopsy. Nevertheless, even without definitive scientific data, CT scan and MRI are considered the main tools for the diagnosis but are not confirmatory.

15. **Answer: B.** *Streptococcus* species are the most common causes for endocarditis specifically *S. viridans*, which comprises about 60% of native valve endocarditis.

16. **Answer: D.** Hyporeflexia and sensory impairment (typically decreased proprioception and loss of vibratory sense) are the most common neurologic findings and are consistent with posterior column deficits.

17. **Answer: C.** Sporadic CJD is the most common prion disease and the mean duration from infection to death is approximately 8 months.

18. **Answer: D.** Classic Ramsay Hunt syndrome is associated with an infection of the geniculate ganglion by HSV type 3 or varicella zoster virus.

19. **Answer: B.** Fever is present in about one third of patients with epidural abscesses. Localized back pain is the most common symptom and is often the presenting sign. There is an increased incidence of epidural abscess in IV drug abusers and immunocompromised patients.

20. **Answer: D.** CSF lactate dehydrogenase appears to be diagnostic and has prognostic value. Lactate dehydrogenase levels that rise sharply often have neurologic sequelae.

21. **Answer: D.** The most common cause of subdural empyema is from extension from the paranasal sinusitis, especially from the frontal and ethmoid sinuses. The others are all possible sources as well.

22. **Answer: A.** Tropical ataxic neuropathy is predominately a sensory neuropathy. It is primarily caused by malnutrition. It is often seen in populations that use large quantities of cassava in their diets. The bitter variety has a high content of cyanide. B-group vitamin deficiencies were initially thought to be the primary cause, however, treatment with B supplementation was unsuccessful.

23. **Answer: B.** HIV coinfection is the strongest risk factor for progression to active TB. This population is also at increased risk for TB meningitis.

24. **Answer: C.** Herpes virus encephalitis carries a mortality rate of 70% in untreated patients and severe sequelae among survivors. Children and young adults are the most common affected groups.

25. **Answer: F.** Dementia, vertical ophthalmoplegia, and myoclonus are part of the triad associated with CNS Whipple's disease. If left untreated, all cases of Whipple's disease are fatal. The cause of Whipple's disease is yet to be determined—if it is caused by direct bacterial invasion or from the inflammatory response of the host due to the bacteria.

CHAPTER
11

Neurogenetics

QUESTIONS

1. Which one of the following is associated with a trinucleotide repeat expansion?

   A. Tuberous sclerosis
   B. McCardle's disease
   C. Myotonic dystrophy
   D. Sjögren's syndrome
   E. Acute intermittent porphyria

2. You examine a child with weakness, wasting of the calf muscles, and diminished ankle reflexes. On nerve conduction study, you find severe slowing of the conduction velocity. Several of the patient's relatives have had similar symptoms, including the patient's father as well as three of her four siblings. This disease is most likely is associated with which chromosome?

   A. 1
   B. 12
   C. 6
   D. 21
   E. X linked

3. A variant of the apolipoprotein E (apoE) gene has been linked with increased risk of Alzheimer's disease. On which chromosome is this gene found?

   A. 1
   B. X
   C. 19
   D. 23
   E. 6

4. A patient is diagnosed with mitochondrial myopathy, encephalopathy, lactic acidosis, and stroke (MELAS), which is a mitochondrial genetic disorder. Which of the following medications should be avoided?
   A. Warfarin
   B. Valproic acid
   C. Aspirin
   D. Gabapentin
   E. Leviteracitam

5. A patient is diagnosed with cerebral autosomal dominant arteriopathy with subcortical infarcts and leukoencephalopathy (CADASIL). Which of the following is true?
   A. Pseudobulbar palsy is a rare complication.
   B. Mutation of the Notch3 gene
   C. Skin biopsy is diagnostic.
   D. Strokes are rare complications.
   E. None of the above

6. The triad of dysmorphic features, periodic paralysis, and cardiac arrhythmias is part of Anderson-Tawil syndrome. This syndrome is associated with what mutation?
   A. Sodium channel gene
   B. Potassium channel gene
   C. Dopamine synthesis gene
   D. Triple repeat disorder
   E. X-linked recessive

7. The majority of inborn errors of metabolism are inherited in what fashion?
   A. X-linked recessive
   B. Autosomal dominant
   C. Sporadic
   D. Autosomal recessive
   E. None of the above

8. Neurofibromatosis type 2 (NF2) is associated with meningiomas and acoustic neuromas (often bilateral). NF1 has better prognosis and is associated with a lower incidence of central nervous system (CNS) tumors. The NF1 gene codes for neurofibromin. What is the function of this protein?

    A. ATPase associated
    B. Tumor suppressor
    C. Pro-oncogene
    D. cAMP associated
    E. None of the above

9. NF1 is inherited in what fashion and is associated with which chromosome?

    A. AR: 15
    B. AD: 17
    C. AD: 22
    D. X-linked
    E. AR: 9

10. Duchenne's muscular dystrophy (DMD) is the most common type of muscular dystrophy. Which statement is true?

    A. Spontaneous transmission is the most common.
    B. Autosomal dominant transmission is the most common.
    C. X-linked transmission is the most common.
    D. The size of the mutation increases the severity of the disease.
    E. Missense mutation is the most common cause of DMD.

11. Which of the following is the most common hereditary ataxia syndrome?

    A. Vitamin E deficiency
    B. Refsum disease
    C. Friedreich's ataxia (FA)
    D. Hereditary motor and sensory neuropathy
    E. None of the above

12. A 20-year-old female with progressive ataxia and gait disturbance is found to have FA. Which of the following is true?

    A. Almost 100% of patients are wheelchair bound by age 45.
    B. It is inherited in an autosomal dominant fashion.
    C. It is most prevalent in the African American populations.
    D. The average age of onset is 40 years old.
    E. None of the above

13. Which chromosome does the frataxin gene expansion occur on?
    A. 2
    B. 9
    C. 12
    D. 21
    E. 14

14. A 30-year-old male with hx of Huntington's disease (HD) has a father who recently passed away at age 50 with the same disease. Which of the following is true?
    A. There will be gross atrophy of the caudate and putamen.
    B. Patients with HD only have chorea and no bradykinesia.
    C. Dementia is a rare complication of HD.
    D. Juvenile HD accounts for the majority of patients with this disease.
    E. None of the above

15. Which of the following is not considered part of the differential diagnosis of HD?
    A. Wilson's disease
    B. Neuroacanthocytosis
    C. Lupus
    D. Thyroid disease
    E. All of the above are part of the differential.

16. A patient with a well-known family history of Alzheimer's dementia (AD) starts developing memory issues. Which of the following is true regarding familial AD?
    A. There have been no genes associated with this disorder.
    B. There are four major loci that have been found associated with AD.
    C. Lipoprotein E epsilon 3 has been a known risk factor.
    D. Down syndrome patients are protected from AD.
    E. None of the above

17. Which of the following statements is true regarding episodic ataxia type 1 and 2?
    A. Episodic ataxia type 1 is associated with continuous myokymia.
    B. Episodic ataxia type 1 and 2 are autosomal recessive disorders.
    C. Episodic ataxia 1 is autosomal recessive, and type 2 is autosomal dominant.
    D. Episodic ataxia type 1 is associated with hemiplegic migraines.
    E. None of the above

18. A 25-year-old female patient presents with cerebellar ataxia, night blindness, and degeneration of the retina. She also has polyneuropathy and sensorineural deafness. A lumbar puncture (LP) is performed, and cerebrospinal fluid (CSF) protein is elevated. Which of the following is true?
    A. Steroid therapy should be instituted immediately.
    B. This is inherited in an autosomal dominant pattern.
    C. There will be elevated phytanic acid in the plasma and urine.
    D. There is no treatment for this disorder.
    E. None of the above

19. What is the most common genetic alteration associated with meningiomas?
    A. Defect on chromosome 1
    B. Loss of NF2 gene on chromosome 22
    C. Trisomy 21
    D. Monosomy 8
    E. None of the above

20. Which of the following is or are part of the differential diagnosis for Kennedy's disease?
    A. Amyotrophic lateral sclerosis (ALS)
    B. Myasthenia gravis
    C. Syphilis
    D. Spinal muscular atrophy
    E. All of the above

21. Which of the following is the most common misdiagnosed disease in Kennedy's disease?
    A. ALS
    B. Myasthenia gravis
    C. Syphilis
    D. Spinal muscular atrophy
    E. Inclusion body myositis

22. A 15-year-old girl presents after having a generalized tonic-clonic seizure. She has noticed that, when she brushes her teeth or combs her hair in the morning, she occasionally experiences a brief jerking movement in her upper extremities. Past medical history is otherwise unremarkable. Her father was also diagnosed with epilepsy as a teenager, and he remains on antiepileptic medication. The patient's examination findings are normal. You obtain an electroencephalogram (EEG), which reveals occasional generalized bilateral polyspikes and spike wave complexes at 4 Hz. Which of the following statements is true?

    A. This disorder has an abnormality on chromosome 2.
    B. This disorder is inherited in an autosomal recessive pattern.
    C. This disorder is not genetic but sporadic.
    D. This disorder is inherited in an autosomal dominant fashion.
    E. None of the above

23. A 21-year-old male presents with confusion, memory difficulty, and psychosis. He is diagnosed with extensive white matter changes, and on magnetic resonance imaging (MRI), he is found to have elevated urine sulfatide. Which of the following is true regarding the genetics of this disorder?

    A. Autosomal dominant
    B. Chromosome 1p
    C. Autosomal recessive
    D. Sporadic
    E. None of the above

24. A 2-month-old boy presents with severe nystagmus, titubation, and weakness. At 3 months, he developed ataxia and cognitive delay. The patient is found to have Pelizaeus-Merzbacher disease. This disease is caused by a mutation on the PLP1 gene. Which chromosome is associated with this gene?

    A. 1
    B. 21
    C. 12
    D. X
    E. None of the above

25. Wilson's disease is inherited in an autosomal recessive fashion and is associated with chromosome 13. Which of the following is true?

    A. Patients have elevated serum copper levels.
    B. Patients have low ceruloplasmin levels.
    C. Patients have decreased urinary copper levels.
    D. The liver function test results are normal.
    E. None of the above

ANSWERS

1. **Answer: C.** Myotonic dystrophy is associated with a CTG repeat expansion. None of the others are triple repeat disorders.

2. **Answer: D.** Charcot-Marie-Tooth (CMT) disease type 2C is a primarily axonal sensorimotor polyneuropathy. CMT type 2C is autosomal dominant and is associated with chromosome 12.

3. **Answer: C.** The apoE gene is located on chromosome 19.

4. **Answer: B.** Valproic acid has been shown to exacerbate symptoms of MELAS. Patients with MELAS typically have ischemic strokes, migraine headaches, hearing loss, growth retardation, and limb weakness/exercise intolerance.

5. **Answer: B.** Mutation of the Notch3 gene is associated with CADASIL. Recurrent strokes, migraines, depression, pseudobulbar palsy, and subcortical dementia are all associated with this disease. Skin biopsy can be helpful but is not diagnostic.

6. **Answer: B.** Anderson-Tawil syndrome is associated with potassium channel mutation. In theory, the gene controls the inward rectifying potassium channel; therefore, mutations are supposed to cause hypokalemia, however, this has not been confirmed.

7. **Answer: D.** Most inborn errors of metabolism are inherited as autosomal recessive conditions.

8. **Answer: B.** Mutation or deletion of the NF gene results in neurofibromatosis. The gene product is neurofibromin, which acts as a tumor suppressor; therefore, a decrease in production or absent levels results in the clinical features.

9. **Answer: B.** NF1 is an autosomal dominant condition, and only one gene needs to be deleted or mutated to result in the condition. The NF1 gene has been localized to chromosome 17.

10. **Answer: C.** DMD is most commonly transmitted in an X-linked fashion. Larger deletions of one or more exons account for most of the causes of DMD (not missense mutations). The size of the mutation does not determine the severity of disease.

11. **Answer: C.** FA is the most common autosomal recessive ataxia and accounts for 50% of all hereditary ataxias.

12. **Answer: A.** More than 95% of patients with FA are wheelchair bound by age 45. It is inherited in an autosomal recessive fashion. It is most prevalent in white populations, and the average age of onset is 10 years of age.

13. **Answer: B.** Gene mutation on chromosome 9 is the classic cause for FA. This results in a mutation that leads to a GAA trinucleotide repeat. The larger the expansion of GAA correlates with earlier onset and a shorter time to becoming wheelchair bound.

14. **Answer: A.** The most amount of atrophy occurs in the neostriatum, which includes the caudate and putamen. Atrophy occurs elsewhere but to varying degrees.

15. **Answer: E.** All of the above are potential mimickers of HD and need to be evaluated when there is no family history. Genetic testing for HD is available as well.

16. **Answer: B.** The familial form of AD accounts for less than 10% of all cases of AD. Four major loci have been found to be associated or responsible for AD: (1) amyloid precursor protein on chromosome 21; (2) presenilin I chromosome 14; (3) presenilin II on chromosome 1; and (4) potential markers on chromosome 12 and 19.

17. **Answer: A.** Episodic ataxia type 1 is associated with continuous myokymia, whereas type 2 is associated with the absence of myokymia.

18. **Answer: C.** The patient has Refsum's disease, which is caused by elevated phytanic acid. The treatment consists of reducing dietary phytanic acid and plasmapheresis. It is inherited in an autosomal recessive pattern.

19. **Answer: B.** The best-described and most common genetic alteration is the loss of the NF2 gene on chromosome 22 (also associated with neurofibromatosis type II).

20. **Answer: E.** The typical symptoms are an insidious onset of fatigue, muscle cramps, and weakness in the limbs. Bulbar muscles are often involved. Cognition is spared. Testicular atrophy and gynecomastia are the most common nonneurological findings.

21. **Answer: A.** Kennedy's disease is most frequently misdiagnosed as ALS.

22. **Answer: D.** The patient has juvenile myoclonic epilepsy. This is inherited in an autosomal dominant fashion, and the abnormality is on chromosome 6.

23. **Answer: C.** The patient has metachromatic leukodystrophy, which is inherited in an autosomal recessive fashion (late onset).

24. **Answer: D.** Pelizaeus-Merzbacher disease is caused by a mutation to the PLP1 gene, which is located on the long arm of the X chromosome.

25. **Answer: B.** Patients with Wilson's disease have low serum copper levels, low ceruloplasmin levels, as well as increased urinary copper levels and liver function tests (ie, transaminases).

CHAPTER

12

Neuro-Oncology

QUESTIONS

1. Which of the following has been associated with polyostotic fibrous dysplasia, hyperpigmented skin macules, and precocious puberty?
   A. Gardner's syndrome
   B. Hand-Schüller-Christian disease
   C. McCune-Albright syndrome
   D. Guillain-Barré syndrome
   E. None of the above

2. Of all primary tumors, which one has the most predilection toward metastasizing to the brain?
   A. Lung
   B. Breast
   C. Melanoma
   D. Colon cancer
   E. Lymphoma

3. Which of the following primary tumors account for the majority of all metastatic brain tumors?
   A. Lung
   B. Breast
   C. Melanoma
   D. Colon cancer
   E. Lymphoma

4. A patient is found to have metastatic cancer to the brain. Which of the following besides headache is the most common presenting symptom?

   A. Stroke
   B. Hemorrhage
   C. Seizure
   D. Nausea
   E. None of the above

5. A patient is found to have a brain stem glioma. More than 75% of these tumors are in patients in what age group?

   A. 0 to 20
   B. 21 to 40
   C. 40 to 60
   D. Over 60
   E. None of the above. They occur in all age groups equally.

6. A 56-year-old Caucasian female is found to have metastatic brain cancer. On imaging studies, the lesions are hemorrhagic. Which of the following would be a possible primary tumor?

   A. Lymphoma
   B. Melanoma
   C. Meningioma
   D. Neurofibroma
   E. Schwannoma

7. Which of the following is the most common endocrine dysfunction seen with craniopharyngiomas?

   A. Adrenal failure
   B. Hypothyroidism
   C. Diabetes insipidus
   D. Diabetes mellitus
   E. None of the above

8. A patient with a retrochiasmal craniopharyngioma is associated with hydrocephalus. Which of the following is also associated?

   A. Horizontal double vision
   B. Seizures
   C. Electrolyte abnormalities
   D. Amenorrhea
   E. Orthostatic hypotension

9. Which of the following treatments for ependymomas is considered the most effective therapy?

    A. Monitor closely
    B. Surgical excision
    C. Chemotherapy
    D. Radiation
    E. None of the above

10. Which of the following is the most common type of primary brain tumor?

    A. Lymphoma
    B. Glioblastoma multiforme (GBM)
    C. Meningioma
    D. Pituitary adenoma
    E. None of the above

11. Which of the following has the highest potential for increasing the risk of secondary glioblastoma?

    A. Hx of whole brain radiation
    B. Hx of multiple computed tomography (CT) scans
    C. Cellular telephone use
    D. Hx of chemotherapy
    E. Hx of head trauma

12. Which of the following is the most common clinical manifestation of glioblastoma multiforme?

    A. Headache
    B. Seizure
    C. Focal neuro deficit
    D. Mental status change
    E. All of the above occur in almost equal frequency.

13. Which of the following tumors most commonly metastasizes to the leptomeninges?

    A. Small cell lung cancer
    B. Adenocarcinoma
    C. Breast
    D. Lymphoma
    E. None of the above

14. A 76-year-old male with a history of adenocarcinoma is found to have leptomeningeal carcinomatosis. The family and the patient decide they do not want any treatment. What is the usual mortality associated with untreated patients?
    A. 1 month
    B. 6 months
    C. 1 year
    D. 5 years
    E. None of the above

15. Patients with known leptomeningeal carcinomatosis usually can have multiple presenting complaints. Which of the following is one of the most common complaints?
    A. Memory loss
    B. Incontinence
    C. Sensory loss
    D. Seizures
    E. All of the above

16. A 68-year-old male with a history of metastatic small cell lung cancer has complaints of headaches, diplopia, as well as neck and back pain with nuchal rigidity. The patient is found to have leptomeningeal carcinomatosis. Which of the following is the most common area of the central nervous system (CNS) that is involved?
    A. Cranial nerves
    B. Spinal root
    C. Cerebral hemisphere
    D. Anterior horn cells
    E. None of the above

17. A 68-year-old male with a history of melanoma cancer is found to have complaints of headaches, diplopia, and neck and back pain with nuchal rigidity. The patient is found to have leptomeningeal carcinomatosis. Which of the following is the next best test to confirm the diagnosis?
    A. Magnetic resonance imaging (MRI)
    B. CT scan
    C. Biopsy
    D. Spinal tap
    E. None of the above

18. Which of the following is probably the most common CT scan finding with oligodendrogliomas?

    A. Fat
    B. Calcifications
    C. Cyst
    D. "Fried egg" appearance
    E. None of the above

19. What percentage of all intracranial tumors are pituitary tumors?

    A. 1%
    B. 15%
    C. 45%
    D. 90%
    E. None of the above

20. Which of the following is the most lethal complication of pituitary tumors?

    A. Excessive prolactin
    B. Decreased growth hormone
    C. Apoplexy
    D. Metastasis
    E. None of the above

21. Which of the following medications can treat a prolactinoma?

    A. Metoclopramide
    B. Fluorouracil (5-FU)
    C. Prednisone
    D. Bromocriptine
    E. None of the above

22. A 33-year-old male with HIV/AIDS develops a brain tumor. He is diagnosed with primary central nervous system (CNS) lymphoma. What is the median survival for this patient if he undergoes radiation alone?

    A. 4 weeks
    B. 4 months
    C. 4 years
    D. 1 year
    E. None of the above

23. Which of the following is the most common malignant skull-based tumor?

    A. Osteosarcoma
    B. Multiple myeloma
    C. Chondrosarcoma
    D. Fibrosarcoma
    E. Ewing's sarcoma

24. Which of the following statements regarding radiation necrosis in the CNS is true?

    A. MRI of the brain can differentiate radiation necrosis from tumor-related changes.
    B. Radiation necrosis only occurs within a few weeks of radiation exposure.
    C. MRI of the brain cannot differentiate radiation necrosis from tumor changes.
    D. A history of diabetes does not increase your risk for radiation necrosis.
    E. None of the above

25. A 56-year-old male with a primary brain tumor has a history of whole brain radiation and presents with new-onset seizures. Which of the following would be a confirmatory test to determine the cause of the seizure?

    A. CT scan
    B. MRI brain
    C. Surgical biopsy
    D. X-ray
    E. None of the above

ANSWERS

1. **Answer: C.** McCune-Albright syndrome consists of the triad of polyostotic fibrous dysplasia, hyperpigmented skin macules, and precocious puberty.

2. **Answer: C.** Approximately 40% of melanomas metastasize to the brain. Twenty-one percent of lung tumors and 9% of breast cancer go the brain.

3. **Answer: A.** Primary lung cancer accounts for half of all metastatic brain tumors.

4. **Answer: C.** Headache (42%) and seizure (21%) are the two most common presenting symptoms.

5. **Answer: A.** Approximately three quarters of patients with brain stem gliomas are under age 20. There is a bimodal distribution to these tumors with the peak incidence occurring in the latter part of the first decade of life and the second peak occurring in the fourth decade of life.

6. **Answer: B.** Melanoma has the highest propensity to be hemorrhagic. There is no cure. Increased survival may be seen if whole brain radiation therapy (WBRT) is used in combination with tumor resection.

7. **Answer: B.** On presentation, approximately 40% of patients have symptoms of hypothyroidism. A quarter of patients have signs of adrenal failure (orthostatic hypotension, hypoglycemia, hypoglycemia), and about 20% have signs of diabetes insipidus.

8. **Answer: A.** With retrochiasmal locations, the patient typically presents with hydrocephalus with signs of increased intracranial pressure such as papilledema and horizontal diplopia.

9. **Answer: B.** Surgery remains the most effective treatment for this tumor. Postoperative radiation therapy improves survival; however, surgery remains the most effective treatment. Chemotherapy is the most disappointing.

10. **Answer: B.** GBM is the most common and unfortunately the most aggressive primary brain tumor. It is highly malignant and infiltrates the brain extensively.

11. **Answer: A.** Patients with an hx of acute lymphocytic leukemia often undergo prophylactic whole brain radiation therapy and therefore they are at a 22-fold increased risk of developing an astrocytoma.

12. **Answer: E.** Headaches occur approximately 30% to 50% of the time; seizures occur about 30% to 60% of the time, focal neurological deficits occur 40% to 60% of the time, and mental status change occurs about 20% to 40% of the time. Essentially, they all occur about the same frequency.

13. **Answer: B.** Adenocarcinoma is the most common tumor type that spreads to the leptomeninges. The incidence of leptomeningeal involvement increases the longer the patient has a primary cancer.

14. **Answer: A.** Without any treatment, most patients have a median survival duration of 4 to 6 weeks due to progressing neurologic dysfunction.

15. **Answer: D.** Seizures and pain are the two most common presenting complaints in patients with leptomeningeal carcinomatosis.

16. **Answer: A.** Cranial nerve deficits are the most frequent sign that occurs with this disease. Approximately 94% of patients have cranial nerve involvement. However, only one-third present with cranial nerve complaints.

17. **Answer: D.** The diagnosis is made and confirmed with a positive CSF cytologic result; therefore, a spinal tap is the next best test to obtain the diagnosis.

18. **Answer: B.** Intratumoral calcification is very common finding. Hemorrhage is noted occasionally. The microscopic finding is often referred to as having a "fried egg" appearance.

19. **Answer: B.** Pituitary tumors represent about 10% to 15% of all intracranial tumors. Incidental pituitary tumors are found in approximately 10% of autopsies.

20. **Answer: C.** Pituitary apoplexy can be a lethal complication. Pituitary apoplexy is characterized by a sudden onset of headache, visual symptoms, altered mental status, and hormonal dysfunction caused by acute hemorrhage or infarction of a pituitary gland.

21. **Answer: D.** A majority of prolactinomas respond to dopamine receptor agonists. Improvement in visual field abnormalities, resolution of symptoms, and visible diminution of mass size can result with treatment.

22. **Answer: B.** With radiation therapy alone, patients with AIDS have a median survival duration of 4 months. A subgroup of patients with AIDS who are able to tolerate chemotherapy and radiation therapy may survive as long as 18 months.

23. **Answer: B.** Multiple myeloma is the most common bone-forming tumor. Osteosarcoma is the second most common, and chondrosarcoma is the third most common type of malignant bone tumor.

24. **Answer: C.** MRI cannot differentiate radiation necrosis changes from tumor-related changes.

25. **Answer: C.** Surgical biopsy provides histologic diagnosis and usually is confirmatory. It also has the benefit of relieving increased intracranial pressure and improves disability. Conservative management is observation with serial MRIs but is not confirmatory.

Movement Disorders

QUESTIONS

1. A 34-year-old female presents with acute psychotic symptoms. She is described as being immobile, mute, and having a waxy flexibility. Which of the following statements is false?

   A. Nonconvulsive status epilepticus is part of the differential.
   B. An accurate history is rarely available from the patient.
   C. Patients with this disorder only have symptoms while an examiner or bystander is present, and they disappear when no one is around.
   D. Grasp reflex is a secondary feature of catatonia.
   E. None of the above

2. A 22-year-old female presents during pregnancy with abnormal movements. There is no family history of any neurologic disorders. She states that during stressful times, the movements become worse, and her husband states that they disappear during sleep. She is noted to have a "milkmaid" grip. Which of the following is true?

   A. This is the most common neurologic disorder during pregnancy.
   B. Rheumatic disease used to be a common cause for this disorder.
   C. This is conversion disorder.
   D. This is essential tremor.
   E. None of the above

3. Chorea is defined as a state of excessive movements that are irregular, do not repeat, and are abrupt in character. Which of the following statements is false?

   A. Huntington's chorea is the most well-studied chorea syndrome.
   B. The basal ganglia is the sight of dysfunction.
   C. Physostigmine cannot overcome anticholinergic-induced chorea.
   D. Decreased gamma-aminobutyric acid (GABA) levels in the basal ganglia is seen in these patients.
   E. None of the above

4. A 75-year-old male develops progressive dementia, Parkinson's features, and limb apraxia. On examination, the patient also has signs of supranuclear palsy. Which of the following is true?

   A. The patient has Lewy-body dementia.
   B. Males develop this disorder more frequently.
   C. Resting tremor is the most common feature.
   D. Hallucinations are not a common feature of this disorder.
   E. None of the above

5. A 56-year-old male presents with complaints of difficulty feeding. He states his hand starts to shake when he brings a utensil to his mouth. Alcohol seems to relieve the problem, and therefore, he has started drinking more frequently. There are no problems when the patient is relaxed and sitting still. Which of the following is false?

   A. The problem is located in the Mollaret triangle near the brain stem.
   B. These symptoms often have isolated head tremor.
   C. Both genders are affected equally.
   D. About half the patients have a strong family history.
   E. None of the above

6. Which of the following medications is the most effective treatment for essential tremor?

   A. Clonidine
   B. Methylpentynol
   C. Ropinirole
   D. Primidone
   E. None of the above

7. Which of the following is not an exclusion criteria for essential tremor?

   A. Primary orthostatic tremor
   B. Isolated voice tremor
   C. Isolated leg tremor
   D. Isolated head tremor
   E. Writing tremor only

8. Friedreich's ataxia (FA) is inherited in what fashion?

   A. Autosomal dominant
   B. X-linked
   C. Sporadic
   D. Autosomal recessive
   E. None of the above

9. What percentage of patients with FA are wheelchair-bound by their mid-fourth decade of life?

    A. 10%
    B. 25%
    C. 50%
    D. 75%
    E. 95%

10. A patient presents with progressive dementia, chorea movements, and abnormal behavior. His father had a similar disease and died at an early age due to suicide. Which of the following statements is true?

    A. This disorder is sporadic in nature.
    B. It is due to an expansion of a cysteine-adenosine-guanine repeat.
    C. It is inherited in an autosomal recessive fashion.
    D. Anticipation is infrequent in this disorder.
    E. None of the above

11. A 65-year-old male presents with gradual gait disturbance, urinary incontinence, and progressive dementia over the past year. The gait is described as shuffling and magnetic. On examination, there is no papilledema, rigidity, or tremor. Magnetic resonance imaging (MRI) is performed and demonstrates some atrophy but markedly enlarged ventricles. Which of the following is the next best step?

    A. Initiate acetylcholinesterase inhibitor
    B. High-volume spinal tap
    C. Initiate carbidopa/levodopa
    D. Urology consult
    E. Transfer the patient to a nursing home for long-term care.

12. A patient with normal pressure hydrocephalus (NPH) is being evaluated for shunt placement. Which of the following statements is true?

    A. A patient with predominant gait difficulty and minimal cognitive deficit is an ideal candidate for shunt placement.
    B. Significant white matter lesions on MRI is of minimal significance.
    C. Cortical atrophy on MRI is a positive prognostic indicator for shunt placement.
    D. Indwelling cerebrospinal fluid (CSF) catheters have no role in this diagnosis.
    E. Reduction of bladder hyperactivity after high-volume LP is a negative prognosis for shunt surgery.

13. Which of the following statements regarding Parkinson's disease (PD) is false?
    A. It is typically asymmetric.
    B. Tremor typically begins in the lower extremity.
    C. Gait difficulty is a later finding.
    D. Sleep disturbances are common.
    E. Resting tremor is one of the best clinical predictors for pathologic diagnosis.

14. Which of the following is not part of the three cardinal signs of PD?
    A. Resting tremor
    B. Bradykinesia
    C. Postural instability
    D. Rigidity
    E. None of the above

15. A 76-year-old male with a 15-year history of PD develops short-term memory difficulty and some visuospatial impairment. The patient's language is completely intact. What percentage of patients develop dementia?
    A. 1%
    B. 25%
    C. 75%
    D. 100%
    E. None of the above

16. A 34-year-old male develops bradykinesia, tremor, shuffling gate, and is diagnosed with PD. Which of the following has been associated with other causes of PD?
    A. Well water
    B. Pesticides
    C. Herbicides
    D. 1-methyl-4-phenyl-1,2,3,6-tetrahydropyridine (MPTP)
    E. All of the above
    F. None of the above

17. Of all causes of PD, what percentage is due to the known genetic causes?
    A. 5%
    B. 25%
    C. 50%
    D. 75%
    E. 99%

18. Which of the following is an FDA-approved treatment for PD?
    A. Pallidotomy
    B. Deep brain stimulation
    C. Protein redistribution diet
    D. Thalamotomy
    E. All of the above

19. A 45-year-old male is found to have increased muscle tone in one limb. Which of the following is part of the classification of dystonia?
    A. Focal
    B. Segmental
    C. Multifocal
    D. Hemidystonia
    E. Generalized
    F. All of the above
    G. None of the above

20. Which of the following disorders is considered an alpha-synucleinopathy as well as a tauopathy?
    A. Multisystem atrophy
    B. Lewy body disease
    C. Progressive supranuclear palsy
    D. PD
    E. Pantothenate kinase 2 deficiency

21. Patients with multisystem atrophy (MSA) go on to develop Parkinsonism, autonomic failure, cerebellar, and pyramidal signs. What percentage of patients develops Parkinson's features?
    A. 1%
    B. 10%
    C. 50%
    D. 90%
    E. 25%

22. Which of the following is not considered an extrapyramidal sign?
    A. Akathisia
    B. Spasticity
    C. Chorea
    D. Athetosis
    E. Stereotypy

23. Tardive dyskinesia typically occurs in patients that have been on which of the following medications for many years?
    A. Metoclopramide
    B. Carbidopa
    C. Ropinirole
    D. Diphenhydramine
    E. None of the above

24. Which of the following tests should be considered when evaluating a patient with tardive dyskinesia?
    A. Calcium level
    B. Serum ceruloplasmin
    C. Thyroid function
    D. Complete blood count
    E. All of the above
    F. None of the above

25. Which of the following is the most common manifestation of Wilson's disease in children?
    A. Neuropsychiatric symptoms
    B. Seizures
    C. Hepatic disease
    D. Kayser-Fleisher rings
    E. All of the above occur equally.

ANSWERS

1. **Answer: C.** The patient has catatonia. This should be present in the setting of the examiner as well as when no one is present. If the symptoms resolve when no one is around, factitious disorder or somatoform disorder should be considered.

2. **Answer: B.** The patient has chorea gravidarum. This is a rare disorder, however, and it used to be more common prior to antibiotic treatment. Rheumatic heart disease used to be the main culprit. Rheumatic fever and antiphospholipid syndrome are the main links to this disorder.

3. **Answer: C.** Chorea develops in patients on anticholinergic medications and can be overcome promptly by administering physostigmine.

4. **Answer: D.** The patient has cortical basal ganglionic degeneration, which has features of PD but typically, the rigidity and dystonia are more prominent. Resting tremor is not a feature. Hallucinations are typical of Lewy-body dementia and not this disorder. There is no gender predilection.

5. **Answer: E.** None of the above.

6. **Answer: D.** Primidone and propranolol are the most effective treatments for essential tremor with a reduction in tremor amplitude in about three quarters of all patients.

7. **Answer: D.** Isolated head tremor but absence of abnormal posturing of the head is an inclusion criterion for essential tremor. The rest of the options are all exclusions.

8. **Answer: D.** FA is the most common of all the autosomal recessive ataxias. Cardinal features include progressive limb and gait ataxia, dysarthria, posterior column deficits, and absent DTRs and positive Babinski's sign.

9. **Answer: E.** FA is a progressive disorder with significant morbidity. Loss of ambulation usually occurs within 15 years of the start of the disease, and more than 95% of patients are wheelchair bound by age 45.

10. **Answer: B.** The patient has Huntington's disease, and the genetic basis for this disorder is the expansion of a CAG repeat (triple repeat) encoding a polyglutamine tract in the N-terminus of the protein huntington. It is transmitted in an autosomal dominant fashion and anticipation is common in this disorder.

11. **Answer: B.** The patient probably has NPH, and a gait and neuropsychological evaluation pre– and post–high-volume spinal tap would be the next best step to determine if placing a shunt would be beneficial.

12. **Answer: A.** Patients with NPH that have primarily just a gait difficulty and minimal cognitive problems are the best candidates and usually improve the most after shunt placement. The other statements are false.

13. **Answer: B.** Typically the tremor begins in the upper extremities. It is asymmetric, and the rest of the statements are true.

14. **Answer: C.** Postural instability is not part of the core cardinal signs for PD; however, it is a fourth cardinal sign that usually emerges later in the disease, typically after 8 or more years with the disease.

15. **Answer: B.** Dementia with PD typically occurs late in the disease, and affects approximately 15% to 30% of patients. If dementia occurs within 1 year of onset of motor features, consider Lewy body disease.

16. **Answer: E.** All of the above have been associated with PD.

17. **Answer: A.** It is estimated that of all the currently known genetic causes of PD account for less than 5% of all cases.

18. **Answer: B.** Deep brain stimulation is an FDA-approved treatment for PD.

19. **Answer: F.** All of the above are part of the classification of dystonias.

20. **Answer: C.** All of the above are alpha-synucleinopathies, but progressive supranuclear palsy is also considered a tauopathy as well.

21. **Answer: D.** Approximately 90% of patients with MSA develop Parkinsonism. Autonomic failure is usually part of all MSA patients and may be the first sign. About 50% of patients develop cerebellar and pyramidal signs.

22. **Answer: B.** Spasticity is considered a pyramidal sign. The others are considered extrapyramidal signs.

23. **Answer: A.** Patients on dopamine antagonists for many years are typically susceptible to developing tardive dyskinesia.

24. **Answer: E.** All of the above are recommended tests to be done when evaluating a patient with tardive dyskinesia.

25. **Answer: C.** Liver disease is the most common initial manifestation in children. In older individuals, neuropsychiatric symptoms are the usual initial symptoms. Kayser-Fleisher rings are almost always present when neurologic symptoms are present.

Neuroimmunology

QUESTIONS

1. Which of the following statements is true regarding acute disseminated encephalomyelitis (ADEM)?
   A. It is indistinguishable from multiple sclerosis.
   B. It is a nonvasculitic demyelinating process.
   C. Genetics probably play no role in this disease.
   D. Multiple sclerosis (MS) is usually a monophasic illness.
   E. None of the above

2. What percentage of patients that develop ADEM occurs in children under the age of 10?
   A. 1%
   B. 25%
   C. 80%
   D. 99%
   E. None of the above

3. Which of the following is helpful in distinguishing ADEM from MS?
   A. Age younger than 12
   B. Fever
   C. Seizures
   D. Recent immunization
   E. All of the above

4. A 17-year-old patient presents with ankylosing spondylitis. Which of the following statements is true?

   A. More females than males are affected.
   B. Uveitis is a possible associated condition.
   C. Approximately 25% of the US population is affected.
   D. The pain associated with this condition is worse in the afternoon and improves in the morning.
   E. None of the above

5. What percentage of patients with ankylosing spondylitis have HLA-B27 antigen?

   A. 1%
   B. 10%
   C. 50%
   D. 75%
   E. 95%

6. What percentage of patients with Bell's palsy have recurrence?

   A. 15%
   B. 30%
   C. 70%
   D. 90%
   E. None of the above

7. Which of the following statements regarding Bell's palsy is true?

   A. Men are more likely to be affected than women.
   B. The lowest incidence is in persons older than age 60.
   C. Pregnant women are three times more likely to be affected than non-pregnant women.
   D. Overall, patients have a poor prognosis with Bell's palsy.
   E. None of the above

8. What percentage of patients with Behçet's disease have an associated oral ulcer?

   A. 1%
   B. 10%
   C. 50%
   D. 75%
   E. 100%

9. Which of the following are hallmark features of MS?

    A. Neurologic deficits usually once in time
    B. Recurrent neurologic deficits that are disseminated by space and time
    C. Seizure disorder
    D. Bilateral optic neuritis and transverse myelitis
    E. None of the above

10. Which of the following is not part of the four standard categories used to describe the clinical course of MS?

    A. Relapsing remitting
    B. Secondary progressive
    C. Progressive relapsing
    D. Primary progressive
    E. All of the above

11. Which of the following subtypes of MS responds the least to treatment?

    A. Relapsing remitting
    B. Secondary progressive
    C. Progressive relapsing
    D. Primary progressive
    E. All of the above

12. Which of the following is the best way to diagnose MS?

    A. Lumbar puncture (LP)
    B. Magnetic resonance imaging (MRI)
    C. Computed tomography (CT) scan
    D. Clinical
    E. Positron emission tomography (PET) scan

13. What percentage of patients with MS have abnormalities detected on CT scan?

    A. 5%
    B. 10%
    C. 33%
    D. 60%
    E. 100%

14. Which of the following is not part of the disease modifying drugs for the treatment of MS?

    A. Interferon beta-1b
    B. Intravenous immunoglobulin (IVIG)
    C. Glatiramer acetate
    D. Interferon beta-1a
    E. Methylprednisolone

15. What percentage of patients with MS will do well for 20 years and therefore would be considered to have benign MS?

    A. 10%
    B. 25%
    C. 46%
    D. 78%
    E. None of the above

16. Which of the following groups is most susceptible to contracting MS?

    A. Caucasian
    B. Asian
    C. Pacific Islander
    D. African American
    E. Ashkenazi Jew

17. Which of the following supports the autoimmune theory?

    A. Elevated eosinophils
    B. Animal model of allergic encephalomyelitis
    C. Response to steroids
    D. All of the above
    E. None of the above

18. What percentage of patients with definite MS have an abnormal response to visual evoked response?

    A. 85%
    B. 50%
    C. 5%
    D. 35%
    E. None of the above

19. Which of the following tests is the most useful in detecting suspected pontine lesions in MS patients?
    A. Brain stem auditory response
    B. Somatosensory response
    C. Nerve conduction study
    D. Visual evoked response
    E. None of the above

20. What is the average survival of patients with primary progressive MS?
    A. 5 years
    B. 1 year
    C. 10 years
    D. 25 years
    E. 35 years

21. Which of the following is suggestive of worse prognosis in MS?
    A. Age of onset <35 years
    B. Acute onset of first symptoms
    C. Cerebellar signs
    D. Onset with sensory symptoms
    E. None of the above

22. Which of the following describes Marchiafava-Bignami disease?
    A. Damage to the mamillary bodies
    B. Bilateral occipital lobe infarctions
    C. Demyelination of the corpus callosum
    D. First noted in Irish men
    E. Rapidly progressive

23. Which of the following viruses have been associated with MS?
    A. Herpes virus type 6 (HSV 6)
    B. Human immunodeficiency virus (HIV)
    C. Measles
    D. Polio
    E. None of the above

24. Which of the following is considered a variant of MS?

    A. Primary progressive MS
    B. Marburg virus
    C. Devic's disease
    D. Schilder's disease
    E. A and C
    F. All of the above

25. Which of the following may develop neutralizing antibodies as a treatment of MS?

    A. Glatiramer acetate
    B. Beta-interferon
    C. Cyclophosphamide
    D. Methotrexate
    E. None of the above

ANSWERS

1. **Answer: B.** ADEM is a nonvasculitic inflammatory demyelinating condition that is very similar to MS but can be differentiated by clinical features and laboratory tests.

2. **Answer: C.** Around 80% of childhood cases of ADEM occur under the age of 10. Less than 20% of cases occur in the second decade of life.

3. **Answer: E.** All of the above help distinguish ADEM from MS. Also, there are often less posterior column abnormalities, which is more common in MS patients.

4. **Answer: B.** Uveitis, iritis, aortitis, pulmonary fibrosis, amyloidosis, and inflammatory bowel disease are all associated conditions. More men are affected than women, and only approximately 1% of the population is affected with this condition.

5. **Answer: E.** Ninety percent to 95% of patients have this antigen. This test is most helpful when the diagnosis is not clear.

6. **Answer: A.** Approximately 10% to 15% of patients can have recurrence of Bell's palsy on the ipsilateral side or the contralateral side of the initial palsy. Recurrence typically occurs in patients with a family history of recurrent Bell's palsy. Some patients with recurrence were found to have tumors of the seventh nerve or inflammatory or demyelinating disease. Patients with diabetes are more likely to have recurrence as well.

7. **Answer: C.** Pregnant women are more likely to be affected. The sexes are equally affected, and the highest incidence is in persons older than age 60.

8. **Answer: E.** All patients with Behçet's disease will have an associated oral aphthous ulceration. Approximately three fourths of patients will have genital aphthous ulceration.

9. **Answer: B.** The clinical hallmark of the disease is the recurrent neurologic deficits that are disseminated in space and time.

10. **Answer: E.** All of the above are part of the standard categories.

11. **Answer: D.** Primary progressive MS is the least responsive subtype of MS.

12. **Answer: D.** MS is a clinical diagnosis. The use of the other tests helps to support the diagnosis.

13. **Answer: C.** Approximately one third of patients with MS can detect abnormalities on CT scan.

14. **Answer: E.** Methylprednisolone is not disease modifying but is used for the acute relapses to hasten clinical recovery.

15. **Answer: A.** Approximately 10% of patients will do well for 20 years. Approximately 70% will develop secondary progression of neurologic deficits.

16. **Answer: A.** Caucasians are the most susceptible to MS. Multiple genes are suspected in the involvement of MS. The lifetime risk of developing MS is 0.00125% in the general population.

17. **Answer: B.** The autoimmune theory is supported by the animal model that demonstrates allergic encephalomyelitis.

18. **Answer: A.** Approximately 85% of patients with definite MS will have an abnormal response to visual evoked response, and approximately 58% of patients with probable MS have an abnormal response.

19. **Answer: A.** This test is the most useful in detecting suspected pontine lesions. Abnormal response is seen in 67% of patients with definite MS.

20. **Answer: E.** Patients with primary progressive usually have 35 years of survival. About 70% of patients after 10 years are not working full time.

21. **Answer: C.** Polysymptomatic onset, cerebellar signs, vertigo, or corticospinal tract signs are all prognostic indicators of worse disease.

22. **Answer: C.** Marchiafava-Bignami disease is demyelination of the corpus callosum without inflammation, and sometimes other areas of the central nervous system may be involved. It was first noted in elderly Italian men who consumed red wine. It is usually slowly progressive and results in death in 3 to 6 years.

23. **Answer: A.** HSV 6 has been implicated and has been seen around acute plaques in some studies.

24. **Answer: F.** Primary progressive MS, Marburg variant, Devic's disease, and Schilder's disease is fulminant MS in children with confluent lesions in both hemispheres.

25. **Answer: B.** Beta-interferon may develop neutralizing antibodies and may make treatment ineffective. Patients may also develop flu-like symptoms early on. Elevation of LFTs may also develop.

Neurology High-Yields

1. The specific pathology of multiple sclerosis (MS) is demyelination with axonal sparing, and the mean age of onset for MS is 32 years.

2. MS is the most common demyelinating illness in the central nervous system (CNS).

3. The disease course for MS usually manifests itself as relapsing and remitting.

4. MS is primarily diagnosed clinically in conjunction with magnetic resonance imaging (MRI) findings typical of the disease (periventricular white matter changes).

5. Ménière's disease consists of vertigo, hearing loss, and a feeling of fullness or blockage in the ear(s).

6. Intractable cases of Ménière's disease may be treated via surgical shunting.

7. The tetrad of narcolepsy consists of excessive daytime sleepiness, cataplexy, hypnagogic or hypnapompic hallucinations, and sleep paralysis.

8. Horner's syndrome consists of ptosis, miosis, and anhidrosis.

9. Subdural hematomas are caused by tearing of the bridging emissary veins.

10. Radiologic manifestation of subdural hematomas are concave or crescentic in shape typically seen on computed tomography (CT) scan.

11. Epidural hematomas are usually caused by skull fractures and result from tearing of the middle meningeal artery.

12. Epidural hematomas are lens shaped on CT scan.

13. Temporal arteritis is a granulomatous arteritis affecting large and medium-sized arteries. Histologic studies demonstrate intimal thickening and lymphocytic infiltration of the media and adventitia.

14. The most common pathogens for bacterial meningitis are *Streptococcus pneumoniae* (most common in adults), *Haemophilus* influenzae, and *Neisseria meningitides*.

15. Typical cerebrospinal fluid (CSF) findings in septic meningitis are neutrophils, high protein, and low glucose versus aseptic meningitis which has lymphocytes, normal glucose, and high protein.

16. Tuberculosis meningitis is rare, however, it should be thought of in patients with the right clinical symptoms and with a history of immunosuppression, alcoholics, intravenous drug abusers, immigrants from endemic areas, or prisoners.

17. Herpes simplex virus (HSV) encephalitis is typically caused by HSV type 1. The CSF findings are lymphocytes, normal glucose, elevated protein, and many high red blood cell counts.

18. A long-term complication of HSV encephalitis is often amnesia.

19. Untreated cases of HSV encephalitis have a mortality rate of 70%.

20. Tabes dorsalis is caused by untreated primary infection with syphilis (treponema pallidum) and usually occurs 10 to 20 years after the initial infection.

21. Progressive multifocal leukodystrophy (PML) is due to reactivation of the John Cunningham (JC) virus. It causes widespread demyelination due to infecting the oligodendrocytes in immunocompromised patients.

22. PML is a subacute course resulting in subcortical dementia, and death usually occurs within 6 months of diagnosis.

23. Lacunar strokes account for approximately one fifth of all strokes.

24. Amaurosis fugax is due to retinal artery occlusion/ischemia and is primarily caused by internal carotid artery stenosis.

25. Carotid endarterectomy for symptomatic artery stenosis (70% to 99%) is the standard of care for stroke prevention.

26. The most common cause for subarachnoid hemorrhage (spontaneous) is rupture of a berry aneurysm.

27. Nimodipine (calcium channel blocker) is thought to be neuroprotective in the case of vasospasm.

28. Treatment of vasospasm includes triple H therapy (hypertension, hypervolemia, and hemodilution).

29. The highest risk for rebleeding after Subarachnoid Hemorrhage (SAH) is within the first 48 hours.

30. The most common sites for hypertensive hemorrhagic stroke are the basal ganglia, thalamus, cerebellum, and pons.

31. Approximately two thirds of hemorrhagic strokes are due to hypertension.

32. Broca's aphasia is a nonfluent (motor) aphasia that results in an inability to speak (broken speech) but comprehension of speech is intact.

33. Wernicke's aphasia is a fluent (sensory/receptive) aphasia in which patients make incomprehensible speech and are usually unaware of their deficit. Comprehension is impaired.

34. Brown-Séquard syndrome is caused by unilateral hemisection of the cord and results in ipsilateral weakness, loss of vibration and proprioception with hyperreflexia, and loss of pain and temperature contralaterally below the lesion.

35. Vitamin B_{12} deficiency can result in neuropathy, weakness, depression, and dementia.

36. Pernicious anemia is a common cause of vitamin B_{12} deficiency.

37. Carpal tunnel syndrome is caused by compression of the median nerve at the wrist under the flexor retinaculum.

38. Tinel's sign is numbness or tingling that occurs while tapping or percussing the wrist over the median nerve.

39. Guillain-Barré syndrome (GBS) is a progressive ascending flaccid paralysis (areflexia) that peaks within 4 weeks of onset.

40. Treatment of choice for GBS is plasmapheresis or intravenous immunoglobulin (IVIG).

41. GBS is classically preceded by gastroenteritis or upper respiratory infection.

42. Amyotrophic lateral sclerosis (ALS) affects the anterior horn cells and the corticospinal tract.

43. SOD1 mutation occurs in familial ALS (rare form).

44. Complicated migraine is a migraine headache with severe or persistent sensorimotor deficits (suggestive of a cerebral infarction).

45. Cluster headache is excruciating, unilateral head pain associated with ipsilateral tearing, conjunctival injection, and nasal congestion.

46. The triad of headache, papilledema, and increased intracranial pressure (ICP) is known as benign intracranial hypertension (pseudotumor cerebri).

47. One third of patients with benign intracranial hypertension have resolution after their first lumbar puncture.

48. Optic nerve sheath fenestration is an option for medically refractive patients with pseudotumor cerebri.

49. The main complication of temporal arteritis is visual loss (ischemic optic neuropathy).

50. Myasthenia gravis can be established with Tensilon test, repetitive nerve stimulation, single-fiber electromyography, and acetylcholine receptor antibodies.

51. About 5% of patients with acute stroke will have early seizure.

52. Alcohol-related seizures usually occur about 24 hours after the last drink but can occur at any time in chronic alcoholics.

53. Antiepileptic drugs are not indicated in pure alcohol-related seizures.

54. Approximately 3% to 6% of patients undergoing supratentorial craniotomy will develop seizures perioperatively.

55. Approximately 5% of patients who have sustained concussion will have an intracranial hemorrhage.

56. Parkinson's disease is a clinical diagnosis with the cardinal features of tremor, rigidity, bradykinesia, and loss of postural reflexes.

57. Toxoplasmosis is the most common opportunistic infection affecting the CNS in patients with AIDS.

58. Wilson's disease diagnosis is supported by Kayser-Fleischer rings, low serum ceruloplasmin level, abnormal liver function tests, or hepatitis.

59. The gene for Wilson's disease is located on chromosome 13.

60. A common gene for idiopathic torsion dystonias, the DYT1 gene, is located on chromosome 9 and is inherited in an autosomal dominant manner with a penetrance as low as 30%.

61. Fifteen percent of strokes are caused by artery-to-artery embolism.

62. Six classic lacunar syndromes are clumsy-hand dysarthria, pure-motor hemiparesis, ataxic hemiparesis, sensorimotor syndrome, and pure hemisensory loss. More than 70 lacunar syndromes have been described.

63. Up to 40% of strokes are cryptogenic.

64. Fifty percent of patients that have a transient ischemic attack (TIA) go on to develop a stroke within the next 5 years. Ten percent of the strokes occur in the first 90 days (if untreated).

65. If no carotid stenosis or cardioembolic source is identified, *acetylsalicylic acid* is the drug of choice.

66. The posterior communicating artery is the most common site of aneurysms.

67. Cigarette smoking is an increased risk factor for aneurysmal bleeding.

68. Surgical resection followed by whole brain radiation therapy is the gold standard for the treatment of solitary brain metastases.

69. Leptomeningeal metastasis is most common from the breast, lung, non-Hodgkin's lymphoma, and malignant melanoma.

70. The prognosis of patients with leptomeningeal metastasis is about 3 to 6 months.

71. Approximately 40% of patients have a solitary metastasis to the brain (usually gastrointestinal and gynecologic).

72. Brain metastasis usually presents with headache, motor weakness, and mental status change.

73. Most highly vascular metastatic cancers are melanoma and renal cell carcinoma.

74. Acoustic neuromas account for approximately 8% to 9% of all primary brain tumors, arise from the eighth cranial nerve, and usually grow at the cerebellopontine angle.

75. Meningiomas account for 20% of all intracranial tumors. They are usually benign tumors that arise from arachnoid cap cells.

76. Patients with olfactory groove meningiomas present with dementia, ipsilateral optic atrophy, or contralateral papilledema (Foster-Kennedy syndrome).

77. Ependymomas account for 60% of spinal cord gliomas. On histopathology, rosettes and pseudorosettes are seen perivascular space.

78. The pathology of oligodendrogliomas contains cells that have a characteristic "fried egg" appearance.

79. Glioblastoma multiforme tumors (grade IV astrocytomas) are the most malignant and common form of the tumor. They represent 50% of tumors.

80. HIV-associated sensory neuropathy is the most common complication of AIDS.

81. Progressive multifocal leukoencephalopathy is caused by the JC virus in immunosuppressed patients (typically AIDS patients), and the median survival is 6 months.

82. Inclusion body myositis differs from polymyositis in that it typically affects distal muscles and causes asymmetric weakness.

83. Critical illness myopathy is seen in patients in the intensive care unit that have been treated with steroids and nondepolarizing paralyzing agents.

84. Neuroleptic malignant syndrome caused by to dopamine blockage and is a rare idiosyncratic reaction with muscle rigidity with rhabdomyolysis, fever, mental status change, and autonomic instability. Creatine kinase levels are always elevated.

85. The treatment of NMS is to stop the offending agent and to provide cooling, dantrolene, and bromocriptine.

86. Malignant hyperthermia is an autosomal dominant condition that predisposes an individual to severe muscle rigidity, rhabdomyolysis, fever, and metabolic acidosis with exposure to inhaled anesthetics or succinylcholine.

87. Duchenne's muscular dystrophy is an X-linked progressive degenerative myopathy. Inability to walk occurs by age 10.

88. Wilson's disease consists of the triad of cirrhosis, neurologic manifestation, and a Kayser-Fleischer ring.

89. Von Hippel-Lindau (VHL) disease is inherited in an autosomal dominant fashion.

90. VHL presents with hemangioblastomas of the retina, cerebellum, brain stem, and spinal cord.

91. Patients with VHL have an increased incidence of renal cell carcinoma.

92. Friedreich's ataxia (FA) is inherited in an autosomal recessive fashion.

93. Classical presentation of FA consists of progressive gait and truncal ataxia, dysarthria, areflexia in the lower extremities, and a positive Babinski sign.

94. Patients who have dementia with Lewy bodies (DLB) present with visual hallucinations, delirium, Parkinson's features, and rapid eye movement sleep behavior disorder.

95. Memory is relatively preserved in patients with DLB.

96. Lewy bodies are intracytoplasmic inclusions in the neurons.

97. Patients with DLB respond well to acetylcholinesterase inhibitors for the treatment of hallucinations.

98. Patients with frontotemporal dementia demonstrate atrophy of the frontal and temporal lobes.

99. Patients with frontotemporal dementia have Pick bodies on histology with silver staining.

100. Patients with frontotemporal dementia typically present clinically with apathy, emotional lability, disinhibition, hyperorality, and lack of insight.

101. Creutzfeldt-Jakob disease (CJD) is a subacute encephalopathy of the spongiform type.

102. CJD is caused by slow virus-like agents called prions that contain no DNA or RNA.

103. Patients with CJD typically present with progressive dementia and associated myoclonus.

104. CJD patients have a 90% mortality rate within the first year.

105. Status epilepticus is a neurologic emergency. Prolonged seizures after 30 minutes show pathologic changes, and after 60 minutes, neurons start to die.

106. The typical treatment of status epilepticus is benzodiazepine initially and then phenytoin (or another intravenous antiepileptic) and if necessary, an anesthetic agent until the seizing stops.

107. About 50% of patients that suffer from new-onset generalized tonic-clonic seizures will go on to have recurrence.

108. About 33% of patients with new-onset seizures will have spontaneous resolution or can be controlled with medication. The remaining patients' seizures will be uncontrolled.

109. Complex partial seizures have an aura and are then followed by impaired consciousness.

110. Complex partial seizures are typically caused by cerebral scar tissue or a focal lesion.

111. Complex partial seizures are more typically seen in males and are the most common in the first decade of life and then after age 60.

112. Absence seizures, also known as petit mal seizures, are inherited in an autosomal recessive fashion.

113. Absence seizures have an abrupt onset and offset.

114. Patients with absence seizures typically stare into space with automatism (e.g., lip smacking or finger movements).

115. Electroencephalogram readings in absence seizures show 3-per-second spike-and-wave activity (often precipitated by hyperventilation).

116. Febrile seizures typically occur from age 6 months to 5 years of age, have no organic cause, and are precipitated by a high fever.

117. Malignancies that metastasize to the brain are lung, breast, melanoma, renal cell, and colon.

118. Temporal arteritis should be suspected in any patient over the age of 50 with new-onset headaches.

119. Patients with temporal arteritis clinically present with headache (usually temporal), jaw pain/claudication, an elevated sedimentation rate (greater than 100), and polymyalgia rheumatica.

120. A classic migraine is described as a throbbing, unilateral/lateralized headache associated with nausea, vomiting, photophobia, and phonophobia.

121. Classic migraine sufferers have associated auras of flashes/scotoma (zig-zag lines) within the visual field.

122. Cluster headaches typically occur in middle-aged men and most often occur at night.

123. Cluster headaches typically last about 2 hours or less, and patients usually have associated symptoms of periorbital headache, ipsilateral nasal congestion, lacrimation, conjunctival injection, and Horner's syndrome.

124. Tension headaches are the most common type of headache, are typically bilateral, and there is no photophobia or vomiting.

125. The classic presentation of pseudotumor cerebri is headache, papilledema, and double vision due to sixth cranial nerve dysfunction in young obese females.

126. Patients with pseudotumor cerebri can suffer from blindness.

127. Pseudotumor cerebri is typically treated with acetazolamide. Serial LPs can be done if medications are not tolerated, in which case, cerebral shunting or optic nerve fenestration is possible.

128. Parkinson's disease is typically caused by a decrease of dopamine neurons in the basal ganglia.

129. The triad of Parkinson's disease is due to resting tremor, rigidity, and bradykinesia. The symptoms typically start asymmetrically.

130. Huntington's disease is inherited in an autosomal dominant fashion with a high penetrance and results in triple repeat disorder.

131. Echopraxia is imitating other people's movements.

132. Coprolalia is use of obscene language.

133. Echolalia is the repetition of other people's speech patterns.

134. Tic disorder often has comorbid conditions of obsessive-compulsive disorder and attention-deficit disorder.

135. Tic disorder has also led to depression and suicide mainly related to social embarrassment.

136. Hemiballismus is caused by damage to the contralateral subthalamic nucleus.

137. Hemiballism is sometimes treatable with dopamine antagonists.

138. Myasthenia gravis (MG) is an autoimmune disorder that results in muscle weakness resulting from blockade at the neuromuscular junction.

139. MG patients worsen with repetitive movements.

140. MG patients typically have antiacetylcholine antibodies.

141. MG can be diagnosed with the Tensilon test.

142. MG patients should have a CT scan of the chest looking for thymomas.

143. Lambert Eaton syndrome (LES) is also an autoimmune disorder usually associated with small cell lung cancer (paraneoplastic).

144. LES is associated with voltage-gated calcium channel antibodies.

145. LES patients on repetitive nerve stimulation have an incremental response, which is the opposite of MG.

146. Botulism results from a toxin produced by the gram-positive bacillus *Clostridium botulinum*.

147. Botulism initially causes oculobulbar paralysis and then progresses in a descending fashion.

148. Botulism toxin binds irreversibly to the presynaptic portion of the neuro-muscular junction leading to flaccid paralysis.

149. Dermatomyositis (DM) is an inflammatory myopathy associated with proximal muscle weakness, rash, and is often associated with a malignancy.

150. DM is associated with an elevated creatine kinase level.

151. DM patients have positive ANA and anti-Jo-1 antibodies and are also as-sociated with interstitial lung disease.

152. DM patients are treated with corticosteroids.

153. Myotonic dystrophy (MD) is inherited in an autosomal dominant fashion.

154. MD also demonstrates anticipation similar to Huntington's disease.

155. MD patients also have myotonia and often have cardiac arrhythmias.

156. MD patients clinically can be noted to have difficulty releasing a hand-grip after a handshake due to myotonia.

157. Benign positional vertigo occurs in adults over 50 years of age.

158. Central causes of vertigo typically do not respond to meclizine.

159. Labyrinthitis, Ménière's disease, and benign positional vertigo are typical peripheral causes for vertigo.

160. Craniopharyngiomas occur in childhood as well as in adulthood and rep-resent approximately 3% of all brain tumors.

161. Germ cell tumors are the most common type of pineal tumor.

162. Brain stem encephalitis is associated with testicular, ovarian, uterine, breast, and small cell lung cancers.

163. Pure sensory neuropathy associated with paraneoplastic syndrome usually shows anti-Hu positivity.

164. Decerebrate or decorticate posturing is incompatible with brain death.

165. A patient must be apneic for brain death criteria.

166. Wernicke-Korsakoff syndrome is a nutritional thiamine deficiency occurring in chronic alcoholics.

167. Treatment for Wernicke-Korsakoff syndrome is thiamine 100 mg per day.

168. Wernicke-Korsakoff syndrome is characterized by anterograde amnesia and patchy long-term memory loss.

169. Patients with Wernicke-Korsakoff syndrome are not worried about their amnesia.

170. Wernicke-Korsakoff syndrome demonstrates cell loss in the thalami, mamillary bodies, periaqueductal gray, and Purkinje cells in the cerebellum.

171. Transient global amnesia recurs about 25% of the time.

172. AIDS dementia complex has shown to respond to AZT treatment.

173. Carpal tunnel syndrome is the most common cause for a mononeuropathy.

174. Bell's palsy is the most common cranial neuropathy.

175. Parsonage-Turner syndrome is also known as idiopathic brachial neuritis (pain is a common feature).

176. Multifocal neuropathy is an immune-mediated motor neuropathy differentiated by the presence of conduction block on nerve conduction studies.

177. Spinal muscular atrophy resembles ALS but is limited to pure lower motor neuron and typically occurs in infancy or childhood.

178. ALS is also known as Lou Gehrig's disease and is the most common motor neuron disease.

179. Ulnar neuropathy is usually due to compression at the medial epicondyle of the humerus (cubital tunnel).

180. Median nerves can also be entrapped at the pronator teres.

181. Radial neuropathy usually occurs at the spiral groove of the humerus.

182. Obturator nerve damage can occur at the obturator foramen.

183. Lateral femoral cutaneous neuropathy is also known as meralgia paresthetica.

184. Posterior tibial neuropathy can occur at the tarsal tunnel.

185. Mononeuropathy multiplex (MM) is a disease that affects multiple peripheral nerves at different sites.

186. MM is sometimes associated with vasculitis, and polyarteritis nodosa is the most common vasculitis that leads to MM.

187. The classic polyneuropathy usually presents with gradual distal, symmetric sensorimotor deficits and hyporeflexia.

188. The most frequent cardiovascular manifestation of dysautonomia of GBS is sustained hypertension and tachycardia.

189. GBS prognosis is poor in advanced age, and patients exhibit very low distal motor amplitudes on nerve conduction studies (NCS), with rapidly progressive weakness occurring over the first week and respiratory failure requiring intubation.

190. In the CSF, GBS demonstrates a dissociation between albumin levels and cytologic findings with elevated protein levels and a normal white blood cell count.

191. GBS is typically treated with plasmapheresis. If the patient is treated within 10 days of symptom onset, the drug course can be shortened.

192. GBS can also be treated with IVIG, which has been shown to be equally effective.

193. Eighty percent of patients with recurrent vasovagal syncope respond to treatment with beta-blockers.

194. Neurologic causes for syncope are rare.

195. Subclavian steal syndrome is an unusual cause of vertebrobasilar insufficiency.

196. Shy-Drager syndrome (multisystem atrophy) is characterized by Parkinson's features and central autonomic failure.

197. Hyperventilation causing hypocapnia can cause syncope.

198. Trigeminal neuralgia caused by to the sensory division of the trigeminal nerve causing pain.

199. Paroxyms of trigeminal neuralgia usually last 1 to 2 minutes.

200. Triggers for trigeminal neuralgia are usually chewing, facial movements, or light touch.

201. Diagnosis of trigeminal neuralgia is based on history and observation (there are usually no objective clinical signs).

202. Postherpetic neuralgia is the persistence of pain after an infection with herpes zoster infection.

203. Shingles is thought to be due to reactivation of a latent infection of the virus in the sensory ganglion cells.

204. The lifetime incidence of shingles is 10% to 20%.

205. Thoracic dermatome is the most common sight for shingles.

206. Brachial neuritis is a rare syndrome that begins with pain localized to the C5 and C6 dermatomes.

207. Brachial neuritis is idiopathic and sporadic and affects men more than women (2:1).

208. The immediate treatment of increased ICP is to elevate the head 30 to 45 degrees and intubation with hyperventilation.

209. Cerebral perfusion pressure is measured by mean arterial blood pressure minus the ICP.

210. At high ICPs, the intracranial space becomes less compliant.

211. ICP waves are known as Lundberg waves. A waves or plateau waves are dangerous elevations of ICP.

212. Lundberg waves are associated with reduced cerebral perfusion pressure and cerebral blood flow with global hypoxic-ischemic injury.

213. Hepatic encephalopathy (HE) usually appears in a patient with liver function already compromised from alcoholic cirrhosis, chronic hepatitis, or malignancy.

214. HE is caused by an increased protein load, such as a gastrointestinal bleed, leading to elevated ammonia levels, which then accumulate in the brain.

215. It is unclear if the high level of ammonia itself or the increase in concentration of its metabolites produce the alterations in consciousness.

216. HE is treated by reducing the protein load with dietary reduction.

217. HE is also treated with neomycin, which reduces the population of ammonia-producing bacteria in the bowel.

218. HE can also be treated with lactulose to induce diarrhea, which may also reduce the intestinal bacteria.

219. Rapid correction of hyponatremia may lead to central pontine myelinolysis (CPM).

220. CPM is an acute demyelinating syndrome occurring mostly in patients with poor nutritional status. It leads to quadriplegia, dysarthria, and pseudobulbar palsy.

221. Symptomatic uremia with renal failure can cause delirium, asterixis, and may necessitate urgent hemodialysis.

222. Nicotine withdrawal delirium can occur in rare instances, and the nicotine patch may improve symptoms in some cases.

223. Diffuse axonal injury is thought to be the single most important cause of persistent disability in patients with traumatic brain damage.

224. Basilar skull fractures occur with more serious trauma and are frequently missed on routine skull x-ray films.

225. Basilar skull fractures may be associated with cranial nerve injury or CSF leakage from the nose or ear.

226. Three major threats to life are epidural hematomas, subdural hematoma, and increased ICP.

227. Concussion refers to the temporary loss of consciousness that occurs at the time of impact.

228. Concussion is usually associated with a short period of amnesia.

229. Concussion patients typically have normal CT or MRI scans.

230. Anton's syndrome is due to a lesion at the bilateral calcarine area.

231. Anton's syndrome results in a bilateral loss of vision in which the patient denies blindness.

232. Balint's syndrome is damage at the bilateral occipitoparietal junction.

233. Balint's syndrome results in simultanagnosia, optic ataxia, and ocular apraxia.

234. Bonnet's syndrome is due to damage either unilaterally or bilaterally at the calcarine fissure.

235. Bonnet's syndrome leads to "Lilliputian" visual hallucinations in the absence of delirium.

236. Dyschromatopsia results from damage at the lingual gyrus.

237. Dyschromatopsia is abnormal color perception contralateral to the lesion.

238. Palinopsia is due to incomplete injury or recovery in the calcarine cortex.

239. Palinopsia is visual persistence of afterimages.

240. Prosopagnosia is the inability to recognize faces due to a lesion in the right lingual gyrus.

241. Transient ischemic attacks are clinically important due to the high incidence of subsequent strokes.

242. The most important etiology for TIA is high-grade carotid stenosis.

243. Patients with Devic's disease have acute bilateral optic neuritis and transverse myelitis.

244. Devic's disease is more common in Asia and India.

245. Patients with acute disseminated encephalomyelitis have a high mortality rate and significant persistent neurologic deficits.

246. Acute necrotizing hemorrhagic encephalomyelitis is the most fulminant demyelinative disease.

247. When central pontine myelinosis affects the basal ganglia, it is referred to as extrapontine myelinolysis.

248. Sarcoidosis is a generalized disease characterized by a granulomatous reaction to an unknown stimulus involving any organ.

249. The cause of sarcoidosis remains unknown and affects the nervous system in a minority of patients.

250. Behçet's disease is an inflammatory disorder of unknown etiology characterized by relapsing iritis and uveitis.

SECTION

II

Psychiatry

Anxiety Disorders

QUESTIONS

1. A 54-year-old male presents for a consultation due to sudden onset of seizures. On examination, the patient is noted to be slightly delirious and is not able to give a coherent history. Collateral information reveals that he was taking diazepam up to 30 mg every day to "calm his nerves." He bought these pills from someone off the street and has not been able to obtain any pills for the past 2 days. His wife mentions that he has been irritable and agitated over the past 12 hours and then had a sudden onset of "seizures" after which she called 911. Cessation of benzodiazepines after chronic use may cause all of the following except:

   A. depersonalization and derealization
   B. perceptual disturbances
   C. anxiety
   D. constipation
   E. rhinorrhea

2. A 24-year-old salesperson is referred for an evaluation because of difficulty dealing with customers because she gets "so nervous and anxious that my mind goes blank." A careful evaluation reveals that she has social phobia. She is motivated to obtain treatment and continue doing her job. All of the following are effective interventions except:

   A. selective serotonin reuptake inhibitors (SSRIs)
   B. flooding
   C. modeling
   D. systematic desensitization
   E. electroconvulsive therapy (ECT)

3. Phobia is an anxiety disorder that can be severe and debilitating. All of the following features are noted in phobias except:

    A. higher incidence of major depressive disorder
    B. patients usually come from stable families
    C. patients tend to have anxious and/or dependent traits
    D. in general, phobias are more common in women
    E. phobias are usually triggered by major life events

4. Anxiety disorders are more common in women compared to men. However, not all phobias (which is an anxiety disorder) are more common in women. All of the following have a higher incidence in women compared to men except:

    A. needle phobia
    B. social phobia
    C. animal phobia
    D. hospital phobia
    E. claustrophobia

5. Numerous theories have been put forward to explain the pathogenesis of phobias. All of the following theories explain phobias to some extent except:

    A. concept of "preparedness"
    B. classical conditioning
    C. neurodevelopmental theory
    D. operant conditioning
    E. observational learning

6. Anxiety is a normal emotional response, and a degree of anxiety is necessary for survival. Pathological anxiety is distinguished from a normal emotional response by all of the following characteristic features except:

    A. autonomy
    B. physical health status
    C. intensity
    D. duration
    E. behavior

7. Which of the following structures is the main source of the brain's adrenergic innervations?
   A. Nucleus raphe
   B. Locus ceruleus
   C. Nucleus of Meynert
   D. Midbrain
   E. Medial temporal lobe

8. According to the Epidemiologic Catchment Area (ECA) study, which of the following is the most common anxiety disorder in the United States?
   A. Panic disorder
   B. Simple phobia
   C. Agoraphobia
   D. Social phobia
   E. Generalized anxiety disorder

9. A 65-year-old male experiences a panic attack for the first time in his life. He had a stroke recently and has other cardiac problems including angina and atrial fibrillation. The treating physician makes a diagnosis of organic anxiety syndrome. All of the following are the features of organic anxiety syndrome except:
   A. onset of symptoms after 35 years of age
   B. family history of anxiety disorders
   C. no history of childhood anxiety disorders
   D. poor response to the usual treatments of panic disorder
   E. no avoidance behavior

10. According to the National Ambulatory Medical Survey, all of the following are true regarding anxiety disorders in primary care settings except:
    A. high rates of anxiety symptoms in patients with chest pain, dyspnea, and dizziness
    B. presenting problem in 11% of patients visiting primary care physicians
    C. a common psychiatric disorder in primary care physicians' office
    D. a majority of these patients have serious medical problems
    E. high utilizers of primary care physicians' time and resources

11. According to the *Diagnostic and Statistical Manual of Mental Disorders*, 4th edition (DSM-IV), patients with generalized anxiety disorder (GAD) have excessive anxiety and worry on more days than not for a period of at least:
    A. 2 weeks
    B. 2 months
    C. 6 weeks
    D. 6 months
    E. 4 weeks

12. All of the following are true about specific phobias except:
    A. If the patient is under 18 years of age, the phobia should last for longer than 6 months.
    B. Natural environment phobias (heights, water) have an onset in childhood.
    C. Situational phobias (elevators, airplanes) have an onset in the mid-50s.
    D. Lifetime prevalence varies between 10% to 11%.
    E. Cognitive behavior therapy (CBT) and other psychological interventions are found to be effective.

13. According to the DSM-IV, all of the following are true regarding posttraumatic stress disorder (PTSD) except:
    A. symptoms should last for more than 1 month
    B. there are four subtypes: acute, subacute, chronic, and delayed onset
    C. the individual is exposed to a traumatic event
    D. the response to the traumatic event involves intense fear, horror, or helplessness
    E. acute stress disorder is a different diagnosis

14. According to the DSM-IV, the diagnostic criteria for acute stress disorder emphasize a group of symptoms that are not included in the criteria for PTSD. These include:
    A. dissociative symptoms
    B. psychotic symptoms
    C. neurotic symptoms
    D. depressive symptoms
    E. cognitive symptoms

15. A 28-year-old female was diagnosed to have PTSD after she was assaulted and raped 6 months ago. Over the next 2 years, despite extensive therapy and pharmacological treatment, the response was suboptimal. She was later diagnosed to have major depressive disorder and substance abuse problems. Which of the following is the most common comorbid condition in women with PTSD?

    A. Substance abuse
    B. Depression
    C. Obsessive compulsive disorder
    D. Psychotic disorders
    E. Eating disorders

16. According to the DSM IV, chronic PTSD cannot be diagnosed unless the patient has PTSD symptoms for a period of at least:

    A. 6 months
    B. 1 year
    C. 2 years
    D. 3 months
    E. 1 month

17. Which of the following medications have been found to be effective in the treatment of PTSD symptoms?

    A. SSRIs
    B. Mood stabilizers
    C. Beta-blockers
    D. Antipsychotics
    E. Benzodiazepines
    F. All of the above

18. Psychological interventions are considered to be equally, if not more important than pharmacological interventions in the treatment of PTSD. All of the following psychological interventions have been found to be effective in the treatment of PTSD except:

    A. supportive psychotherapy
    B. psychoanalytic psychotherapy
    C. cognitive behavioral therapy
    D. group therapy
    E. eye movement desensitization and reprocessing therapy

19. According to the DSM-IV, all of the following are included in the diagnostic criteria for somatization disorder except:

    A. four pain symptoms
    B. two gastrointestinal symptoms other than pain
    C. one sexual symptom
    D. one pseudoneurologic symptom
    E. symptoms beginning after the age of 30 years

20. A 35-year-old woman is seen by a neurologist for impaired coordination. However, a detailed neurologic examination reveals nothing abnormal. A careful history reveals that starting at the age of 18, she has been having multiple physical symptoms including pain symptoms, gastrointestinal symptoms, and irregular menstruation. Despite extensive tests, however, nothing abnormal was detected. All of the following are more likely suggestive of a somatization disorder except:

    A. family history of histrionic personality
    B. early onset of symptoms
    C. chronic course
    D. multiorgan system involvement
    E. absence of laboratory, radiologic, and physical abnormalities

21. Which of the following is the most common somatoform disorder?

    A. Conversion disorder
    B. Somatization disorder
    C. Pain disorder
    D. Hypochondriasis
    E. Body dysmorphic disorder

22. All of the following are recognized subtypes of conversion disorder except:

    A. gastrointestinal problems
    B. motor symptoms or deficit
    C. sensory symptoms or deficit
    D. seizures or convulsions
    E. mixed presentation

23. All of the following are characteristic features of conversion disorder except:

    A. patients are usually suggestible
    B. symptoms appear or exacerbated following severe stress
    C. patients believe that they have serious underlying illness
    D. symptoms are not feigned
    E. usually occurs between the age of 10 to 35 years

24. A 34-year-old female is admitted to the neurology in-patient unit for further assessment and management of "episodes of shaking of whole body followed by drooling of saliva and eyes rolling upward." An extensive workup including an admission to an epilepsy monitoring unit at an outside hospital did not find anything abnormal. There is no family history of seizure disorder, but one of her neighbors was diagnosed with seizure disorder recently. Collateral information reveals that the patient is under a lot of stress because of a recent divorce and problems at her workplace. The psychiatry consult team believes the patient has conversion disorder. All of the following are true about conversion disorders except:

    A. usual age of onset is between 10 to 35 years.
    B. the symptoms tend to conform to the patient's own idea of illness
    C. paralysis, aphonia, and blindness are associated with bad prognosis
    D. remission is usually noticed within 2 weeks after hospitalization
    E. recurrence rate is as high as 20% to 25% within the first year

25. According to the DSM-IV, to make a diagnosis of hypochondriasis, the symptoms should last for at least:

    A. 2 weeks
    B. 2 months
    C. 6 weeks
    D. 6 months
    E. 1 month

26. All of the following are true about hypochondriasis except:

    A. more common in women
    B. onset in early adulthood
    C. course is chronic with waxing and waning of symptoms
    D. the belief of having a serious illness is not of delusional intensity
    E. the symptoms can involve more than one organ system

27. Factitious disorder with predominant physical signs and symptoms is also known as:

   A. hypochondriasis
   B. Münchhausen syndrome
   C. Münchhausen syndrome by proxy
   D. somatoform disorder
   E. Factitious disorder not otherwise specified

28. According to the DSM-IV, all of the following are required to diagnose factitious disorder except:

   A. intentional production or feigning of physical or psychological signs or symptoms
   B. motivation for the behavior is to assume the sick role
   C. external incentives for the behavior are absent
   D. medical tests are negative

29. A 30-year-old male is seen in the ED for acute abdominal pain, nausea, vomiting, and diarrhea. He mentions that he has not been able to "keep anything down for the past 4 days." On examination, however, he is not dehydrated, and his vital signs are normal. On examination of the abdomen, the patient complains of tenderness and screams at deep palpation. Review of old medical records indicates that he has been seen in the ED at least four times in the past 3 months for similar symptoms. The ED physician strongly suspects factitious disorder. All of the following are true about factitious disorders except:

   A. a desire to assume a sick role
   B. no external incentives for the behavior
   C. good prognosis, once the condition is diagnosed
   D. intentional production of signs and symptoms
   E. exact prevalence is unknown

30. The average number of personality states in dissociative identity disorder is:

   A. 3
   B. 13
   C. 30
   D. 33
   E. 10

31. The relationship between mitral valve prolapse (MVP) and panic disorder can be best described as:

    A. important to recognize and treat MVP in panic disorder
    B. high clinical relevance
    C. patients with panic disorder are predisposed to develop MVP
    D. higher incidence of MVP in patients with panic disorder
    E. panic disorder is very well controlled if MVP is corrected

32. A 46-year-old male is admitted to a general medical unit for unexplained recurrent episodes of hypoglycemia. The primary team requests a psychiatry consultation because the patient's story "just does not add up." The patient is not too happy to see someone from the psychiatry department, but he was more than willing to talk to many doctors from other specialties. He reluctantly agrees to see a psychiatrist and tells him how sick he is and appears quite familiar with medical terminology. He appears to have above average intelligence with strong dependency traits. The nurse interrupts the psychiatrist and tells him that she found insulin-filled syringes underneath the patient's bed. The patient is very upset and decides to leave the hospital. The most likely diagnosis in this patient is:

    A. somatization disorder
    B. hypochondriasis
    C. factitious disorder
    D. malingering
    E. Münchhausen syndrome by proxy

33. A 34-year-old male is brought to the emergency department (ED) by police for "found wandering in the road and not knowing his name or address." The ED requests both neurology and psychiatry consultations because of the patient's "bizarre presentation." The patient is neither able to recall his personal information nor is he able to explain if he even lives in that city. The social worker somehow manages to obtain collateral information. She states that he is from a nearby town, and according to the family members, he was "normal" until a severe earthquake hit the town recently; there is no history of any substance abuse, and family members are concerned. What is the most likely diagnosis?

    A. Dissociative amnesia
    B. Dissociative fugue
    C. Transient global amnesia
    D. Malingering
    E. Dissociative identity disorder

34. All of the following are true about depersonalization disorder except:
    A. more common in women than men
    B. onset is usually in late adolescence or early adulthood
    C. may last from days to weeks
    D. reality testing is impaired
    E. up to 50% of people have transient depersonalization symptoms at some point

35. Anxiety disorders are common and patients present with different clusters of symptoms. The DSM IV-Text Revision (TR) lists how many anxiety disorders?
    A. 10
    B. 12
    C. 6
    D. 4
    E. 13

36. Social stressors can be precipitating or perpetuating factors in the pathogenesis of many anxiety disorders. In panic disorders, however, this is not necessarily the case. What is the only social factor that has been identified as contributing to the development of panic disorder?
    A. Recent history of death in the family
    B. Recent history of separation or divorce
    C. Lack of friends
    D. Unsupportive family
    E. Recent history of witnessing a panic attack

37. SSRIs are considered first-line treatment in PTSD. However, several different classes of medicines are also used in the treatment of PTSD. All of the following medications are considered to be useful in the treatment of PTSD except:
    A. anticonvulsants
    B. monoamine oxidase inhibitors (MAOIs)
    C. melatonin
    D. propranolol
    E. antipsychotics

38. Genetic influence is considered to be important in various anxiety disorders. Which of the following phobias show a strong familial tendency?
    A. Blood-injection-injury
    B. Animal
    C. Heights/elevators
    D. Spiders/insects
    E. Social

39. Which of the following is true about blood-injection-injury phobia?
    A. Twice as common in women than men
    B. Low familial inheritance
    C. Severe tachycardia and hypertensive response
    D. Easily treated
    E. Bradycardia and hypotension often follow the initial tachycardia

40. A 42-year-old male with severe, debilitating obsessive-compulsive disorder (OCD) has tried all options for OCD but none of them were helpful. He has seen several psychiatrists who found the patient to be resistant to pharmacotherapy, psychotherapy, and ECT. Psychosurgery was considered to be the next step. What is the most common psychosurgical procedure for OCD?
    A. Cingulotomy
    B. Subcaudate tractotomy
    C. Caudate nucleus ablation
    D. Internal capsule stimulation
    E. Frontal tractotomy

41. A 56-year-old male is seen by a neurologist for "severe tension headaches." The neurologist finds the patient to be anxious and holding his muscles taut. The patient further mentions that he was involved in a car accident and was trapped in his car for several hours before he was rescued. This happened 5 months ago, and since then, he has not been able to drive because he is "scared" and has nightmares about the accident. He also complains of difficulty in sleeping, inability to concentrate at work, and feels nervous and on edge all the time and cannot relax his muscles. He avoids watching movies or television shows that involve automobile accidents. What is this patient's most likely diagnosis?
    A. Acute PTSD
    B. Acute stress disorder
    C. Chronic PTSD
    D. Major depressive disorder
    E. Panic disorder

42. All of the following are true about phobias in children except:
    A. phobias are a persistent and compulsive dread of and preoccupation with the feared object or situation
    B. the DSM-IV classifies phobias as anxiety disorders
    C. the number of fears typically peaks at age 11 years
    D. parental education is an important aspect in the management of childhood phobias
    E. situational types of phobias have an onset in the fourth decade of life

43. All of the following are true about the psychological profile of patients with factitious disorder except:
    A. problems with self-identity
    B. dependence traits
    C. self-importance
    D. no formal thought disorder
    E. high frustration tolerance

44. Which of the following helps in distinguishing malingering and factitious disorders?
    A. Age of onset
    B. Secondary gain
    C. Deliberate production of symptoms
    D. Course of illness
    E. Response to confrontation

45. The condition brainwashing included in the DSM-IV under the category of "dissociative disorders, not otherwise specified" is characterized by all of the following except:
    A. occurs mostly in the setting of political reforms
    B. often seen in people subjected to prolonged and intense coercive persuasion
    C. confrontation of the brainwashed subject is found to be helpful in treatment
    D. coercive techniques include isolation and induction of fear
    E. validation is an important tool in the treatment

46. Body dysmorphic disorder is associated with all of the following defense mechanisms except:

   A. denial
   B. repression
   C. distortion
   D. symbolization
   E. dissociation

47. Factitious disorder is associated with all of the following defense mechanisms except:

   A. repression
   B. identification
   C. sublimation
   D. symbolization
   E. regression

48. Brain imaging studies have shown certain abnormalities in anxiety disorders. One of the consistent abnormalities found in patients with posttraumatic stress disorder (PTSD) is with the:

   A. hippocampus
   B. frontal lobe
   C. occipital lobe
   D. brain stem
   E. parietal lobe

49. Cynophobia refers to:

   A. fear of cats
   B. fear of dogs
   C. fear of spiders
   D. fear of caffeine
   E. fear of enclosed places

50. Kinetophobia refers to:

   A. fear of kites
   B. fear of standing
   C. fear of falling
   D. fear of movement
   E. fear of running

51. A 30-year-old female with GAD and panic disorder complains of palpitations and "hearing" her own heartbeats all the time. Cardiac studies in subjects with anxiety disorders have shown all of the following abnormalities except:
    A. decreased deceleration after stress
    B. high beat-to-beat fluctuation
    C. higher baseline heart rate
    D. higher subjective awareness of heartbeats
    E. increased deceleration after stress

52. The following neurotransmitter abnormalities are detected in anxiety disorders except:
    A. increased platelet MAO activity
    B. increased activity of central noradrenaline
    C. increased central gamma-aminobutyric acid (GABA) activity
    D. increased circulating adrenaline
    E. increased circulating noradrenaline

53. In patients with anxiety spectrum disorders, all of the following abnormalities have been found except:
    A. decreased skin conductance
    B. panic response to sodium lactate infusion
    C. increased cutaneous blood flow
    D. decreased splanchnic blood flow
    E. decreased habituation following electrodermal stimulation

54. Several studies have shown an association between MVP and panic disorder. All of the following are true about MVP and panic disorder except:
    A. the incidence of MVP in the general population is 5% to 20%
    B. the incidence of MVP in patients with panic disorder is up to 40% to 50%
    C. MVP causes panic attacks
    D. MVP and panic may represent a part of primary autonomic syndrome

55. A 22-year-old anxious female is referred to a psychologist by her neurologist for specific phobia. The patient would like to know if there are any factors that would result in less than ideal response in her case. All of the following are predictors of a good response except:

A. good relaxation response
B. free-floating anxiety
C. good motivation
D. no secondary gain from the phobia
E. willing to practice relaxation

56. A 46-year-old woman is frustrated and angry with her neurologist because he recommended a psychiatry evaluation for what she describes as "medical problems." She complains of dizziness, nausea, palpitations, abdominal pain, and sweating, but no one is able to give her the right treatment. She was seen by an ear specialist, a cardiologist, and a gastroenterologist, but nothing abnormal was detected. She was hoping that a neurologist would find a cause for her symptoms. She also states that these symptoms occur in episodes without any precipitating factors, last for 20 to 30 minutes, and she feels as if she is "about to die." The most probable diagnosis in this woman is:

A. GAD
B. major depressive disorder
C. MVP
D. panic disorder
E. Ménière's disease

57. A 56-year-old anxious executive calls 911 at 5:00 AM because he woke up with chest tightness and shortness of breath. He was scared that he was having a heart attack, and he also reported feeling dizzy, trembling, and his heart was pounding. He thought he was going to die. The symptoms subsided in 20 minutes, however, and by the time the emergency medical services arrived, he was sitting in his living room and in no distress. The patient's electrocardiogram reading was normal, and his cardiac enzymes were also found to be normal. What is the most likely diagnosis?

A. Nocturnal panic attack
B. PTSD
C. Psychophysiological insomnia
D. Somatization disorder
E. Myocardial infarction

58. Of all the different phobias, specific phobias are the most common phobias. All of the following are false about specific phobias except:
    A. more common in men
    B. more common in women
    C. phobic avoidance is uncommon
    D. onset in adult life
    E. treatment is usually not effective

59. Buspirone is an effective drug used to treat anxiety disorders. What is its main mechanism of action?
    A. 5HT-1A antagonist
    B. 5HT-2C antagonist
    C. 5HT-1A agonist
    D. Norepinephrine reuptake inhibition
    E. MAOI

60. The term *rupophobia* refers to:
    A. fear of being raped
    B. fear of reptiles
    C. fear of dirt
    D. fear of falling
    E. fear of traveling

ANSWERS

1. **Answer: E.** Benzodiazepine withdrawal symptoms can be serious and sometimes fatal. They last for many days. Apart from anxiety, delirium, depersonalization, and derealization, the withdrawal symptoms can also result in seizures. Both constipation and diarrhea are recognized features of benzodiazepine withdrawal. Rhinorrhea is a feature of opiate withdrawal.

2. **Answer: E.** ECT is most commonly indicated for severe depression not responding to medications. Social phobia is an anxiety disorder that responds well to psychological interventions. Flooding, modeling, systematic desensitization, and relaxation techniques have all been found to be effective. The pharmacological treatments that have been found to be effective include SSRIs and MAOIs.

3. **Answer: A.** The incidence of major depressive disorder is no more common in phobia patients than in the general population. There is also a known association between phobias and childhood enuresis. Subjects with phobia have anxious/dependent traits, and they usually come from stable families.

4. **Answer: B.** Although all anxiety spectrum disorders are more common in women, social phobia is equally common in men and women, and in some studies, it was found to be more common in men than in women.

5. **Answer: C.** The theories of classical conditioning, operant conditioning, observational learning, and the concept of "preparedness" try to explain the pathogenesis of phobias. Neurodevelopmental theory was proposed to explain the etiology of schizophrenia.

6. **Answer: B.** Certain characteristic features distinguish pathological anxiety from normal emotional response. Pathological anxiety is autonomous (i.e., it may or may not have a trigger). The intensity and duration of anxiety are out of proportion to the real or imagined stressor, and behavior is impaired. Physical health status is not a criterion used to distinguish normal fear from pathological anxiety.

7. **Answer: B.** The locus ceruleus is a small retropontine structure and is the main source of the brain's adrenergic innervations. In experimental studies, stimulation of the nucleus ceruleus caused severe anxiety and panic attacks, and the blockade of locus ceruleus efferents decreased anxiety and panic attacks. The raphe nucleus is the main source of serotonin.

8. **Answer: D.** The ECA study collected data on the prevalence and incidence of mental disorders and on the use of and need for services by the mentally ill. In this study, social phobia is the most common anxiety disorder with a lifetime prevalence of 13.3%. This is closely followed by simple phobia at 11.3%.

9. **Answer: B.** Patients with organic anxiety syndrome usually do not have a family history of anxiety disorders. All of the other features above are commonly seen in patients with organic anxiety disorder. One other feature, which helps to distinguish organic anxiety syndrome from primary panic disorder, is the absence of triggering factors for the anxiety syndrome.

10. **Answer: D.** The National Ambulatory Medical Care Survey is a national probability sample survey conducted by the National Center for Health Statistics, which annually collects information on the use of ambulatory medical services provided by office-based physicians in the United States. Anxiety disorders are very common in primary care settings. A majority of these patients do not have any serious medical problems.

11. **Answer: D.** According to the DSM-IV, patients with GAD have symptoms of excessive worry and anxiety on most days for at least 6 months. They find it hard to control worrying and must have three out of the following six symptoms to make a diagnosis of GAD: muscle tension, restlessness, easy fatigability, difficulty concentrating, irritability, and insomnia.

12. **Answer: C.** Situational phobia typically has a bimodal onset with one peak in childhood and the other in mid-20s. All of the specific phobias are more common in women, and evidence suggests aggregation within families by the type of phobia. In situational phobias, the phobic situation is avoided or else is endured with intense anxiety or distress.

13. **Answer: B.** There are three subtypes of PTSD based on duration criteria: (1) acute: symptoms last for less than 3 months; (2) chronic: symptoms last for more than 3 months; and (3) delayed onset: symptoms appear more than 6 months after the traumatic event. In acute stress disorder, symptoms occur within 4 weeks of the traumatic event and last for a minimum of 2 days but resolve within 4 weeks.

14. **Answer: A.** According to the DSM-IV, the diagnostic criteria for acute stress disorder emphasize dissociative symptoms such as depersonalization, derealization, and dissociative amnesia, while experiencing or after experiencing the distressing event. This set of symptoms is not included in the diagnostic criteria for PTSD. In acute stress disorder, symptoms occur within 4 weeks of the traumatic event and last for a minimum of 2 days but resolve within 4 weeks.

15. **Answer: B.** PTSD is associated with significant comorbidities. The most common comorbid condition in women is depression (49%), and the most common comorbid condition in men is substance abuse (52%).

16. **Answer: D.** There are three subtypes of PTSD based on duration criteria: (1) acute: symptoms last for less than 3 months; (2) chronic: symptoms last for more than 3 months; and (3) delayed onset: symptoms appear more than 6 months after the traumatic event. In acute stress disorder, symptoms occur within 4 weeks of the traumatic event and last for a minimum of 2 days but resolve within 4 weeks.

17. **Answer: F.** Various medications have been tried to treat different groups of symptoms in patients with PTSD, and all of the above have some utility. SSRIs, however, are found to be most effective, and these are often used as first-line treatments. Other medicines that have been tried in PTSD include clonidine, anticonvulsants, and MAOIs.

18. **Answer: B.** Psychological interventions are an essential component in the treatment of PTSD. Most of the evidence is for cognitive behavioral therapy. However, group therapy is being increasingly utilized at the present time.

19. **Answer: E.** According to the DSM-IV, for the diagnosis of somatization disorder, the onset of symptoms should be before the age of 30 years. The multiple, recurring, physical symptoms usually start in adolescence, and the diagnostic criteria are usually met by 25 years of age. The multiple symptoms can occur at any time during the course of the illness, resulting in treatment-seeking behavior and significant impairment in functioning.

20. **Answer: A.** Patients with somatization disorders often have a family history of somatization disorder. In fact, 10% to 20% of first-degree female relatives of female patients with somatization disorder develop somatization disorder. The male relatives of women with somatization disorder show an increased risk of antisocial personality disorder and substance-related disorders.

21. **Answer: C.** Pain disorder is relatively more common. The prevalence of conversion disorder varies widely from 11 to 300 out of 100,000. The prevalence of hypochondriasis in general medical practice is reported to be between 4% to 9%.

22. **Answer: A.** One of the diagnostic features of conversion disorder is the presence of one or more symptoms or deficits affecting voluntary motor or sensory function that suggest a neurological or general medical condition. The DSM-IV has four subtypes, and they are listed above.

23. **Answer: C.** Patients with conversion disorder are more focused on the presenting symptom, and there may be *la belle indifference*. In contrast, patients with hypochondriasis are preoccupied with having serious underlying illness.

24. **Answer: C.** Paralysis, aphonia, and blindness are associated with good prognosis, whereas tremors and seizures are associated with a bad prognosis. Onset of conversion disorder is rare after 35 years. The likelihood of occult neurological or general medical condition is high in someone who develops conversion disorder for the first time in middle or old age.

25. **Answer: D.** For hypochondriasis, the symptoms should last for at least 6 months, and the symptoms cannot be accounted for by another mental disorder.

26. **Answer: A.** The incidence of hypochondriasis is equal in both men and women. The prevalence of hypochondriasis in general medical practice is reported to be between 4% and 9%.

27. **Answer: B.** Factitious disorder has three subtypes: (1) with predominantly psychological signs and symptoms; (2) with predominantly physical signs and symptoms; and (3) with combined psychological and physical signs and symptoms. Factitious disorder with predominant physical signs and symptoms is more commonly known as Münchhausen syndrome. Here, the patient's goal is get admitted or stay in the hospital. This is usually a more severe form and accounts for 10% of individuals with factitious disorder. In factitious disorder, the signs and symptoms are feigned, whereas in hypochondriasis, they exaggerate a real and usually minor health problem.

28. **Answer: D.** The DSM-IV does not mention anything about medical tests in these patients. In conversion disorders, the medical tests are negative. In factitious disorder, however, sometimes, the subjects go to great lengths to feign the disease, and certain test results such as in hematuria can be "positive."

29. **Answer: C.** The prognosis in factitious disorder is poor, as patients have little insight and go from one hospital to another; the goal for the behavior is to assume a sick role. External incentives for the behavior such as economic gain are typically absent. In the absence of a thorough knowledge of the patient's history, physicians are sometimes reluctant to diagnose factitious disorder. The prevalence of factitious disorder is not known.

30. **Answer: B.** The average number of personality states in dissociative identity disorder is 13; however, they vary from one to 50.

31. **Answer: D.** Historically there was a lot of debate and interest associated with MVP and panic disorder. The incidence of MVP in the general population is 5% to 20% and is as high as 40% to 50% in subjects with panic disorder. Despite a high association between panic disorder and MVP, there is no evidence to prove MVP causes or predisposes patients to have panic attacks.

32. **Answer: C.** This patient has most of the features of factitious disorder such as intentional production of signs and symptoms as well as assuming a sick role and no obvious secondary gain (at least from the information available). There are also other supporting features such as dependency traits and leaving the hospital as soon as deception is discovered.

33. **Answer: B.** The most likely diagnosis in this patient is dissociative fugue. It is commonly seen after natural disasters and is seen in men in their second to fourth decades of life. Dissociative fugue is associated with travel to distant places with the inability to recall one's past.

    In dissociative amnesia, there is no history of travel away from one's home. In dissociative identity disorder, there are two or more distinct personalities, and finally, malingering is unlikely given this patient's history.

34. **Answer: D.** Reality testing is intact in depersonalization disorders, which is an important distinction from other psychotic disorders. Although depersonalization disorder is more common in women, transient depersonalization symptoms are equally common in both men and women.

35. **Answer: B.** The DSM IV-TR lists 12 different types of anxiety disorders: (1) panic disorder with agoraphobia; (2) panic disorder without agoraphobia; (3) agoraphobia without history of panic disorder; (4) specific phobia; (5) social phobia; (6) OCD; (7) posttraumatic stress disorder; (8) acute stress disorder; (9) GAD; (10) anxiety disorder caused by a general medical condition; (11) substance-induced anxiety disorder; and (12) Anxiety disorder, NOS.

36. **Answer: B.** Apart from a recent history of separation or divorce, no other social factor is identified as a contributory factor for the development of panic disorder. Panic disorder is two to three times more common in women and occurs equally among all races.

37. **Answer: C.** Several different classes of medicines are used in the treatment of PTSD. Antidepressants, anticonvulsants, antipsychotics, and beta-blockers are used for the treatment of various symptoms. There is no evidence, however, to show that melatonin is effective in PTSD.

38. **Answer: A.** The blood-injection-injury phobia has a particularly high familial tendency, and studies have shown that at least two thirds to three fourths of the affected probands have at least one first-degree relative with specific phobia of the same type.

39. **Answer: E.** Blood-injection-injury phobia is unique from other phobic disorders in that bradycardia and hypotension follow initial tachycardia. This condition is almost equally common in both men and women and has a high familial inheritance. It is also one of the most difficult conditions to treat.

40. **Answer: A.** Cingulotomy is the most common psychosurgical procedure performed for treatment-resistant OCD. It is found to be effective in 25% to 30% of otherwise treatment- resistant OCD. The most common complication of this procedure is seizures.

41. **Answer: C.** The patient has most of the signs and symptoms suggestive of PTSD including a history of life-threatening trauma, re-experiencing, avoidance, etc. Acute and chronic PTSD are differentiated by duration criteria of 3 months. In acute stress disorder, the symptoms last for less than 4 weeks. Major depressive disorder and panic disorder are not the right choices, as the patient does not meet the criteria.

42. **Answer: E.** The DSM-IV describes phobias as anxiety disorders and lists three different types of phobias: specific phobia (formerly called *simple phobia*), social phobia, and agoraphobia. The number of fears typically peak at 11 years of age, and the onset of situational phobias (e.g., airplanes, enclosed spaces) have a bimodal onset (one peaks in childhood and the other in mid-20s).

43. **Answer: E.** Factitious disorders are conditions in which a person acts as if he or she has an illness by deliberately producing, feigning, or exaggerating symptoms. Patients with factitious disorder have low frustration tolerance, normal or above-average intelligence, dependency traits, sense of self-importance, and no formal thought disorder.

44. **Answer: B.** In malingering, there is an obvious, recognizable secondary gain that is expected in response to signs and symptoms. Both conditions are characterized by signs and symptoms that are produced intentionally. The goal in patients with factitious disorder is to assume a sick role, and there is no obvious secondary gain as in malingering. Confrontation is not helpful most of the time in both factitious disorders and malingering.

45. **Answer: C.** Validation of traumatic experience and cognitive reframing of the traumatic experiences will help in the treatment of this condition.

46. **Answer: A.** Denial is not one of the defense mechanisms used in subjects with body dysmorphic disorder. According to the psychodynamic theory, body dysmorphic disorder results from the displacement of a sexual or emotional conflict onto a nonrelated body part.

47. **Answer: C.** Sublimation is a mature defense mechanism in which unacceptable aggressive ideas/wishes are rechanneled into another form, which are accepted and appreciated by society. This is not one of the defense mechanism used in factitious disorders.

48. **Answer: A.** The brain imaging studies in PTSD have consistently shown abnormal hippocampus. Studies in acute PTSDs show a hyperactive hippocampus, and in chronic PTSD, the hippocampus is found to be hypoactive and shrunken in size.

49. **Answer: B.** Cynophobia refers to fear of dogs, ailurophobia is fear of cats, arachnophobia is fear of spiders, and claustrophobia is fear of enclosed places.

50. **Answer: D.** Kinetophobia refers to fear of movement or action.

51. **Answer: E.** Patients with anxiety disorders have a higher baseline heart rate and continue to have higher rates after stress. Therefore, they have decreased deceleration and not increased deceleration after stress.

52. **Answer: C.** Patients with anxiety disorders have increased levels of activating neurotransmitters such as adrenaline and noradrenaline and decreased levels of GABA.

53. **Answer: A.** Patients with anxiety spectrum disorders have numerous electrodermal abnormalities including increased cutaneous blood flow, increased skin conductance, and decreased habituation.

54. **Answer: C.** Despite a high association between panic disorder and MVP, there is no evidence to prove MVP causes or predisposes patients to have panic attacks.

55. **Answer: B.** Psychological treatments have been found to be very effective in the treatment of anxiety spectrum disorders. However, the presence of free-floating anxiety is a predictor of a poor response, as it does not allow the patient to relax or divert attention from the phobic stimulus.

56. **Answer: D.** Panic attacks are characterized by the sudden onset of intense apprehension, fear, or terror and by the abrupt development of specific somatic, cognitive, and affective symptoms. The symptoms this patient is reporting are all features of a panic attack.

57. **Answer: A.** The symptoms are typical of panic attacks. The acute onset of intense symptoms and quick resolution are characteristic of panic attacks. There is no evidence in the patient's history to suggest that he was having a nightmare or underwent trauma to suggest PTSD. He does not meet the criteria for somatization disorder or psychophysiological insomnia. Myocardial infarction was ruled out by appropriate medical tests in this patient.

58. **Answer: B.** Specific phobias are the most common phobias. These are more common in women than in men. By definition, avoidance should be present to meet the diagnostic criteria for phobia. Psychological treatments including systematic desensitization, exposure, and response prevention have been found to be effective treatments.

59. **Answer: C.** Buspirone, an effective antianxiety agent, exerts its effect by 5HT-1A agonist effect.

60. **Answer: C.** The term *rupophobia* refers to the fear of dirt, and it is often seen in individuals with OCD.

Mood Disorders

QUESTIONS

1. A 76-year-old male patient is admitted to an acute psychiatric unit for severe suicidal ideation. He admits to feeling hopeless and refuses to contract for safety. He has a history of noncompliance with treatment and is refusing to take any medicines. He has severe psychomotor retardation and stops eating and drinking. A reasonable choice of treatment in this patient would be:

    A. persuade the patient to take antidepressants
    B. wait and watch for the patient to change his mind
    C. consider feeding against his will
    D. electroconvulsive treatment (ECT)
    E. intensive psychotherapy

2. A 22-year-old female is self-referred for an evaluation to rule out bipolar disorder. She complains of rapid mood swings with uncontrollable anger and irritability. During the assessment, it is noted that she has not had any sustained relationships for many years and feels empty. She fears abandonment by her friends and blames others for making her feel angry. What is the most important differential diagnosis in this patient?

    A. Major depressive disorder
    B. Borderline personality disorder
    C. Histrionic personality
    D. Depressive personality
    E. Generalized anxiety disorder

3. A 56-year-old female is admitted to an acute psychiatric inpatient unit for severe depression. The patient was ruminating about suicide and guilt feelings that were distressing her. She is "convinced" that she has committed sin and deserved to be punished, although there was nothing in her history to justify this. The resident doctor thinks that the patient is obsessed with thoughts of guilt and feels that the patient has a primary obsessional disorder. A trial of antidepressant medication was not helpful despite trying a high dose. The attending physician explains that patient is not obsessional but severely depressed because:
   A. she has suicidal ideation
   B. she has indeed committed sin and is now depressed
   C. she is distressed by the guilt feelings and is "convinced" of the sin
   D. the attending physician thinks so
   E. antidepressants alone were not effective

4. A 62-year-old female with seasonal affective disorder prefers "nonmedical" treatment for depression. She tried cognitive behavioral therapy with limited success. She likes the idea of bright light therapy and is willing to spend 30 to 40 minutes every morning in front of the light therapy unit. For light therapy to be effective, the intensity of the light should ideally be:
   A. 1,000 lux
   B. 10,000 lux
   C. 100,000 lux
   D. 500 lux
   E. 5,000 lux

5. All of the following support the norepinephrine deficiency hypothesis for depression except:
   A. decreased norepinephrine-mediated release of growth hormone in response to clonidine
   B. decreased cyclic adenosine monophosphate (cAMP) turnover in platelets following stimulation with clonidine
   C. increased platelet alpha 2-adrenergic receptor binding
   D. increased beta-adrenergic receptors in depression and subjects who committed suicide
   E. decreased levels of cAMP in cerebrospinal fluid (CSF)

6. Several biomarkers were investigated for depression, but none of them had a high specificity. One of the consistent findings in depression, however, is abnormally elevated cortisol levels. This is thought to be secondary to:
   A. primary hypersecretion of cortisol
   B. primary hypersecretion of adrenocorticotropic hormone (ACTH)
   C. primary hypersecretion of corticotrophin-releasing factor (CRF) by the hypothalamus
   D. higher incidence of diabetes in depression
   E. higher incidence of adrenal tumors in depression

7. A 56-year-old male with a history of chronic recurrent depression is bothered by a recent news article that mentions increased mortality in patients with depression because of increased incidence of a variety of health problems and infections. He would like to know if this is true. According to the psychoimmunology theory, the higher incidence of infections and other chronic conditions is because:
   A. patients with depression do not take care of themselves
   B. patients with depression do not receive adequate care because they have mental illness
   C. antibiotics are not as effective in depressed patients compared to others without depression
   D. hypothalamic-pituitary-adrenal (HPA) dysfunction causes immune suppression
   E. increased T-cell replication

8. Research in subjects with depression has revealed several immunological abnormalities that are in turn responsible for increased morbidity and mortality. All of the following findings are true except:
   A. decreased natural killer cells
   B. decreased interleukin-2
   C. decreased absolute neutrophil count
   D. decreased T-cell replication
   E. increased monocyte activity

9. A 63-year-old male with major depressive disorder complains of difficulty falling asleep and early morning awakenings. He is otherwise healthy and does not have any physical health problems. He is referred for a sleep study. The sleep architecture in this patient is likely to show all of the following except:
   A. decrease in sleep efficiency (total duration of sleep/total duration of time in bed multiplied by 100 or the percentage of time in bed spent asleep)
   B. increase in the total duration of rapid eye movement (REM) sleep
   C. decrease in the latency to the onset of REM sleep
   D. increased latency to the onset of REM sleep
   E. impaired sleep continuity

10. Brain imaging studies in depression have revealed some interesting facts that have enhanced our understanding of the pathophysiology of depression. All of the following were found in brain imaging studies in subjects with depression except:
    A. decreased volume of parietal lobes
    B. decreased volume of frontotemporal lobes
    C. decreased caudate size
    D. increased ventricular size
    E. decreased blood flow in the dorsolateral prefrontal cortex

11. One of the criteria for the diagnosis of major depressive disorder is weight loss that is unintentional. The criteria for weight loss specify that:
    A. loss of any amount of weight is significant
    B. loss of 5% or more of the body weight in the past 1 month
    C. loss of 10% or more of body weight in the past 1 month
    D. loss of 10% of body weight in the past 2 weeks
    E. loss of 5% of the body weight in the past 2 weeks

12. The manifestation of depression symptoms are slightly different in different age groups and also in men and women. *Agitated depression* is a term more commonly used to describe depression in which group of patients?
    A. Young children
    B. Adolescents
    C. Adults
    D. Women
    E. Elderly

13. A 32-year-old female presents with low mood and lack of interests. After careful history and extensive collateral information, the treating psychiatrist makes a diagnosis of atypical depression. All of the following are the features of atypical depression except:

  A. intense, unstable emotions
  B. increased appetite
  C. increased sleep
  D. mood reactivity
  E. rejection sensitivity
  F. leaden paralysis

14. The term *double depression* is used to describe:

  A. major depressive disorder superimposed on grief reaction
  B. major depressive disorder superimposed on dysthymia
  C. major depressive disorder; patient not responding to treatment
  D. major depressive disorder with psychosis
  E. major depressive disorder with anxiety

15. A 36-year-old Caucasian male is stable on lithium for bipolar disorder for the past 4 years. During his routine visit with his family physician, he complains of fatigue and lack of motivation. He is also feeling very cold during this winter and has gained weight. He wonders if he is getting depressed again. What is the next most appropriate step to take in this case?

  A. Diagnose depression, and start the patient on antidepressants.
  B. Obtain the patient's lithium levels.
  C. Check the patient's thyroid-stimulating hormone (TSH) levels.
  D. Discontinue lithium.
  E. Consider ECT.

16. All of the following are true regarding suicide risk except:

  A. high in single men living alone
  B. high in alcohol abuse/dependence
  C. low in patients with schizophrenia
  D. high in mixed anxiety-depressive disorder
  E. high in subjects with hopelessness

17. Seasonal affective disorder is characterized by all of the following except:
    A. depression in winter months
    B. hypomania or even mania can occur in summer months
    C. associated with hypersomnia
    D. associated with anorexia
    E. response to bright light therapy in some patients

18. Mania can be associated with all of the following features except:
    A. sometimes associated with depression symptoms
    B. can be triggered by antidepressants
    C. irritability is a recognized symptom
    D. is always followed by depression
    E. can occur during bereavement

19. A 46-year-old female who is 6 weeks postpartum complains of feeling low in her mood and having crying spells, lack of motivation, and feelings of hopelessness for the past 4 weeks. She is diagnosed to have postpartum depression. Which of the following is true about postpartum depression?
    A. Risk of infanticide is minimal.
    B. Selective serotonin reuptake inhibitors (SSRIs) are contraindicated.
    C. Risk of depression during subsequent pregnancies is increased.
    D. Suicide risk is low.
    E. Hospital admission is rarely required.

20. All of the following are features of bipolar affective disorder except:
    A. has a genetic basis
    B. associated with increased risk of suicide
    C. women tend to have more manic episodes than depression episodes
    D. more common in men than in women
    E. equally common in all social classes

21. All of the following drugs are associated with depression except:
    A. levetiracetam
    B. propranolol
    C. fenfluramine
    D. corticosteroids
    E. isoniazid

22. All of the following are true about depression in the elderly except:
    A. may present as dementia
    B. more common in the early stages of dementia
    C. can present as agitation
    D. does not respond to SSRIs
    E. can be associated with cerebrovascular disease

23. All of the following are suggestive of depressive pseudodementia rather than dementia except:
    A. anhedonia
    B. nihilistic delusions.
    C. disorientation to time
    D. lack of appetite
    E. worthlessness

24. All of the following psychotropic medications are likely to cause sedation except:
    A. haloperidol
    B. mirtazapine
    C. quetiapine
    D. venlafaxine
    E. olanzapine

25. Which of the following conditions are associated with a higher risk of depression?
    A. Hypothyroidism
    B. Alzheimer's disease
    C. Parkinson's disease
    D. Stroke
    E. All of the above

26. All of the following are true about depression except:
    A. more common in women than in men
    B. higher incidence in first-degree relatives of patients with bipolar disorder
    C. more common in prepubertal girls compared with prepubertal boys
    D. bright light therapy is effective in some patients with seasonal affective disorder
    E. ECT is a considered a safe and effective treatment

27. All of the following are true regarding major depressive disorder, severe with psychosis except:
    A. high risk of suicide
    B. responds well to ECT
    C. can present with paranoia
    D. nihilistic delusions are often present
    E. antipsychotics are not effective

28. All of the following are features of lithium toxicity except:
    A. fine tremors
    B. disorientation
    C. diarrhea
    D. vomiting
    E. drowsiness

29. All of the following are used as augmenting agents in the treatment of depression except:
    A. thyroxine
    B. propranolol
    C. pindolol
    D. lithium
    E. bright light therapy

30. Which of the following SSRIs is least likely to cause serotonin discontinuation syndrome?
    A. Paroxetine
    B. Citalopram
    C. Escitalopram
    D. Fluoxetine
    E. Sertraline

31. Of all the tricyclic antidepressants, which of the following has the most potent serotonin reuptake inhibition activity?
    A. Clomipramine
    B. Imipramine
    C. Amitriptyline
    D. Nortriptyline
    E. Desipramine

32. In the diagnosis of major depressive disorder, one of the criteria is weight loss. According to the *Diagnostic and Statistical Manual of Mental Disorders*, 4th edition (DSM-IV), what is considered as weight loss?

    A. Loss of at least 10 lbs.
    B. Loss of at least 5 lbs.
    C. Loss of at least 10% of body weight in the past 1 month
    D. Loss of at least 5% of body weight in the past 1 month
    E. Loss of at least 5% of body weight in the past 2 weeks

33. Which of the following symptoms has to be present to diagnose major depressive disorder?

    A. Depressed mood or loss of interest/pleasure
    B. Lack of energy or motivation
    C. Lack of appetite
    D. Hopelessness
    E. Guilt or worthlessness

34. What is the relapse rate for major depressive disorder after two episodes?

    A. 50%
    B. 50% to 70%
    C. 70% to 90%
    D. 100%
    E. 30%

35. A 22-year-old female with major depressive disorder refuses to take any antidepressant medications because she is not interested in any "mind-altering medicines." She is willing to try St. John's wort, however, because it is a "natural herbal supplement." All of the following are true about St. John's wort except:

    A. can cause serotonin syndrome
    B. found to be effective in moderate-to-severe depression
    C. effective in mild depression
    D. can lower the levels of oral contraceptive pills
    E. possible mechanism of action is by inhibiting the serotonin reuptake

ANSWERS

1. **Answer: D.** This elderly male has major depressive disorder, severe with suicidal ideation. Although antidepressants are helpful, it will take a few weeks before response is noted. Severe depression and suicidal ideation needs immediate treatment. To obtain response quickly, ECT is a reasonable option in this patient.

2. **Answer: B.** Borderline personality disorder is characterized by pervasive instability in moods, interpersonal relationships, self-image, and behavior. This instability often disrupts family and work life, long-term planning, and the individual's sense of self-identity. It affects about 2% of adults, mostly young women. There is a high rate of self-injury without suicide intent, as well as a significant rate of suicide attempts and completed suicide in severe cases.

3. **Answer: C.** This patient is "convinced" that she has committed sin and has guilt feelings about it, despite no evidence to the contrary. This is suggestive of a delusion probably secondary to depression. In obsessional disorder, the patients are not delusional, and however bizarre the obsessions and compulsions are, they have insight into their condition. In patients who are depressed and delusional like this, a low-dose antipsychotic is often necessary.

4. **Answer: B.** Although lower light intensity has also been found to be effective in some studies, 10,000 lux was found to be most effective.

5. **Answer: E.** There is no evidence for deficiency of cAMP in CSF in subjects with depression. The rest of the facts support the norepinephrine deficiency hypothesis for depression.

6. **Answer: C.** Primary hypersecretion of CRF by the hypothalamus results in increased secretion of ACTH. This in turn leads to elevated cortisol levels. There is no evidence to suggest a primary hypersecretion of either ACTH or cortisol. Results of the dexamethasone suppression test are positive in 50% of depressed patients because of increased cortisol levels. There is no evidence for a higher incidence of adrenal tumors in depression.

7. **Answer: D.** HPA axis dysfunction leads to increased cortisol levels, which is thought to be responsible for various immune system abnormalities noticed in depression. There is no evidence to show that patients with depression are any less motivated in taking care of themselves when compared to patients with other chronic illness.

8. **Answer: C.** Absolute neutrophil count is found to be in the normal range in depressed patients. All the other abnormalities mentioned are thought to be secondary to abnormal HPA axis.

9. **Answer: D.** There is a decrease in the latency to the onset of REM sleep, an increase in the total duration of REM sleep, and an increase in REM density (number of rapid eye movements per epoch of REM sleep). Sleep continuity is disrupted, resulting in decreased sleep efficiency.

10. **Answer: A.** All of these findings are noted in brain-imaging studies of subjects with depression, except that no consistent abnormalities have been found in parietal lobes.

11. **Answer: B.** The weight loss criteria for depression specifies that it should be 5% or more of the total body weight in the past 1 month.

12. **Answer: E.** The manifestations of depression symptoms are slightly different in different age groups and also in men and women. Irritability is sometimes the predominant symptom in adolescents, whereas agitation is a common symptom in the elderly.

13. **Answer: A.** Intense, unstable emotions are more characteristic of borderline personality disorder than atypical depression. Atypical features are two to three times more common in women and individuals report earlier age of onset of depressive episodes. Episodes of atypical features are more common in patients with bipolar I disorder, bipolar II disorder, and in major depressive disorder, recurrent, occurring in a seasonal pattern.

14. **Answer: B.** Double depression refers to major depressive disorder superimposed on dysthymia.

15. **Answer: C.** Before patients are placed on lithium, they should have their TSH levels tested and then re-tested at regular intervals thereafter, as lithium can cause hypothyroidism. The possibility of recurrence of depression should also be considered, but cold intolerance is more likely secondary to hypothyroidism, and it is not a typical symptom of depression.

16. **Answer: C.** Suicide risk is relatively higher if a person has comorbid physical or mental illness, has poor social support, feels hopeless, is jobless, or has alcohol/substance abuse problems.

17. **Answer: D.** Seasonal affective disorder is characterized by depression mainly in winter months and euthymia in summer months. However, hypomania and even mania in summer months has been reported. It is associated with hyperphagia and hypersomnia. Response to bright light therapy is noted in a significant number of patients.

18. **Answer: D.** Mania is not always followed by depression. To diagnose bipolar, type I, an episode of mania is all that is required. In mania with mixed features, symptoms of both depression and mania are present.

19. **Answer: C.** Postpartum depression is a medical and psychiatric emergency, especially if it is associated with suicide/infanticide ideation. Admission to a psychiatric unit and if necessary, an involuntary admission is warranted if the patient is at risk of suicide/homicide/neglect or deterioration of mental health.

20. **Answer: C.** Bipolar affective disorder has a strong genetic component and is equally common among both men and women and across all social classes. In bipolar disorder, women tend to have more depressive episodes, and men are more likely to have more hypomanic or manic episodes.

21. **Answer: E.** Isoniazid, an antituberculosis medication is found to have a mild antidepressant effect. Fenfluramine, a monoamine-depleting agent is associated with depression. Levetiracetam, an antiepileptic drug is associated with increased risk of depression.

22. **Answer: D.** Depression in the elderly can sometimes present as dementia (pseudo-dementia). SSRIs have been found to be safe and effective in the treatment of depression in the elderly.

23. **Answer: C.** Depressive pseudodementia is sometimes very difficult to differentiate from true dementia. Anhedonia (lack of any feelings), lack of appetite, and worthlessness are more common in depression as are nihilistic delusions (delusions of negation).

24. **Answer: D.** Venlafaxine, a selective serotonin and norepinephrine reuptake inhibitor is activating rather than sedating. The other drugs listed all have sedating properties.

25. **Answer: E.** All of the conditions listed are associated with increased risk of depression.

26. **Answer: C.** Prior to puberty and after menopause, depression is found to be equally common in males and females. From puberty to menopause, the prevalence of depression is twice as common in women than in men. Relatives of patients with unipolar depression are at a higher risk of depression, whereas relatives of patients with bipolar disorder are at a higher risk of both depression and mania.

27. **Answer: E.** In major depressive disorder, severe with psychosis, antipsychotics are often administered along with antidepressants. Psychosis in the form of delusions, hallucinations, and paranoia is common, and ECT is often very effective in these patients.

28. **Answer: A.** Lithium toxicity is characterized by coarse tremors and not fine tremors. Lithium has a narrow therapeutic index, and toxicity can be life-threatening. Hemodialysis to remove the circulating lithium from blood is an effective treatment.

29. **Answer: B.** Propranolol, a beta-blocker is associated with increased risk of depression. Pindolol, by its central 5HT-1A receptor antagonistic properties enhances the postsynaptic serotonin concentration and therefore helps with depression.

30. **Answer: D.** Of all the SSRIs, fluoxetine has a relatively long half-life and is least likely to cause discontinuation syndrome. The half-life of fluoxetine is 2 to 4 days, and its active metabolite, norfluoxetine has a half-life of up to 2 weeks.

31. **Answer: A.** Of all the tricyclic antidepressants, clomipramine has the most potent serotonin reuptake inhibition activity.

32. **Answer: D.** According to the DSM-IV criteria for the diagnosis of major depressive disorder, weight loss is considered to be present if the individual loses at least 5% of his or her body weight in the past 1 month.

33. **Answer: B.** According to the DSM-IV, to diagnose major depressive disorder, the subject must have at least five of the nine symptoms of depression over a 2-week period. At least one of the symptoms should be either depressed mood or loss of interest or pleasure.

34. **Answer: C.** The rate of relapse with major depression disorder is very high. The relapse rate following one episode of depression is about 50%, and after two episodes, the relapse rate is about 70% to 90%.

35. **Answer: B.** St. John's wort is used as an antidepressant in many European countries (mainly Germany) and the United States. Although the exact mechanism of action is not known, it is thought to inhibit the reuptake of serotonin. Therefore, before prescribing an SSRI, it is important to know if the patient is taking St. John's wort, to prevent the occurrence of serotonin syndrome. St. John's wort also interacts with different drugs and can lower the levels of oral contraceptive pills, thereby increasing the risk of pregnancy.

Psychosis

QUESTIONS

1. What is the most common form of thought disorder in patients with schizophrenia?

   A. Loose associations
   B. Circumstantiality
   C. Tangentiality
   D. Flight of ideas
   E. Prolixity

2. A 46-year-old male with treatment-resistant schizophrenia is started on clozapine after unsuccessful trials of two other atypical antipsychotics and one typical antipsychotic. He shows signs of response but unfortunately develops seizures when be begins taking a higher dose. What is the incidence of seizures in patients taking clozapine at a dose greater than 600 mg per day?

   A. 1%
   B. 10%
   C. 5%
   D. 15%
   E. 25%

3. All of the following drugs can cause psychotic symptoms similar to schizophrenia except:

   A. ecstasy
   B. opiates
   C. phencyclidine
   D. ketamine
   E. lysergic acid diethylamide (LSD)

4. All of the following are considered to be risk factors for neuroleptic-induced tardive dyskinesia except:
   A. male gender
   B. brain injury
   C. mood disorder
   D. old age
   E. long duration of treatment

5. All of the following are characteristic features of a delusion except:
   A. firmly held belief
   B. consistent with an individual's cultural context
   C. no basis in reality
   D. believed by the subject despite evidence to the contrary
   E. all of the above

6. Bleuler's four A's of schizophrenia include all of the following except:
   A. loosening of associations
   B. inappropriate affect
   C. altruism
   D. autism
   E. ambivalence

7. Which of the following illicit drugs can lead to a full range of symptoms similar to that seen in patients with schizophrenia?
   A. Ecstasy
   B. Alcohol
   C. Marijuana
   D. Phencyclidine
   E. Opiates

8. The first rank-symptoms of schizophrenia were described by:
   A. Schneider
   B. Bleuler
   C. Kraepelin
   D. Freud
   E. Jung

9. According to the *Diagnostic and Statistical Manual of Mental Disorders*, 4th edition (DSM-IV), the duration criteria to make a diagnosis of schizophrenia is:
   A. 1 month
   B. 6 months
   C. 2 months
   D. 2 weeks
   E. 6 weeks

10. The prevalence of schizophrenia is:
    A. 10%
    B. 1%
    C. 5%
    D. 0.1%
    E. 2%

11. All of the following are true about schizophrenia except:
    A. stressful life events appear to trigger schizophrenia at an earlier age in vulnerable individuals
    B. equally prevalent in both men and women
    C. females have an earlier age of onset compared to males
    D. in the northern hemisphere, schizophrenic patients are more likely to have been born between January and April
    E. substance abuse is common in patients with schizophrenia

12. A 32-year-old male with chronic paranoid schizophrenia, in full remission is married and living a productive life. He and his wife decide to have children, but would like to know the probability of his children developing schizophrenia. Which of the following statements is correct?
    A. The risk is similar to that of general population (1%).
    B. The risk is about 50%.
    C. The risk is much lower than the general population because he will be able to recognize the early signs of schizophrenia and seek prompt treatment for his child.
    D. The risk is about 10%.
    E. The risk is about 100%.

13. All of the following support the theory of dopamine hyperactivity in schizophrenia except:
    A. dopamine receptor antagonists are effective antipsychotic agents
    B. dopamine-releasing agents such as cocaine produce psychosis
    C. atypical antipsychotics such as quetiapine act at serotonin receptors and decrease psychotic symptoms
    D. all of the above
    E. none of the above

14. Which of the following theories has been proposed to explain the etiology of schizophrenia?
    A. Viral infection during pregnancy
    B. Serotonin dysfunction
    C. Dopamine hyperactivity
    D. Diathesis and stress model
    E. All of the above

15. All of the following are considered as negative symptoms of schizophrenia except:
    A. alogia
    B. apathy
    C. affect flattening
    D. paranoia
    E. anhedonia

16. All of the following features predict a good prognosis in patients with schizophrenia except:
    A. acute onset
    B. later age of onset
    C. negative symptoms
    D. female gender
    E. good social support

17. The suicide rate of patients with schizophrenia is:
    A. 10%
    B. 20%
    C. the same as the general population (11/100,000)
    D. 50%
    E. 5%

18. Which of the following is true about expressed emotions (EE) in schizophrenia?
    A. High EE is associated with bad prognosis.
    B. Family therapy is useful.
    C. Criticism, hostility, and overinvolvement are considered to be high EE.
    D. All of the above
    E. None of the above

19. A 24-year-old male is admitted to a psychiatry in-patient unit for social isolation, lack of emotions, and alogia. The resident doctor considers a diagnosis of schizophrenia because of these negative symptoms. However, he also realizes that he has to consider other causes of negative symptoms in this patient before attributing all of those symptoms to schizophrenia. All of the following should be considered in the differential diagnosis of negative symptoms of schizophrenia except:
    A. depression
    B. side effects of typical antipsychotics
    C. drug abuse
    D. generalized anxiety disorder (GAD)
    E. hypothyroidism

20. According to the DSM-IV, all of the following are recognized subtypes of schizophrenia except:
    A. paranoid type
    B. disorganized type
    C. delusional type
    D. catatonic type
    E. undifferentiated type

21. According to the DSM-IV, all of the following are recognized subtypes of delusional disorder except:
    A. persecutory type
    B. somatic type
    C. jealous type
    D. grandiose type
    E. disorganized type

22. According to the DSM-IV, the duration criteria for brief psychotic disorder is:
    A. at least 1 day but less than 1 month
    B. at least 1 week but less than 1 month
    C. at least 6 months
    D. minimum of 2 months
    E. minimum of 6 hours

23. Which of the following subtypes of schizophrenia has the worst prognosis?
    A. Paranoid type
    B. Disorganized type
    C. Catatonic type
    D. All of the above

24. Which of the following abnormalities are often seen in patients with schizophrenia?
    A. Decreased neuronal density
    B. Decreased brain volume
    C. Increased sizes of lateral and third ventricles
    D. Decreased size of temporal lobe
    E. All of the above

25. All of the following psychological interventions have been found to be helpful in patients with schizophrenia except:
    A. psychodynamic psychotherapy
    B. family therapy
    C. supportive psychotherapy
    D. group therapy
    E. cognitive behavioral therapy

26. A 56-year-old chronic schizophrenic patient who is on haloperidol for more than 30 years would like to know more about "atypical" antipsychotics. He mentions that one of his friends at the group home was recently prescribed this medication, and his psychiatrist told the other patient that these "new" medicines are better than haloperidol. Which of the following statements about atypical antipsychotics is true?
    A. They have antagonistic properties at both dopamine and serotonin receptors.
    B. They are also known as second-generation antipsychotics.
    C. There is a decreased incidence of extrapyramidal side effects.
    D. There is a decreased elevation of prolactin levels.
    E. All of the above

27. All of the following are atypical antipsychotics except:
    A. aripiprazole
    B. risperidone
    C. ziprasidone
    D. fluphenazine
    E. quetiapine

28. One of the common side effects associated with antipsychotics, both typical and atypical, is weight gain. Of all the typical antipsychotics, which of the following is considered as "weight-neutral"?
    A. molindone
    B. perphenazine
    C. haloperidol
    D. chlorpromazine
    E. pimozide

29. A 48-year-old chronic schizophrenic male is admitted to the in-patient unit again for relapse. He is known to be noncompliant with medicines necessitating the fourth admission in the past 6 months. He is homeless again, and all efforts to find assisted living failed because he just walks out of these facilities and prefers to stay on the streets. Which of the following interventions are reasonable in a patient like this?
    A. Consider depot antipsychotics.
    B. Consider referral to Assertive Community Treatment (ACT) program.
    C. Consider compliance therapy.
    D. All of the above
    E. None of the above

30. A 46-year-old male is stable on low-dose haloperidol for chronic schizophrenia. Recently, he was diagnosed to have comorbid depression and was started on fluoxetine 20 mg. He calls the physician with complaints of stiffness in his arms and legs. What is the possible cause for this symptom?
    A. Malingering: the patient would like to stop taking antidepressant medicine.
    B. Increased levels of haloperidol because of fluoxetine
    C. Fluoxetine is causing extrapyramidal side effects.
    D. Decreased levels of haloperidol are causing extrapyramidal side effects.
    E. Increased levels of fluoxetine because of haloperidol

ANSWERS

1. **Answer: A.** Loose associations are the most common form of thought disorder seen in patients with schizophrenia. It is present in about 45% of patients with schizophrenia.

2. **Answer: C.** The incidence of seizures in patients taking more than 600 mg per day of clozapine is around 5%. Therefore, some psychiatrists tend to start seizure prophylaxis in patients who need at least 600 mg or more of clozapine every day.

3. **Answer: B.** Ecstasy, phencyclidine, ketamine and LSD can all cause psychotic symptoms similar to schizophrenia. Opiates are rarely associated with any psychotic symptoms.

4. **Answer: A.** Female gender is associated with a higher incidence of neuroleptic-induced tardive dyskinesia, not male gender. All the other risk factors mentioned increase the risk of neuroleptic-induced tardive dyskinesia.

5. **Answer: B.** Delusion is a fixed, firmly held belief that has no basis in reality and persists despite evidence to the contrary. It is out of character of a person's social or cultural background.

6. **Answer: C.** Bleuler made great contributions to the understanding of schizophrenia. He believed that schizophrenia has four fundamental symptoms including loosening of associations, inappropriate affect, autism, and ambivalence.

7. **Answer: D.** Although many illicit drugs including ecstasy, LSD, and ketamine can cause symptoms similar to schizophrenia, only phencyclidine is associated with the full range of symptoms as seen in patients with schizophrenia.

8. **Answer: A.** Schneider described the first-rank symptoms of schizophrenia. The 11 symptoms describing different types of hallucinations (including passivity symptoms) were thought to be important in the diagnosis of schizophrenia. We now know that these symptoms are not always present in schizophrenia, however, and that they can be present in other conditions such as mania.

9. **Answer: B.** According to the DSM-IV, to diagnose schizophrenia, the total duration of illness (including prodromal or residual phases) should last at least 6 months.

10. **Answer: B.** The prevalence of schizophrenia worldwide is about 1%.

11. **Answer: C.** Males tend to have earlier onset of illness compared to females (18 to 25 years vs 26 to 45 years). Also, males tend to be more symptomatic and have a poorer prognosis compared to females, in general.

12. **Answer: D.** The risk of schizophrenia for a child of a schizophrenic patient is 10%. Genetic contribution is considered to play a role based on various genetic studies in schizophrenia. Monozygotic twins have a higher rate of schizophrenia (45% to 50%) compared to dizygotic twins (10% to 15%).

13. **Answer: C.** One of the proposed theories of the etiology of schizophrenia is dopamine hyperactivity. The facts that dopamine antagonists are used to treat psychosis and dopamine agonists are associated with psychosis support this theory. However, the atypical antipsychotics have minimal action at dopamine receptors and mainly act at serotonin receptors. This suggests possible serotonin dysfunction in schizophrenia rather than just dopamine hyperactivity.

14. **Answer: E.** Various theories have been proposed to explain the etiology of schizophrenia including dopamine hyperactivity, serotonin dysfunction, viral infection during pregnancy (influenza), diathesis, stress model (environmental stressor in individuals with genetic vulnerability), and N-methyl-D-aspartic acid receptor antagonism (phencyclidine, ketamine).

15. **Answer: D.** Negative symptoms of schizophrenia indicate a poor prognosis and are often resistant to treatment. These symptoms include alogia, apathy, flattening of affect, anhedonia, and asociality. Paranoia is a positive symptom of schizophrenia.

16. **Answer: C.** Studies have shown that some features in schizophrenia are associated with a better prognosis, including later age of onset, female gender, positive symptoms, early diagnosis and treatment of index episode, good response to medications during the first episode, good social support, presence of affective symptoms, good premorbid function, married, and patients living in developing countries.

17. **Answer: A.** The suicide rate in patients with schizophrenia is 10%, which is much higher than the general population.

18. **Answer: D.** Criticism, hostility, and overinvolvement are considered high EE in schizophrenia. These are associated with poor prognosis, and family therapy has been found to be helpful in these situations.

19. **Answer: D.** It is necessary to make sure there are no other causes (especially treatable causes) for negative symptoms. Some of the important conditions to consider are comorbid depression, drug abuse, akinesia, or Parkinsonism symptoms induced by neuroleptics, hypothyroidism, or head injury. GAD is characterized by fidgeting, inability to control worrying, difficulty with relaxation, sleep disturbances, and sweating.

20. **Answer: C.** According to the DSM-IV, there are five different subtypes of schizophrenia: paranoid type, disorganized type, catatonic type, undifferentiated type, and residual type.

21. **Answer: E.** Delusional disorder has various subtypes including erotomanic type, grandiose type, jealous type, persecutory type, somatic type, mixed type, and unspecified type. Disorganized type is a subtype of schizophrenia.

22. **Answer: A.** According to the DSM-IV, the duration criteria specifies that one of the four symptoms (delusions, hallucinations, disorganized speech, disorganized behavior) should last for at least 1 day but less than 1 month, with eventual full return to premorbid function.

23. **Answer: B.** The disorganized type of schizophrenia is associated with the worst prognosis. This type of schizophrenia has a continuous course with no significant remissions.

24. **Answer: E.** Schizophrenia is associated with various biologic abnormalities. The importance of these abnormalities is not entirely known, but these findings support the neurodegenerative theory of schizophrenia.

25. **Answer: A.** Psychological interventions have been found to be effective in patients with schizophrenia. There is no evidence to show that psychodynamic psychotherapy is helpful in schizophrenia, however.

26. **Answer: E.** Atypical antipsychotics, also known as second-generation antipsychotics have predominantly 5-HT_2 receptor antagonistic properties. They are associated with a lower incidence of extrapyramidal side effects and hyperprolactinemia. They are thought be effective against negative symptoms of schizophrenia as well, but the evidence for this is not strong.

27. **Answer: D.** The six atypical antipsychotics approved by the Food and Drug Administration (FDA) are clozapine, risperidone, olanzapine, quetiapine, aripiprazole, and ziprasidone. Of all these agents, risperidone resembles typical antipsychotics more than the others.

28. **Answer: A.** Of all the typical antipsychotics, molindone is least likely to cause weight gain and of all the typical antipsychotics, ziprasidone is associated with the least weight gain.

29. **Answer: D.** A proportion of patients with chronic mental illness require more intensive support. Depot medications administered by the case manager or visiting nurse is one way of making sure the patient is medication compliant. The ACT program was specifically designed to take care of patients who require a lot of assistance. Compliance therapy aims to enhance compliance with treatment by educating the patient and understanding the reasons for non-compliance.

30. **Answer: B.** Fluoxetine inhibits CYP 450 2D6 enzymes, thereby increasing the levels of haloperidol, which in turn results in extrapyramidal side effects.

Substance Abuse

QUESTIONS

1. A young couple that recently adopted a child finds out that the child's father was an alcoholic. Although they do not know everything about the child's family, they are concerned about the risk for the child to become an alcoholic. All of the following are known to increase the risk for alcoholism except:

   A. biological relative with alcohol problems
   B. history of posttraumatic stress disorder (PTSD)
   C. male gender
   D. adoptive parents with alcohol problems
   E. history of benzodiazepine abuse

2. Alcohol withdrawal symptoms can result in serious medical complications, which can be life threatening. All of the following are recognized medical complications of alcohol withdrawal except:

   A. seizures
   B. coma
   C. hypertension
   D. hypomagnesemia
   E. hyperglycemia

3. Motivational interview is often used to determine the patient's motivation to change in the treatment of substance abuse/dependence disorders. All of the following are stages in the theory of change except:

   A. action
   B. maintenance
   C. contemplation
   D. precontemplation
   E. reaction

4. All of the following are associated with opiate withdrawal except:
   A. rhinorrhea
   B. lacrimation
   C. yawning
   D. flashbacks
   E. sweating

5. All of the following are features of hallucinogen perceptions persisting disorder (HPPD) except:
   A. it is recognized by the *Diagnostic and Statistical Manual of Mental Disorders*, 4th edition (DSM-IV)
   B. characterized by persisting perception disturbances
   C. mainly visual perceptions are affected
   D. can persist for years after hallucinogen abuse is stopped
   E. risperidone is found to be effective

6. What is the characteristic feature of chronic marijuana abuse?
   A. Amotivational syndrome
   B. Seizures
   C. Wernicke's encephalopathy
   D. HPPD
   E. Stroke

7. A 32-year-old male is brought to the emergency department (ED) by the emergency medical service (EMS) after they received a call about this young man who was found lying unresponsive at a bus stop. The patient is found to have pinpoint pupils, and the ED resident notices needle stick marks on the left forearm, leg, and on both femoral vein areas in the groin. He suspects opiate intoxication. All of the following are features of opiate intoxication except:
   A. constipation
   B. miosis
   C. tachycardia
   D. pruritis
   E. anorexia

8. A 24-year-old male is brought to the ED by the EMS after his friends call 911 following his complaints of chest pain. The patient describes a "crushing chest pain" around the left side of the chest and denies ever having had similar pain. He also denies any drugs use but soon admits to using amphetamines. All of the following are features of amphetamine abuse except:

   A. miosis
   B. seizures
   C. delirium
   D. myocardial ischemia
   E. stroke

9. A 24-year-old male is found to be delirious walking on the street and screaming. When police approach him, he becomes extremely violent. He is restrained and brought to the hospital where he is sedated with a combination of haloperidol and lorazepam. A sample of urine is obtained by catheterization, and analysis shows phencyclidine (PCP) and marijuana. All of the following are seen in PCP intoxication except:

   A. paranoia
   B. unpredictable intermittent violence
   C. decreased pain threshold
   D. hyperacusis
   E. agitation

10. All of the following are true about PCP except:

   A. do not try to talk the patient down unless PCP is cleared
   B. dose-dependent effects are noted
   C. acts as an N-methyl-D-aspartic acid (NMDA) receptor agonist
   D. detected in blood/urine for up to 1 week
   E. agitation is common

11. All of the following can be seen in patients with chronic alcohol abuse except:

   A. optic atrophy
   B. hepatic cirrhosis
   C. flapping tremors
   D. Campbell de Morgan spots
   E. brain atrophy

12. A 36-year-old Asian immigrant comes to the ED with complaints of heart racing, nausea, and feeling sick. He also mentions that he had some alcohol to drink with his friends, and this is the first time he has had alcohol in his life. He spent all his life in China and moved to the United States only 2 weeks ago. On examination, his face is flushed red. His urine toxicology screen is negative for any other illicit drugs. What is the most likely cause of this patient's presentation?
    A. Alcohol dehydrogenase deficiency
    B. Aldehyde dehydrogenase deficiency
    C. Illicit drug use that did not show up on the urine toxicology screen
    D. Malingering
    E. Panic attack

13. A 42-year-old male who is on disulfiram for alcohol dependence would like to stop taking it because he believes he has developed sufficient "inner strength" and does not want to depend on a pill to keep him sober. If he does relapse, how long should he avoid alcohol after stopping disulfiram?
    A. 1 month
    B. 2 days
    C. 1 week
    D. 6 months
    E. 1 year

14. All of the following are true about methadone maintenance programs except:
    A. pregnant women are eligible for methadone maintenance if they are physically dependent on opiates
    B. special licensure is required for the facility where methadone is dispensed for opiate dependence
    C. the half-life of methadone is 48 hours
    D. federal regulations allow a maximum methadone dose of 120 mg per day
    E. methadone maintenance programs have been found to be beneficial not just for the individuals with opiate abuse problems but also for society as a whole

15. Which of the following statements is true about opiate abuse/dependence?
    A. Heroin abuse and dependence is six times more common in men than in women.
    B. Twin studies have shown that monozygotic twins are more likely to be concordant for opiate abuse than dizygotic twins.
    C. Comorbid psychiatric disorders are very common in individuals with opiate dependence.
    D. Opiate dependence is associated with a higher mortality rate compared with the general population.
    E. All of the above

16. Which of the following is associated with fetal alcohol syndrome?
    A. Small for gestational age
    B. Learning disabilities
    C. Hyperactive behavior
    D. Cardiac defects
    E. All of the above

17. All of the following are features of caffeine withdrawal except:
    A. headache
    B. sleep disturbances
    C. nervousness
    D. irritability
    E. paranoia

18. A 32-year-old alcoholic was started on disulfiram after he requests his psychiatrist to start him on this medication because he wants to stop drinking alcohol forever. However, he relapses within few days and comes to the ED with severe nausea, vomiting, and complaints of feeling dizzy. What is the mechanism of action of disulfiram?
    A. Central nervous system stimulant
    B. Aldehyde dehydrogenase inhibitor
    C. Alcohol dehydrogenase inhibitor
    D. Acetyl-coenzyme A inhibitor
    E. Mechanism of action is not known

19. A 72-year-old male is brought to the ED following a 911 call by his wife. She mentions that her husband had a "seizure-like" episode that lasted for few minutes. She also tells the ED physician that her husband has substance abuse problems, but about a day ago, he decided to quit cold turkey. All of the following statements about alcohol withdrawal seizures are true except:

    A. rarely proceed to status epilepticus
    B. occur within 24 to 48 hours after the last drink
    C. generalized tonic-clonic seizures
    D. second seizure is a rule rather than exception
    E. benzodiazepines are often used for treatment of seizures

20. All of the following features help differentiate alcohol hallucinosis from delirium tremens except:

    A. normal pupillary reaction
    B. visual hallucinations
    C. lack of tremors
    D. clear consciousness
    E. rapid onset

21. One of the management strategies involved in the treatment of alcoholism is to make an intervention at an appropriate time. All of the following are stages involved in behavioral change except:

    A. contemplation
    B. action
    C. reaction
    D. precontemplation
    E. relapse

22. All of the following are used in opiate detoxification except:

    A. buprenorphine
    B. clonidine
    C. methadone
    D. lofexidine
    E. chlordiazepoxide

23. All of the following are true regarding naltrexone except:
    A. used in long-term treatment of opiate abuse
    B. acts as an opiate antagonist
    C. major side effect is hepatotoxicity
    D. liver functions should be checked once every 3 months after starting naltrexone
    E. need to discontinue the medicine for at least 5 days if narcotic analgesia is necessary

24. A 52-year-old male is admitted to a medical unit for an ulcer on his foot. Two days after admission, he was found to tolerate the intravenous antibiotics well and has no fever. However, he becomes restless and appears slightly confused. He also complains of insomnia, and the nurse notices that he is diaphoretic, with an elevated heart rate and blood pressure. Physical examination reveals a course tremor of the upper extremities, and his reflexes are described as "brisk." What is the most likely diagnosis?
    A. Alcohol withdrawal
    B. Opiate withdrawal
    C. Methamphetamine withdrawal
    D. Nicotine withdrawal
    E. Marijuana withdrawal

25. A 36-year-old pregnant woman is admitted to the medical unit for possible infection associated with intravenous heroin injection. She admits to heroin dependency. She is now 5 months into her pregnancy and would like to "quit heroin for good." What is the best course of action in this patient?
    A. Allow her to continue to use heroin, as withdrawal can be dangerous.
    B. Methadone maintenance
    C. Naltrexone
    D. Advise her to stop heroin and start supportive therapy.
    E. Buprenorphine

26. A 52-year-old male is seen in the ED for acute exacerbation of chronic schizophrenia. He is fairly compliant with quetiapine 600 mg and takes it every night. He mentions that he has a problem with polysubstance use, and whenever he uses drugs, he will miss quetiapine for few days and end up in the ED. He is noticed to be internally stimulated and appears to be motivated to seek help. What is the ideal course of action in this patient?

    A. Admit him to an acute psychiatric in-patient unit.
    B. Admit him to a chemical-dependency unit.
    C. Admit him to a dual-diagnosis unit.
    D. Start him on an intensive outpatient treatment program.
    E. Restart quetiapine, and discharge him from the ED.

27. An intern on the neurology in-patient unit wonders if there is a good scale to monitor heroin withdrawal in a patient he is taking care of for suspected multiple sclerosis. Which of the following is a good instrument to monitor opioid withdrawal?

    A. Cut down, annoyed, guilt, eye-opener (CAGE)
    B. Michigan Alcohol Screening Test (MAST)
    C. Beck Depression Inventory (BDI)
    D. Alcohol Use Disorders Identification Test (AUDIT)
    E. Clinical Opioid Withdrawal Scale (COWS)

28. Which of the following has the most reinforcing effects, that is, the greatest potential to become addicted?

    A. Cocaine
    B. Alcohol
    C. Marijuana
    D. Heroin
    E. Nicotine

29. A 23-year-old female is diagnosed with first-episode depression following several stressors in her life. She is willing to start medication and wonders if there is a medication that will also help her to quit smoking. Which of the following medications have been found to be effective in both depression and nicotine addiction?

    A. Bupropion
    B. Buprenorphine
    C. Duloxetine
    D. Paroxetine
    E. Sertraline

30. The wife of a 53-year-old alcoholic states that it is becoming increasingly hard for her and her children to cope with the consequences of her alcoholic husband. She wonders if she can find some support as she goes through this process until her husband is sober again. Which of the following is a good option for her?

    A. Alcoholics Anonymous
    B. Al-Anon
    C. Narcotics Anonymous
    D. Adult Children Anonymous
    E. All of the above

ANSWERS

1. **Answer: D.** Alcohol abuse/dependence is thought to result from the interaction of genetic and environmental factors. History of alcohol problems in biological relatives increases the risk of alcoholism even when nonalcoholic parents raise them. If the biological relatives of a child are nonalcoholics, however, the risk is not increased if the adoptive parents are alcoholics. History of other substance abuse, PTSD, and attention-deficit hyperactivity disorder is found to increase the risk of alcohol abuse or dependence.

2. **Answer: E.** Alcohol withdrawal symptoms can result in serious medical complications, which can be life threatening. Some of the recognized medical complications include tremors, delirium, seizures, hypertension, hypomagnesemia, coma, agitation, and autonomic hyperactivity. Hypoglycemia (hyperglycemia) is commonly seen in patients with alcohol intoxication and withdrawal.

3. **Answer: E.** Miller and Rollnick proposed the motivational interview to assess the patient's motivation to change, which is often used in the treatment of subjects with substance abuse/dependence. According to this theory, there are five stages that help to understand patient's reasons for seeking treatment and help clinicians make effective interventions. The stages are precontemplation, contemplation, determination, action, and maintenance.

4. **Answer: D.** Opiate withdrawal symptoms can be very uncomfortable with symptoms of rhinorrhea, lacrimation, nausea, vomiting, diarrhea, yawning, sweating, and irritability. Flashbacks, however, is not a symptom of opiate withdrawal. It is associated with hallucinogen abuse.

5. **Answer: E.** HPPD is recognized in the DSM-IV and has a distinct code. It is a rare disorder characterized by persisting perceptual disturbances following hallucinogen abuse in some individuals. The exact cause of persistence of perception problems (sometimes for years) is unknown. Visual problems are often reported and consist of halos/hues around objects. Visualization of vivid floaters as well as trails on following a moving object are also often reported. Interestingly, risperidone is found to make the symptoms worse in some individuals. Benzodiazepines are often found to be helpful.

6. **Answer: A.** Amotivational syndrome is a recognized feature of chronic marijuana use. It is characterized by severe fatigue, a lack of motivation and energy, as well as a lack of interests. Seizures are associated with acute alcohol withdrawal, and Wernicke's encephalopathy is associated with chronic alcohol abuse. HPPD is associated with hallucinogen abuse in some individuals, and stroke is associated with abuse of stimulants such as cocaine and amphetamines.

7. **Answer: C.** Opiate intoxication is characterized by decreased level of consciousness, stupor, coma, pruritus, anorexia, miosis, and constipation. Bradycardia and not tachycardia is a feature of opiate intoxication.

8. **Answer: A.** Amphetamines and other stimulants such as cocaine abuse can lead to life-threatening complications including seizures, stroke, and myocardial ischemia. Mydriasis is a feature of amphetamine abuse (not miosis).

9. **Answer: C.** PCP intoxication can lead to violent behavior and paranoia. Often, these individuals smoke marijuana to control the agitation associated with PCP. Hyperacusis and increased pain threshold (i.e., decreased response to pain) are also noted.

10. **Answer: C.** PCP abuse intoxication is associated with paranoia and extreme, unpredictable violence. Hence, until PCP is cleared out of the system, it is wise not to talk the patient down. When these patients are admitted to an inpatient unit, they should be monitored closely, and the room should not be shared with other patients (again, because of extreme, intermittent undirected violence associated with PCP). PCP acts as an NMDA receptor antagonist.

11. **Answer: D.** Campbell de Morgan spots are small red spots that tend to occur in people older than 40 years. They are also called cherry angioma or hemangioma. They are usually not removed unless they bleed recurrently or if they are unsightly. All of the other features listed are associated with chronic alcoholism.

12. **Answer: B.** Alcohol flush reaction, caused by aldehyde dehydrogenase deficiency is common in Asians but also occurs in some Caucasians. Degrees of flushing can range from slightly pink to bright red. The reaction has been found to be caused by a mutation in the structural gene for the mitochondrial aldehyde dehydrogenase. In addition to flushing of the face, other unpleasant effects can also occur. These include tachycardia or increased heart rate, low blood pressure, headache, hyperventilation, and nausea.

13. **Answer: C.** Once disulfiram is stopped, the liver has to produce enough acetaldehyde dehydrogenase to convert acetaldehyde to acetic acid. This process usually requires about 1 week after disulfiram is stopped.

14. **Answer: C.** Methadone maintenance programs have been operated successfully for a number of years with great benefits for opiate-dependent patients and for society as a whole by reducing criminal behaviors and decreasing the incidence of infections contracted by sharing needles. The half-life of methadone is 24 to 36 hours, and therefore, it has to be given once every day. The other statements are true.

15. **Answer: E.** Opiate abuse and dependence is a common problem. According to the National Comorbid Survey (NCS, 1994), 7.5% of individuals who used opiates for nonmedical reasons and 23% of individuals who used heroin eventually became dependent on opiates. Heroin abuse is much more common in men than in women. The majority of individuals with opiate dependence had comorbid psychiatric disorders, mainly depression. Opiate dependence is associated with a high mortality rate, which is mainly caused by overdose, infections (AIDS, hepatitis B and C) from sharing needles, and violence associated with obtaining drugs on the streets.

16. **Answer: E.** Fetal alcohol syndrome presents with a spectrum of effects that can occur when a woman drinks during pregnancy. Fetal death is the most extreme outcome. Fetal alcohol syndrome is characterized by abnormal facial features, growth retardation, and central nervous system problems. Various features include microcephaly, epicanthic folds, thin upper lip, atrial and ventricular septal defects, renal hypoplasia, mental retardation, and hyperactivity and behavioral problems.

17. **Answer: E.** Caffeine withdrawal is benign and lasts for less than a few days. It usually begins within 24 hours after the last use and is characterized by headache, nervousness, irritability, sleep disturbances, impaired concentration, and yawning.

18. **Answer: B.** Disulfiram acts by inhibiting aldehyde dehydrogenase leading to accumulation of acetaldehyde in the body. Accumulation of acetaldehyde in the blood produces flushing, throbbing in the head and neck, throbbing headache, respiratory difficulty, nausea, copious vomiting, sweating, thirst, chest pain, palpitation, dyspnea, hyperventilation, tachycardia, hypotension, syncope, marked uneasiness, weakness, vertigo, blurred vision, and confusion and in some cases, even death.

19. **Answer: D.** Seizures following abrupt discontinuation of alcohol in alcohol dependents is not uncommon. However, status epilepticus and a second seizure are uncommon. The seizure is usually a generalized tonic-clonic event, occurs within 24 to 48 hours after the last drink, and the patient responds well to intravenous benzodiazepine.

20. **Answer: B.** Clinically sometimes it might be difficult to differentiate delirium tremens from alcohol hallucinosis. Delirium tremens is characterized by confusion, elevated heart rate, and blood pressure, tremors, visual hallucinations, and the onset is gradual. Alcohol hallucinosis, on the other hand, has a rapid onset and occurs in patients with clear consciousness. It is characterized by auditory hallucinations, vitals are usually in the normal range, and the patient's pupils react normally.

21. **Answer: C.** Miller and Rollnick provided stages of behavioral change that help understand a person's behavior in addictive disorders. The six stages of behavioral change are precontemplation, contemplation, preparation, action, maintenance, and relapse.

22. **Answer: E.** Various drugs are used in opiate detoxification. The most common agent is methadone. Many facilities are now also using buprenorphine, which has been found to be safe in accidental/deliberate overdose due to its "ceiling effect." The other drugs that are used include clonidine, clonidine-naltrexone combination, and lofexidine (in the UK).

23. **Answer: D.** Naltrexone has been used to prevent relapse of opiate use after patients are detoxified of opiates. The major side effect is hepatotoxicity. The patient's liver function tests should be normal before starting naltrexone. Once naltrexone is started, liver functions should be checked every 2 weeks for the first month and then monthly for the next 6 months. If for any reason, these patients require narcotic analgesia, they should discontinue naltrexone at least 5 days before the anticipated need.

24. **Answer: A.** The appearance of symptoms about 2 days after admission associated with coarse tremors and brisk reflexes is typical of alcohol or other sedative (such as benzodiazepine) withdrawal. Opiate withdrawal is characterized by rhinorrhea, yawning, stomach cramps, and diarrhea. Amphetamine withdrawal is mainly characterized by hypersomnia. Nicotine and marihuana withdrawal, although uncomfortable, does not cause significant elevation of heart rate or blood pressure and causes brisk reflexes.

25. **Answer: B.** Methadone maintenance is the best option in this patient. It is important to avoid opiate withdrawal during pregnancy because of the risks to the fetus. Allowing her to continue heroin use, however, is also dangerous because of the associated health risks both to the mother and the fetus. Naltrexone is contraindicated in pregnancy because of the risk of spontaneous abortion. Supportive therapy alone will not help someone who is dependent on heroin. Finally, there is not enough clinical experience to recommend the use of buprenorphine in pregnant women.

26. **Answer: C.** This patient will be best served with an admission to a dual-diagnosis unit where the treatment team has expertise in both psychiatric and substance abuse problems. Although admission to either psychiatric inpatient unit or chemical dependency unit alone will still help him, this might not be ideal for a patient with mental illness and substance abuse. Intensive outpatient treatment programs might be an option after he is stabilized in an inpatient unit. Discharging the patient from the ED when he is psychotic is not an option.

27. **Answer: E.** The COWS is a good instrument to monitor opioid withdrawal. CAGE, AUDIT, and MAST are all screening instruments for alcohol use disorders. BDI is a screening tool for depression.

28. **Answer: A.** Cocaine has been found to have the highest reinforcing effects in animal studies in laboratories. The other choices listed do have some reinforcing effects, and all of them are potentially capable of inducing dependency, but none of them are as addictive as cocaine.

29. **Answer: A.** Bupropion is an effective antidepressant medication that has also been approved for nicotine addiction. Buprenorphine is used in opioid dependence. Duloxetine is an antidepressant medication that has efficacy in pain symptoms as well. Paroxetine and sertraline are serotonin reuptake inhibitors and have antidepressant effects but are not helpful in nicotine dependence.

30. **Answer: B.** Al-Anon is a worldwide organization that offers self-help recovery programs for families and friends of alcoholics whether or not the alcoholic seeks help or even recognizes the existence of a drinking problem. Alcoholics Anonymous is a fellowship of men and women who share their experience, strength, and hope with each other that they may solve their common problem and help others to recover from alcoholism. Narcotics Anonymous is a fellowship of men and women for whom drugs have become a major problem. Adult Children Anonymous (formerly known as Adult Children of Alcoholics or ACOA) is a twelve-step program of women and men who grew up in alcoholic or otherwise dysfunctional homes.

Forensic Psychiatry

QUESTIONS

1. Which of the following statements about exhibitionism is true?
   - A. Equally common in men and women
   - B. Low recidivism following a first conviction.
   - C. Common in the elderly
   - D. None of the above

2. Pathological fire setting or arson behavior is associated with all of the following except:
   - A. antisocial behaviors
   - B. psychotic disorders
   - C. sexual pleasure in some
   - D. multiple personality or dissociative identity disorder
   - E. all of the above.

3. What proportion of people commit suicide after committing a homicide?
   - A. One-third
   - B. Two-thirds
   - C. Three-fourths
   - D. One-fifth
   - E. Two-fifths

4. All of the following are false about transvestites except:
   - A. strong desire to be a female
   - B. they are usually homosexuals
   - C. have gender identity disorder
   - D. usually married
   - E. cross dress in public

5. An arsonist is more likely to reoffend if:
   A. the offender is psychotic
   B. the offender has a learning disability
   C. sexual excitement is associated with arson behavior
   D. all of the above
   E. none of the above

6. The most important predictor of future violence is:
   A. male gender
   B. low social class
   C. past history of violence
   D. access to guns
   E. alcohol abuse

7. All of the following are true about people with seizure disorder and violence except:
   A. more likely to be aggressive against people who they know rather than strangers
   B. more likely to be aggressive within the first few hours to days after seizure onset
   C. among violent offenders, the prevalence of seizure disorder is no higher than in the general population
   D. all of the above
   E. none of the above

8. All of the following are true about transsexualism except:
   A. disorder of gender identity
   B. convinced that they are of the opposite sex
   C. wish to alter the external genitalia and physical features
   D. disorder of gender role behavior

9. Testamentary capacity refers to:
   A. ability to decide on health-related issues
   B. ability to make a legal will
   C. ability to consent for treatment
   D. all of the above
   E. none of the above

10. Which of the following are the essential components of informed consent?
    A. Knowledge of the risks and benefits of the proposed interventions
    B. Knowledge of the risks and benefits of the alternative interventions
    C. Knowledge of the risks and benefits of no intervention
    D. Ability to understand that consent is a voluntary process
    E. All of the above

11. Tarasoff's law deals with:
    A. informed consent
    B. duty to warn
    C. protection of confidentiality
    D. first do no harm
    E. ability to form intent

12. Tarasoff's II law deals with:
    A. informed consent
    B. duty to warn
    C. duty to protect a potential victim
    D. first do no harm
    E. ability to form intent

13. *Habeas corpus* deals with:
    A. ability to form intent
    B. protection of confidentiality
    C. informed consent
    D. duty to warn
    E. curtailment of liberty

14. A 56-year-old female with multiple sclerosis decides to file a malpractice suit against her neurologist and psychiatrist for negligence. She believes that her physicians missed the diagnosis for a number of years until now. To prove dereliction of duty, the plaintiff has to show that:
    A. physician had a duty to care
    B. deviation from standard practice of care occurred
    C. deviation from the standard practice of care caused the damage
    D. damage to her health resulted directly from action/inaction of the physician
    E. all of the above

15. An 82-year-old female with stroke is admitted to the neurology intensive care unit. She requests discharge to home instead of going to the rehabilitation center as recommended by the neurologist. A psychiatrist is consulted to determine if the patient is competent to make the decision about her health. To determine if a person is competent to make a particular decision, all of the following criteria are important except:

    A. understanding of the information
    B. appreciation of the risks and benefits
    C. ability to arrive at the decision after rational thinking
    D. ability to communicate the decision
    E. all of the above

16. A 32-year-old male is charged with assaulting another patient without any provocation, in an inpatient unit. His lawyer, however, makes an argument that the patient is not competent to stand trial because of all of the following reasons. Which of the following reasons given by his lawyer make this person incompetent to stand trial?

    A. Lack of capacity to understand the charges brought against him
    B. Has depression that is only in partial remission
    C. Has mild mental retardation
    D. Has substance abuse problems
    E. All of the above

17. A 30-year-old male is prosecuted for assaulting a teenager with a knife. His lawyer argues that his client is diagnosed with schizophrenia and was "psychotic" when the incident occurred. The patient's lawyer then mentions the Right-Wrong Test, which is also known as:

    A. Model Penal Code
    B. Tarasoff's I law
    C. Tarasoff's II law
    D. Guilty but insane
    E. Incompetent to stand trial

18. A 26-year-old female is arrested for shoplifting and assaulting the cashier. Her lawyer pleads insanity defense because of chronic mental illness. All of the following are associated with increased criminal/aggressive behavior except:
    A. antisocial personality disorder
    B. alcohol abuse
    C. illicit drug abuse
    D. some patients with schizophrenia
    E. panic disorder

19. Which of the following statements are true about violence and schizophrenia?
    A. Increases with comorbid substance abuse
    B. Untreated patients, especially with paranoia are at a higher risk for violence
    C. Majority of patients are not violent
    D. Violence is not a symptom of schizophrenia
    E. All of the above

20. A 32-year-old female is charged with first-degree murder for drowning her two children aged 4 and 2 years old. The defense pleads "not guilty by reason of insanity" because the defendant was suffering from postpartum psychosis. All of the following are true about postpartum psychosis except:
    A. incidence: one in 1,000 child births
    B. follows first childbirth, majority of the times
    C. risk of suicide and infanticide is high
    D. risk of recurrence is high
    E. all of the above

ANSWERS

1. **Answer: B.** Exhibitionism, a mental disorder is characterized by a compulsion to display one's genitals to an unsuspecting stranger. In the *Diagnostic and Statistical Manual of Mental Disorders*, 4th edition (DSM-IV), it is classified under paraphilias. It is more common in middle-aged men, and recidivism rates following a first conviction are low.

2. **Answer: E.** Pathological fire setting or arson behavior has been found to have a high association with other antisocial behaviors, psychotic disorders, and dissociative identity disorders. Some individuals report deriving sexual pleasure from arson behavior.

3. **Answer: A.** Approximately one third of individuals commit suicide after committing a homicide.

4. **Answer: D.** Transvestism is the practice of cross-dressing, which is wearing the clothing of the opposite sex. The majority of these individuals are married and cross-dress in private. They do not have gender identity disorder, do not have any desire to be of the opposite sex, and are heterosexuals.

5. **Answer: D.** Arson behavior is more common if the offender is psychotic, has a learning disability, and if he or she experiences sexual pleasure with arson behavior.

6. **Answer: C.** Past history of violence is the most important predictor of future violence.

7. **Answer: C.** Among violent offenders, the prevalence of seizure disorder is higher than in the general population.

8. **Answer: D.** Transsexualism is a disorder of gender identity in which the individual is convinced that he or she belongs to the opposite sex than that indicated by external genitalia. Transvestism is a disorder of gender role behavior.

9. **Answer: B.** Testamentary capacity refers to the ability to make a legal will.

10. **Answer: E.** All of the above are essential components of informed consent.

11. **Answer: B.** Tarasoff's law deals with the duty to warn. The law states that a physician has a duty to warn third parties of possible serious harm to them by a patient if they are readily identifiable and if the risk of harm is substantial and imminent.

12. **Answer: C.** Tarasoff's II law deals with the duty to protect a potential victim. The law states that a psychiatrist has a duty not only to warn but also the duty to protect the identified victim from a patient that they believe is dangerous.

13. **Answer: E.** *Habeas corpus* is a petition that individuals can file in a court of law if they believe that they have been illegally deprived of their liberty (e.g., involuntary commitment in a hospital).

14. **Answer: E.** To prove malpractice, the plaintiff has to satisfy the "four D's" in a court of law: (1) duty to care existed, (2) deviation from the standard practice of care, (3) damage, and (4) damage resulting directly from the deviation from the standard practice of care.

15. **Answer: E.** Competency to make decisions is issue specific. All of the above criteria have to be satisfied before a person is deemed to be competent to make a particular decision.

16. **Answer: A.** For a person to stand trial, he or she should be able to understand the charges against him or her, be able to understand the procedures of the court, be able to help his or her lawyers in preparing a defense, and be able to testify.

17. **Answer: A.** The Model Penal Code states that, "A person is not responsible for the criminal conduct if, at the time of such conduct, as a result of mental disease or defect, they lacked substantial capacity either to appreciate the criminality of their conduct or to confirm their conduct to the requirement of the law."

18. **Answer: E.** Antisocial personality disorder, alcohol, and substance abuse are associated with increased criminal and aggressive behavior. Overall, patients with mental illness are not likely to be involved in criminal or aggressive behavior except in some cases of mental retardation (inability to understand right from wrong) and schizophrenia (particularly paranoid type and patients with command hallucinations).

19. **Answer: E.** Although the common public perception is that schizophrenic patients are violent, research does not support this view. The majority of patients with schizophrenia are not violent.

20. **Answer: E.** Postpartum psychosis, classified as psychosis not otherwise specified in the DSM-IV is associated with a high risk of suicide and infanticide. It is a psychiatric emergency.

Eating Disorders

QUESTIONS

1. According to the *Diagnostic and Statistical Manual of Mental Disorders*, 4th edition (DSM-IV), all of the following are the characteristic features of anorexia nervosa except:

   A. body mass index (BMI) of less than 19
   B. intense fear of gaining weight
   C. body image disturbance
   D. amenorrhea

2. According to the DSM-IV, all of the following are the characteristic features of bulimia nervosa except:

   A. recurrent episodes of binge eating
   B. recurrent inappropriate compensatory behavior to prevent weight gain
   C. binge eating and compensatory behaviors occur at least twice a week for 6 months
   D. self-evaluation unduly influenced by body weight and shape
   E. the disturbance does not occur exclusively during episodes of anorexia nervosa

3. All of the following are the characteristic features of binge eating disorder except:

   A. recurrent episodes of binge eating for at least 2 days per week in the last 6 months
   B. absence of inappropriate compensatory behavior to prevent weight gain
   C. binge eating episodes are associated with marked distress
   D. BMI greater than 40
   E. the disturbance does not occur exclusively during episodes of anorexia nervosa

4. A 23-year-old female with anorexia nervosa is admitted to the hospital for the third time in the past 12 years for electrolyte imbalance. Her worried parents want to know more about the course of the disorder and the mortality rate for anorexia nervosa. Which of the following is NOT TRUE about eating disorders?

   A. The annual mortality rate for anorexia nervosa is 5%.
   B. Full recovery in anorexia nervosa is 50%.
   C. Full recovery in bulimia nervosa is 50%.
   D. Twenty percent of patients with an eating disorder have a chronic course.
   E. Patients with a binge eating disorder have a more favorable outcome compared to patients with other eating disorders.

5. All of the following electrolyte abnormalities are commonly found in anorexia nervosa except:

   A. hyperchloremia
   B. hypokalemia
   C. elevated blood urea nitrogen
   D. hypomagnesemia
   E. hypophosphatemia

6. A 19-year-old female's parents are worried that the physicians have made an incorrect diagnosis of anorexia nervosa. They insist that their daughter's weight loss is because of something "neurological" because they believe the weight loss occurred only after she had a head injury 3 years ago. However, the patient has all the characteristic features of anorexia nervosa, and the treating physician orders a brain magnetic resonance imaging (MRI) scan just to make sure he is not missing anything. What is the most likely finding on a brain MRI in patients with anorexia nervosa?

   A. No abnormalities on brain MRI
   B. Atrophy of appetite center in hypothalamus
   C. Hypertrophy of satiety center in hypothalamus
   D. Increased ventricular-brain ratio
   E. Frontal lobe atrophy

7. All of the following are true regarding anorexia nervosa except:

   A. mean age of onset is 17 years
   B. prevalence in late adolescence and early adulthood is 0.5% to 1.0%
   C. about 70% of anorexia nervosa patients are females
   D. genetic and environmental factors are responsible
   E. more common in industrial countries

8. All of the following are true about bulimia nervosa except:
   A. usually begins in adolescence or early adult life
   B. prevalence in adolescence and young adult females is 1% to 3%
   C. about 90% of bulimia nervosa patients are female
   D. patients are typically obese
   E. two subtypes: purging and nonpurging type

9. Cognitive behavioral therapy (CBT) has been found to be most effective in which of the following eating disorders?
   A. Bulimia nervosa and binge eating disorder
   B. Anorexia nervosa and bulimia nervosa
   C. Anorexia nervosa
   D. Anorexia nervosa and binge eating disorder
   E. None of the above

10. The only FDA-approved medication for the treatment of eating disorders is:
    A. sertraline
    B. paroxetine
    C. citalopram
    D. fluoxetine
    E. escitalopram

11. Which of the following antidepressants is contraindicated in patients with eating disorders?
    A. Effexor
    B. Bupropion
    C. Duloxetine
    D. Fluoxetine
    E. Citalopram

12. Which of the following is found in patients with bulimia nervosa?
    A. Higher incidence of substance abuse
    B. Higher incidence of depression
    C. Impulsivity
    D. Enlarged parotid glands
    E. All of the above

13. It is not uncommon to see patients with more than one eating disorder. What percentage of patients with anorexia nervosa go on to develop bulimia nervosa?
    A. 50%
    B. 90%
    C. 10%
    D. 25%
    E. 75%

14. Substance abuse is found to be associated with eating disorders, especially bulimia nervosa. Which of the following is the most commonly abused substance in patients with bulimia nervosa?
    A. Amphetamines
    B. Opiates
    C. Alcohol
    D. Cannabis
    E. Cocaine

15. Amenorrhea is one of the diagnostic features of anorexia nervosa. Which of the following sexual hormonal abnormalities is found in patients with anorexia nervosa?
    A. Estrogen
    B. Luteinizing hormone
    C. Gonadotropin-releasing hormone
    D. Follicles-stimulating hormone
    E. All of the above

16. Which of the following is considered to be a poor prognostic factor in patients with anorexia nervosa?
    A. Late age of onset
    B. Family members open to participate in patient care
    C. Early age of onset
    D. No suicidal behavior
    E. No previous hospitalization

17. A 23-year-old female with bulimia nervosa who induces vomiting almost every day visits a dentist for "teeth problems." Which of the following is commonly seen on oral examination of bulimia patients?

  A. Loss of teeth
  B. Smoothening of molar occlusion surface
  C. Erosion of fillings
  D. Enamel erosions on the lingual surface of incisors
  E. All of the above

18. Which of the following psychotherapeutic techniques have been found to have the most beneficial effects in patients with bulimia nervosa with no comorbid conditions?

  A. Cognitive behavioral therapy
  B. Psychodynamic psychotherapy
  C. Solution-focused therapy
  D. Psychoanalytic psychotherapy
  E. All of the above

19. Which of the following is the only Food and Drug Administration (FDA)-approved medication for the treatment of bulimia nervosa?

  A. Paroxetine
  B. Bupropion
  C. Citalopram
  D. Mirtazapine
  E. Fluoxetine

20. Which of the following is true about eating disorders?

  A. Anorexia nervosa is more common in women than in men.
  B. Anorexia nervosa is associated with a high mortality rate.
  C. Bulimia nervosa is often seen in association with cluster B personality traits.
  D. Reports of sexual abuse are more common in patients with eating disorders.
  E. All of the above

ANSWERS

1. **Answer: A.** The essential features of anorexia nervosa are that the individual refuses to maintain a minimal body weight, is intensely afraid of gaining weight, and exhibits a significant disturbance in the perception of the shape or size of his or her body. Amenorrhea is noted in postmenarcheal females. A BMI of less than 17.5 (or less than 85% of weight for the height) is considered as one of the features of anorexia nervosa.

2. **Answer: C.** The essential features of bulimia nervosa are binge eating and inappropriate compensatory methods to prevent weight gain. The self-evaluation of individuals is excessively influenced by body shape and weight. The binge eating and compensatory behaviors must occur, on average, at least twice a week for 3 months.

3. **Answer: D.** Binge eating disorder is characterized by recurrent episodes of binge eating in the absence of inappropriate compensatory behaviors. The binge eating episodes are associated with marked distress. Although many of these individuals are overweight or obese, there is no BMI criteria for this disorder.

4. **Answer: A.** The annual mortality rate for anorexia nervosa is 0.6%. About 50% of individuals with anorexia nervosa and bulimia nervosa make a full recovery. About 30% make partial recovery, and the other 20% follow a chronic course.

5. **Answer: A.** Several electrolyte abnormalities are commonly found in patients with anorexia nervosa. Low zinc levels are also found. Hypochloremia (not hyperchloremia) is noted because of induced vomiting causing loss of hydrochloric acid.

6. **Answer: D.** An increase in ventricular-brain ratio secondary to starvation is often seen in patients with anorexia nervosa.

7. **Answer: C.** Anorexia nervosa is more prevalent in industrial countries where attractiveness for females is linked to being thin. The mean age of onset is 17 years, and it is rare over the age of 40 years. Anorexia nervosa is mainly seen in females, and in fact, more than 90% of the patients are female.

8. **Answer: D.** Bulimia nervosa is more common than anorexia nervosa and typically begins in adolescence or early adult life. It is far more common in females than in males. Patients with bulimia nervosa are typically in the normal weight range, although some may be slightly underweight or overweight.

9. **Answer: A.** CBT is found to be very effective in the treatment of bulimia nervosa and binge eating disorder. In fact, in some studies, CBT has been found to be more effective than medications in these two disorders. Family therapy is found to be more effective in anorexia nervosa, especially in adolescents and young adults.

10. **Answer: D.** Fluoxetine is the only medication that is approved by the FDA for the treatment of bulimia nervosa. The recommended dosage is 60 mg/day. Fluoxetine in high doses has also been found to be helpful in stabilizing weight-recovered individuals with anorexia nervosa.

11. **Answer: B.** Bupropion is contraindicated in the treatment of eating disorders, especially patients with bulimia nervosa. Studies have shown elevated risk of seizures in patients with bulimia nervosa.

12. **Answer: E.** Bulimia nervosa is associated with a higher incidence of depression, anxiety, impulsivity, and substance abuse disorders. Repeated induced vomiting is thought to cause enlarged parotid glands and erosion of tooth enamel.

13. **Answer: A.** Studies have shown that approximately 50% of patients with anorexia nervosa go on to develop bulimia nervosa.

14. **Answer: C.** Alcohol is the most commonly abused substance in patients with bulimia nervosa. Patients with eating disorders are often found to abuse illicit drugs such as amphetamines and cocaine, to control weight.

15. **Answer: E.** Anorexia nervosa is characterized by amenorrhea. In patients with anorexia nervosa, decreased secretion of gonadotropin-releasing hormone is noted, and this in turn causes decreased levels of estrogen, luteinizing hormone, and follicle-stimulating hormone levels.

16. **Answer: A.** Late age of onset is considered to be a poor prognostic factor in anorexia nervosa. Early age of onset, no purging behavior, absence of comorbid psychiatric and substance abuse disorder, no previous hospitalization, and supportive family members are all associated with good prognosis.

17. **Answer: D.** Enamel erosions on the lingual surface of incisors are a very common finding in bulimia nervosa patients who induce vomiting. Loss of teeth is not a feature of bulimia nervosa, and smoothening of the molar occlusion surface is commonly seen in bruxism. Dental fillings are relatively resistant to the effects of gastric acid.

18. **Answer: A.** In the absence of any other comorbid conditions, cognitive behavioral therapy has been found to have the most beneficial effects in patients with bulimia nervosa.

19. **Answer: E.** Although all selective serotonin reuptake inhibitors at relatively high doses are believed to be effective in treating bulimia nervosa, fluoxetine is the only medication that has been approved by the FDA. Relatively higher doses (60 mg/day) are found to be much more effective than the lower doses. Bupropion is contraindicated in bulimia nervosa because of the higher risk of seizures.

20. **Answer: E.** Anorexia nervosa is associated with a high mortality rate. In some studies, the mortality rate is as high as 5.6% per decade of illness. Female anorexia nervosa patients are reportedly 12 times more likely to die than women of a similar age in the general population. The most common causes of death are suicide and starvation-related effects. All the other statements are true.

Psychiatric Emergencies

QUESTIONS

1. A 56-year-old male is brought to the emergency department (ED) by the emergency medical Services (EMS) from a methadone clinic. According to the methadone clinic nurse, the patient walked in with opiate withdrawal symptoms and mentioned that he has missed methadone for 3 days and that he usually takes 80 mg of methadone per day. The patient became drowsy and unarousable when he was given 80 mg of methadone. What should the methadone clinic have done prior to administering methadone?

   A. Examine the patient, and make sure he is having opiate withdrawal.
   B. Try to contact the methadone clinic from where he gets methadone and confirm the dose.
   C. If not able to contact the program, give a low dose of methadone and titrate according to withdrawal symptoms.
   D. Monitor the patient after he receives methadone.
   E. All of the above

2. The number of suicides per 100,000 population per year in the United States is:

   A. 100
   B. 11
   C. 21
   D. 30
   E. 1,000

3. A 32-year-old female is brought to the ED by the EMS following a 911 call by her husband. He mentions to the ED physician that his wife delivered a healthy baby girl 3 weeks ago. She was sad and tearful and felt "gloomy" for the first few days after delivery. Over the past 2 weeks, however, she appears to be suspicious of visitors including her mother and sister who recently visited her. She has started "staring at the baby" and gets distressed. A urine toxicology screen is negative, and the patient has no past psychiatric history. She has no significant medical problems. When the ED physician asks her how she feels about the baby, she starts crying. What is the most important first step in the management of this patient?

   A. Start the patient on antidepressant medication and discharge home.
   B. Start the patient on antipsychotic medication and discharge home.
   C. Give her clonazepam and discharge home.
   D. Admit the patient immediately to the psychiatry inpatient unit.
   E. The patient is just stressed; reassure and discharge her home.

4. Which of the following statements about suicide and gender is true?

   A. Gunshots are the number one cause of death in suicide in both men and women.
   B. Although women attempt suicide more often, men are four times more likely to complete suicide.
   C. Women attempt suicide twice as often as men.
   D. Most suicides are preventable.
   E. All of the above

5. All of the following statements about bipolar disorder and suicide are true except:

   A. 25% to 50% of patients with bipolar disorder attempt suicide at least once
   B. the suicide rate in the first year off lithium treatment is 20 times that during treatment
   C. most bipolar patients who die by suicide do not communicate their suicidal state to others
   D. lithium has shown to decrease the suicide behaviors associated with bipolar disorder
   E. history of suicide attempt is a good predictor of a future suicide attempt

6. Alcohol is a factor in what percentage of suicides?

   A. 10%
   B. 30%
   C. 50%
   D. 5%
   E. 15%

7. Approximately what percentage of patients with schizophrenia commit suicide?

   A. 10%
   B. 20%
   C. 40%
   D. 5%
   E. 25%

8. A 36-year-old female is brought to the ED by her boyfriend after she told him that she took a "handful of Valium (diazepam)" after an argument with him. On examination, the patient responds mildly to even a painful stimulus, and her respiratory rate is 6 breaths per minute. Which of the following is helpful in reversing the effects of benzodiazepines in this patient?

   A. Naloxone
   B. Pralidoxime
   C. Benztropine
   D. Flumazenil
   E. N-acetylcysteine

9. An 82-year-old male is brought in by the EMS to the ED for agitation and confusion. He was noted to be talking to himself and misperceived the nurse as a "thug trying to steal" from him and punched him in the face. An urgent psychiatric consultation was requested. Further workup reveals that he has a urinary tract infection. Over the next 3 days, as the urinary tract infection cleared, the patient returned to his usual pleasant demeanor and apologized to the nurse. Which of the following other medical conditions can present as psychiatric emergencies?

   A. Hypercalcemia
   B. Addison's disease
   C. Cushing's syndrome
   D. Thyrotoxicosis
   E. All of the above

10. Which of the following neurotransmitters is implicated in violent behavior?

   A. Serotonin
   B. Dopamine
   C. Norepinephrine
   D. Acetylcholine
   E. All of the above

11. Which of the following is the most significant risk factor for suicide?

   A. Psychiatric disorder
   B. Death of a loved one
   C. Loss of job
   D. Lack of home
   E. Conflicts at work

12. Which of the following disorders is associated with increased risk of mood disorders and suicide?

   A. Multiple sclerosis
   B. Huntington's disease
   C. Epilepsy
   D. Brain injury
   E. All of the above

13. Which of the following medical disorders is associated with the highest risk of suicide?

   A. Epilepsy
   B. Huntington's disease
   C. AIDS
   D. Cancer
   E. Brain injury

14. The risk of suicide is highest among which of the following professionals?

   A. Dentists
   B. Police officers
   C. Physicians
   D. Nurses
   E. Social workers

15. Which of the following increases the risk of suicide?
    A. Comorbid substance abuse
    B. History of childhood sexual abuse
    C. Impulsivity and aggression
    D. Old age
    E. All of the above

ANSWERS

1. **Answer: E.** When a patient not known to the service walks in with complaints of opiate withdrawal, it is important to make sure the patient is in fact having opiate withdrawal and not any other symptoms. Tolerance to opiates varies from one individual to the other, and the dose should be confirmed. If not, titrate the dose of methadone based on withdrawal symptoms and monitor the patient.

2. **Answer: B.** The number of suicides per 100,000 population per year in the United States is about 11. It is higher in the elderly (17 per 100,000 in the age group of 75+ years).

3. **Answer: D.** The history is suggestive of postpartum psychosis. The most important fist step in this situation is to safeguard the health of the mother and the baby. Ideally, she should be admitted to a mother-baby psychiatry unit that is specifically designed for postpartum depression and postpartum psychosis. The patient might require antipsychotics or other medicines depending on further assessment. Discharging a patient to home in this situation can be very dangerous.

4. **Answer: E.** A majority of suicides are preventable. The key is early recognition and treatment of mental illness, substance/alcohol abuse, and close follow-up.

5. **Answer: C.** Studies show that most bipolar patients who die by suicide actually communicate their suicidal thoughts/intent to others.

6. **Answer: B.** Alcohol is a factor in about 30% of suicides. In fact, more than 90% of alcoholics who die by suicide continue to abuse alcohol up to the end of their lives, and 7% of individuals with alcohol dependence will eventually commit suicide.

7. **Answer: A.** Approximately 10% of patients with schizophrenia commit suicide. About 20% to 40% of patients with schizophrenia attempt suicide. Depression is probably the most important risk factor for suicide in schizophrenia. Only 4% of those with schizophrenia who exhibit suicidal behavior do so in response to command hallucinations telling them to kill themselves.

8. **Answer: D.** Flumazenil is the specific antidote for benzodiazepines. It reverses the effects of benzodiazepines by competitive inhibition at the benzodiazepine binding site on the gamma-aminobutyric acid A (GABA$_A$) receptors. The onset of action is rapid, and effects are usually seen within 1 to 2 minutes.

9. **Answer: E.** Many medical conditions can cause frank psychotic symptoms and present as psychiatric emergencies. It is important to make sure all patients undergo a thorough medical workup and to ensure that all the causes of delirium and other psychiatric conditions are treated.

10. **Answer: E.** Serotonin, dopamine, norepinephrine and acetylcholine are implicated in violent behaviors. Specifically, low levels of central serotonin have been found to be associated with impulsivity and increased risk of violent behavior.

11. **Answer: A.** Of all the factors listed, having a psychiatric disorder carries the highest risk for suicide. The other factors can increase the risk of suicide when present in combination with certain other factors such as a history of suicide attempt, feelings of hopelessness, and substance abuse.

12. **Answer: E.** The presence of a comorbid medical disorder increases the risk of suicide both directly and indirectly by the psychological effects of the comorbid medical conditions. In particular, neurological disorders are found to increase the risk of mood disorders and suicide.

13. **Answer: C.** According to a meta-analysis by Harris and Barraclough, AIDS was associated with the highest standardized mortality ratio (SMR). The SMRs for various disorders were as follows: AIDS (6.58), epilepsy (5.11), spinal cord injury (3.82), brain injury (3.50), Huntington's chorea (2.8), and cancer (1.90).

14. **Answer: A.** Various studies have shown that certain occupations are associated with a higher suicide risk. Dentists were found to have the highest risk followed by physicians. The risk of suicide in police officers was not higher than the general population after age and gender matching.

15. **Answer: E.** Various demographic, physical, and psychological factors have been found to influence the risk of suicide. All of the factors listed have been associated with increased suicide risk.

Mental Retardation

QUESTIONS

1. According to the *Diagnostic and Statistical Manual of Mental Disorders*, 4th edition (DSM- IV), which one of the following is a diagnostic criterion for mental retardation?

   A. Onset before age 12 years
   B. Onset before age 18 years
   C. Deficit in at least one area of adaptive functioning
   D. IQ below 60
   E. Absence of a mental illness

2. An adult with moderate mental retardation has the mental age of a person with a chronological age of:

   A. 3 years
   B. 6 years
   C. 9 years
   D. 12 years
   E. 15 years

3. Mild mental retardation is thought to be much more common in general population but is often undiagnosed. Which of the following is true about mild mental retardation?

   A. It is diagnosed when the IQ is <70 but more than 55.
   B. Subjects can only perform simple elementary tasks.
   C. Most people with this condition live in supported supervised care settings.
   D. They constitute about 3% to 4% of those classified as mentally retarded.
   E. They never learn to read or write.

4. Mental retardation is associated with various other physical and mental health problems. Which of the following conditions are more frequently seen in patients with mental retardation?
   A. Visual impairment
   B. Speech problems
   C. Hearing difficulty
   D. Cerebral palsy
   E. All of the above

5. Seizure disorders are often seen in individuals with mental retardation. The prevalence of seizures in individuals with severe mental retardation can be up to:
   A. 5% to 10%
   B. 10% to 15%
   C. 30% to 50%
   D. 70% to80%
   E. 90%

6. What is the most common cause of mental retardation in the general population?
   A. Fragile X syndrome
   B. Down's syndrome
   C. Central nervous system (CNS) trauma
   D. Edward's syndrome
   E. Alcoholism in mother

7. What is the most common inherited cause of mental retardation?
   A. Fragile X syndrome
   B. Down's syndrome
   C. CNS trauma
   D. Edward's syndrome
   E. Alcoholism in mother

8. Down's syndrome is associated with various physical and mental abnormalities. Which of the following is NOT a feature of Down's syndrome?
   A. Single palmar crease
   B. Atlantoaxial instability
   C. Long thin hands
   D. Early dementia
   E. Oblique palpebral fissures

9. Fragile X syndrome is associated with various physical and mental abnormalities. Which of the following is NOT a feature of Fragile X syndrome?
   A. Large head
   B. Short stature
   C. Hyperextensible joins
   D. Macro-orchidism
   E. Cat-like cry

10. All of the following are features of Prader-Willi syndrome except:
    A. hyperphagia
    B. hypotonia
    C. hypersexual behavior
    D. mental retardation
    E. small hands and feet

11. Which of the following is NOT a feature of Rett syndrome?
    A. Normal development in the first 1 to 2 years of life
    B. Autistic traits
    C. Characteristic hand movements
    D. More common in males
    E. Increased incidence of seizure disorder

12. Which of the following is a feature of Lesch-Nyhan syndrome?
    A. Macrocephaly
    B. Micrognathia
    C. Self-mutilation
    D. Compulsive overeating
    E. Café-au-lait spots

13. All of the following are seen in individuals with Asperger's syndrome except:
    A. stilted speech
    B. eccentric lifestyle
    C. above average intelligence
    D. unusual speech
    E. restricted interests and behaviors

14. Individuals with mental retardation have a higher incidence of certain mental health problems. However, which of the following conditions is rarely seen in individuals with mental retardation?
    A. Anxiety
    B. Behavioral problems
    C. Schizophrenia
    D. Anorexia nervosa
    E. Epilepsy

15. Seizure disorders are common in individuals with mental retardation, particularly in severe mental retardation. Which of the following is NOT true regarding seizure disorder in these patients?
    A. It is often difficult to achieve good control of seizures.
    B. It frequently causes schizophrenia-like psychosis.
    C. It can accelerate intellectual deterioration.
    D. Polypharmacy is often required for adequate control.
    E. It rarely results in violence.

16. A 30-year-old normally pleasant male with Down's syndrome, who has a relatively good quality of life and reasonable social/occupational skills, is found to be aloof, frustrated, and not functioning well. What is the differential diagnosis for this presentation?
    A. Depression
    B. Hypothyroidism
    C. Dementia
    D. Hearing loss
    E. All of the above

17. A 13-year-old patient with Down's syndrome with moderate mental retardation tests positive for a sexually transmitted disease. The treating physician suspects abuse at the group home, and reports the incident to child protective services for further investigation. Which of the following is true about children with mental retardation and sexual abuse?
    A. They are at equal risk of being abused as children with normal intelligence.
    B. Sex education should be discouraged.
    C. They do not benefit from supportive psychotherapy.
    D. They may not disclose if they have been abused.
    E. They should be discouraged from talking about their abusive experiences.

18. Sexual abuse in children with mental retardation is common but under-reported. Which of the following is NOT a feature of sexual abuse in children with mental retardation?

    A. It can result in disruptive behavior.
    B. It can result in stereotyped behaviors.
    C. It presents in the same way as children without mental retardation.
    D. Regression of abilities is sometimes noticed.
    E. It can result in sophisticated sexualized behaviors.

19. Depression in individuals with mental retardation can present with all of the following except:

    A. self-injurious behavior
    B. limited interaction with others
    C. euphoria
    D. tearfulness
    E. appetite disturbance

20. Individuals with mental retardation present with unique challenges when it comes to the diagnosis and treatment of physical and mental health problems. Which of the following techniques has been found to be helpful in assessing individuals with mental retardation?

    A. Leading questions are unhelpful.
    B. Collateral information from more than one source is often helpful.
    C. More than one interview session is sometimes required.
    D. Some individuals are more comfortable in writing or drawing their problems.
    E. All of the above.

21. Physical aggression is sometimes common in certain individuals with mental retardation. All of the following techniques have been found to be helpful in treating aggressive behaviors in patients with mental retardation except:

    A. multidisciplinary approach is most useful
    B. it can be done either on an inpatient or outpatient basis
    C. pharmacotherapy should be avoided
    D. simultaneous introduction of two treatment modalities should be avoided
    E. treatment should focus on the underlying etiology

22. All of the following are true about Asperger's syndrome except:
    A. stereotyped behaviors
    B. verbal deficits are more common than nonverbal deficits
    C. relatives are at a higher risk for schizophrenia
    D. motor coordination problems may be seen
    E. limited social skills

23. Which of the following statements regarding Asperger's syndrome is true?
    A. It can easily be differentiated from autism.
    B. Prevalence is less than classic autism.
    C. No genetic contribution
    D. It resolves in adulthood.
    E. It can be associated with attention-deficit hyperactivity disorder (ADHD).

24. Individuals with Down's syndrome often develop dementia in their 40s. The proportion of people with Down's syndrome who develop neurofibrillary tangles in the brain by the age of 50 is approximately:
    A. 25%
    B. 35%
    C. 50%
    D. 75%
    E. 100%

25. The chromosomal abnormality in Down's syndrome is located on:
    A. 21
    B. 5
    C. 20
    D. 18
    E. 6

ANSWERS

1. **Answer: B.** Mental retardation is characterized by (1) significantly below-average intellectual functioning with an IQ of 70 or below, (2) onset before 18 years of age, and (3) significant limitations in adaptive functioning in at least two of the following skill areas: communication, self-care, home living, social interpersonal skills, use of community resources, self-direction, functional academic skills, work, leisure, health, and safety. Mental illness may or may not be present.

2. **Answer: C.** Moderate mental retardation accounts for about 10% of the total mental retardation population. Most individuals with this level of mental retardation acquire communication skills during early childhood years and benefit from vocational training. During adolescence, their difficulties in recognizing social conventions may interfere with peer relationships. In their adult years, the majority are able to perform unskilled or semiskilled work under supervision in shelter workshops or in the general workforce. They have the approximate mental age of a 9-year-old child.

3. **Answer: A.** Mild mental retardation is characterized by an IQ of 55 to 70. These individuals account for about 85% of the population with mental retardation. They typically develop social and communication skills during preschool years, have minimal impairment in sensorimotor areas, and are often not distinguishable from children without mental retardation until a later age. By their late teens, they can acquire academic skills up to approximately the sixth grade level. During their adult years, they usually achieve social and vocational skills adequate for self-support. Some may need supervision, guidance, and assistance, however, especially when under unusual social or economic stress. With appropriate support, individuals with mild mental retardation can usually live successfully in the community either independently or in supervised settings.

4. **Answer: E.** Mental retardation is associated with various other physical and mental health problems. All of the conditions mentioned are seen more often in individuals with mental retardation. Psychiatric conditions such as ADHD, anxiety disorders, and psychosis are also more common in individuals with mental retardation than in the general population.

5. **Answer: C.** The prevalence of seizure disorder in individuals with mental retardation varies with the severity of mental retardation. Those with mild mental retardation have a prevalence of 15% to 20%, whereas those with severe mental retardation have a prevalence of 30% to 50%.

6. **Answer: B.** Down's syndrome is the most common cause of mental retardation in the general population. The risk of Down's syndrome increases with increasing maternal age. Fragile X syndrome is the most common inherited cause of mental retardation.

7. **Answer: A.** Fragile X syndrome is the most common inherited cause of mental retardation.

8. **Answer: C.** Down's syndrome is characterized by short stature, brachy-cephaly, epicanthic folds, Brushfield spots, single palmar crease, high arched palate, protruded tongue, syndactyly, short hands, and atlantoaxial instability. These individuals often develop dementia in their early 40s.

9. **Answer: E.** Fragile X syndrome accounts for half of all the X-linked mental retardation cases. The genetic abnormalities are caused by an abnormal trinucleotide CGG repeat at a fragile site on the X chromosome. People with Fragile X syndrome have a short stature, macro-orchidism, large head, high arched palate, hyperextensible joints, flat feet, inguinal and hiatal hernia, enlarged aortic root, and mitral valve prolapse. Seizures may be seen in up to 25% of individuals. Cat-like cry is a feature of cri-du-chat syndrome caused by deletion of the short arm on chromosome 5.

10. **Answer: C.** The main features of Prader-Willi syndrome are hypotonia, hypogonadism, hypomentia, and obesity. The majority of these individuals have mild-to-moderate mental retardation and develop hyperphagia between the age of 1 and 4 years. They also have small hands and feet, cleft palate, incurved foot, congenital hip dislocation, scoliosis, heart disease, and deafness. Hypersexual behavior is not a feature of Prader-Willi syndrome.

11. **Answer: D.** Rett syndrome is exclusively seen in females. After 1 to 2 years of age, a normally developing child begins to slow or regress and develops unusual characteristic hand movements. Loss of developmental skill occurs, and head growth decelerates. As individuals with Rett syndrome approach adolescence, they develop increased spasticity, scoliosis, bruxism, hyperventilation, sleep apnea, and seizures.

12. **Answer: C.** Lesch-Nyhan syndrome is an X-linked recessive condition. It is characterized by hypertonia, spasticity, ataxia, and choreoathetosis. Most of the affected children have severe mental retardation, and half develop seizures. Microcephaly and macrognathia may be present. Individuals with this syndrome also show physical and verbal aggression, and about 80% to 90% of those affected have self-mutilating behavior.

13. **Answer: C.** The essential features of Asperger's syndrome are significant impairments in social interaction and the development of restricted, repetitive patterns of behavior, interests, and activities. Affected individuals often exhibit an eccentric social lifestyle. Certain aspects of communication may become deviant over time, for example, with poor prosody and unusual rate of speech. Cognitive functions are often characterized by areas of relative strengths (auditory and verbal skills and rote learning), and weakness (visuomotor and visuoperceptual skills).

14. **Answer: D.** Although mental retardation is associated with a high incidence of other mental health problems, anorexia nervosa is very rare in mental retardation.

15. **Answer: B.** Seizure disorder in individuals with mental retardation is common. It is often difficult to control and may need polypharmacy. The seizures per se rarely result in violence, and over a period of time, comorbid seizure disorders can accelerate the intellectual deterioration in patients with mental retardation. Seizure disorder in mental retardation is not frequently associated with schizophrenia-like psychosis.

16. **Answer: E.** A wide variety of conditions can cause a loss of acquired skills, and patients present with the symptoms mentioned. Some of the common causes for this presentation include depression, psychosis, anxiety, hypothyroidism, dementia, and hearing loss.

17. **Answer: D.** Children with mental retardation may not disclose sexual abuse because of inability to verbalize their experiences, lack of understanding, or fear. They are at high risk of sexual abuse compared to children with normal intelligence. People with mental retardation do benefit from supportive psychotherapy and should not be discouraged from talking about their abusive experiences.

18. **Answer: C.** Sexual abuse of children with mental retardation is common and can present as an increase in disruptive behavior, stereotyped movements, depression, or anxiety. It can also result in regression of abilities and sophisticated or new sexual behaviors. The presentation is very different in children with mental retardation because of their limited ability to understand and verbalize.

19. **Answer: C.** Depression in individuals with mental retardation may present with an increase in self-injurious behavior, tearfulness, psychomotor retardation, self-absorption, loss of interest in usual activities, as well as sleep and appetite disturbance. They do not usually complain of depressed mood or anhedonia. Euphoria is suggestive of hypomania or mania.

20. **Answer: E.** Different interviewing techniques have to be used in people with mental retardation. The interview should begin with open questions, and sometimes, more than one or two sessions is required. Collateral information from more than one source is sometimes required. It is sometimes helpful for patients to write or draw their feelings.

21. **Answer: C.** In the treatment of aggressive behavior in mental retardation, a multidisciplinary approach has been found to be the best method. It can be done both as an inpatient or outpatient, and a combination of pharmacotherapy and behavioral intervention is most helpful. Treatment should focus on the underlying etiology, and pharmacotherapy has a very useful role in treatment.

22. **Answer: C.** Some patients with Asperger's syndrome have problems with motor coordination. Verbal deficits are more common than nonverbal deficits, and patients have limited social skills. Relatives of individuals with Asperger's syndrome are not at increased risk of schizophrenia.

23. **Answer: E.** Asperger's syndrome is much more common than autism and is thought to affect one in 200 individuals. Genetics is thought to play a role because of a higher incidence of Asperger-like symptoms in first-degree relatives. Asperger's syndrome is sometimes difficult to distinguish from autism, especially high-functioning autism. Asperger's syndrome is a life-long disorder.

24. **Answer: E.** Neurofibrillary tangles, which are formed by hyperphosphorylation of tau protein is one of the characteristic features of Alzheimer's disease. Almost all individuals with Down's syndrome are found to have neurofibrillary tangles by the age of 50.

25. **Answer: A.** Down's syndrome is a chromosomal abnormality characterized by the presence of an extra copy of genetic material on chromosome 21, either in full (Trisomy 21) or part.

CHAPTER

24

Consultation-Liaison Psychiatry

QUESTIONS

1. A 45-year-old female admitted to a general medical unit is found to be anxious and has tremors. A psychiatry and neurology consultation is requested. The consultation teams suspect hyperthyroidism as the cause of both anxiety and tremors. What is the most common cause of hyperthyroidism?
   A. Hashimoto's disease
   B. Grave's disease
   C. Administration of exogenous thyroid
   D. Thyroid-stimulating hormone (TSH) secreting pituitary adenoma

2. Mental health problems are not uncommon in rehabilitation patients. What is the most common reason for psychiatric consultation in rehabilitation medicine?
   A. Anxiety
   B. Pain
   C. Depression
   D. Psychosis
   E. Posttraumatic stress disorder

3. Cortisol has a significant impact on mood, and Cushing's syndrome is often associated with psychiatric disturbances. What is the most common psychiatric manifestation in patients with Cushing's syndrome?
   A. Mania
   B. Psychosis
   C. Anxiety
   D. Panic attacks
   E. Depression

4. What is the most common psychiatric condition seen in patients with hyperparathyroidism?

   A. Mania
   B. Depression
   C. Psychosis
   D. Anxiety
   E. Panic attacks

5. Which of the following percentages represent the most likely prevalence of psychiatric problems in patients with diabetes mellitus?

   A. 50%
   B. 30% to 70%
   C. 20%
   D. 80%
   E. 100%

6. Which of the following is NOT a psychiatric manifestation of hyperthyroidism?

   A. Depression
   B. Anxiety
   C. Psychosis
   D. Opiate dependence
   E. Cognitive impairment

7. A 56-year-old male with inflammatory bowel disease is prescribed a course of steroids. She is reluctant to take them, however, because one of her friends "became crazy and was admitted to the hospital" after taking steroids for rheumatoid arthritis. All of the following are associated with increased risk of psychiatric problems with steroid treatment except:

   A. male gender
   B. higher dose
   C. longer duration of therapy
   D. previous psychiatric illness
   E. depressed mood

8. Which of the following is TRUE regarding selective serotonin reuptake inhibitors (SSRIs) in premenstrual dysphoric disorder (PMDD)?

    A. They cannot be combined with hormonal treatments.
    B. They are poorly tolerated by patients with PMDD.
    C. They inhibit ovulation.
    D. They can be used exclusively in the luteal phase.
    E. They have fewer side effects in premenstrual dysphoric disorder.

9. Vitamin B_{12} deficiency is implicated in a variety of disorders. All of the following are true about vitamin B_{12} deficiency except:

    A. macrocytic anemia
    B. strongly associated with depression
    C. polyneuropathy
    D. dementia
    E. memory impairment

10. Wilson's disease is characterized by both neurologic and psychiatric symptoms. All of the following are true about Wilson's disease except:

    A. cognitive impairment
    B. autosomal dominant disorder
    C. seizures
    D. changes in personality
    E. rigidity and dystonia

11. According to the *Diagnostic and Statistical Manual of Mental Disorders*, 4th edition (DSM-IV) criteria, all of the following are features of PMDD except:

    A. pelvic discomfort
    B. irritability
    C. symptoms begin soon after menstruation
    D. carbohydrate craving
    E. symptoms present for 2 consecutive months

12. Which of the following is true about PMDD?

    A. It has a prevalence of 30%.
    B. PMDD indicates abnormal ovarian function.
    C. Symptoms are more severe in middle-aged women.
    D. It is linked to abnormal serotonergic function.
    E. It is not associated with sexual abuse.

13. Porphyria disorders are characterized by neurologic and psychiatric manifestations, and the diagnosis is often a challenge unless the clinician has a high index of suspicion. All of the following are true of porphyria disorders except:

    A. peripheral neuropathy may be seen
    B. elevated ceruloplasmin is diagnostic
    C. benzodiazepines may be used for treatment
    D. symptoms may sometimes resemble schizophrenia
    E. acute intermittent porphyria is the most common form

14. Prion disorders are characterized by a variety of neuropsychiatric features. Which of the following is true about prion disorders?

    A. They are more common in men than women.
    B. Patients have a normal electroencephalogram (EEG) reading.
    C. The onset of Creutzfeldt-Jakob disease (CJD) is typically in adolescence.
    D. Human prion disorders are always inherited.
    E. The familial form is autosomal recessive.

15. Patients with end-stage renal disease (ESRD) are at a high risk of psychiatric disorders and often present a challenge regarding diagnosis and management. All of the following are true in patients with ESRD undergoing dialysis except:

    A. adjustment disorder can lead to behavioral problems
    B. major depression is the most common psychiatric diagnosis
    C. adjustment disorders can influence physical outcome
    D. restless legs are common
    E. lack of energy and insomnia are less indicative of depression than in nondialysis patients

16. Which of the following is NOT true about cognitive therapy in hospital consultation-liaison settings?

    A. It helps with cognitive restructuring.
    B. It helps modify negative automatic thoughts about physical illness.
    C. It helps patients regain control of their illness.
    D. It tries to explore the psychodynamic issues.
    E. Empathy is an important aspect.

17. Depression is characterized by both biological and psychological symptoms. Patients with medical illness often have certain symptoms that are also noticed in depression. Which of the following is NOT useful in diagnosing depression in the patient on a medical inpatient unit?
    A. Hopelessness
    B. Inappropriate guilt feelings
    C. Depressed mood
    D. Sleep disturbance
    E. Suicidal thoughts

18. Psychiatric disorders are more common in patients with diabetes mellitus than in the general population. All of the following are true in patients with diabetes mellitus except:
    A. treatment of comorbid psychiatric conditions leads to better outcomes
    B. SSRIs cause severe hyperglycemia
    C. lithium has been used safely in patients without renal disease
    D. sodium valproate can give false-positive urine tests for glucose
    E. amitriptyline is sometimes used in the treatment of diabetic neuropathy

19. A majority of the psychotropic medications are metabolized in the liver, and therefore, psychiatric treatment in patients with hepatic failure presents with unique challenges. Which of the following statements is true regarding the treatment of depression in hepatic disease?
    A. Fluoxetine is not cleared by hepatic enzymes.
    B. Lithium is the mood stabilizer of choice in the presence of hepatic failure.
    C. SSRIs are contraindicated in liver disease.
    D. Paroxetine causes minimal inhibition of hepatic enzymes.
    E. Half-lives of drugs are reduced in liver disease.

20. Delirium in hospital settings is associated with increased morbidity and mortality rates. Which of the following is true about delirium?
    A. It rarely involves mood symptoms.
    B. It includes a narrow range of psychiatric symptoms.
    C. Clouding of consciousness is sufficient for the diagnosis.
    D. Attention disturbance is the core cognitive disturbance.
    E. The sleep-wake cycle is preserved.

21. Delirium, characterized by waxing and waning of consciousness can present in hyperactive/agitated and hypoactive forms. Which of the following is true of hypoactive delirium?
    A. Psychotic symptoms are rare.
    B. Poor response to antipsychotics
    C. Frequently missed in practice
    D. Better prognosis than agitated delirium
    E. The patient is commonly unarousable.

22. All of the following are true regarding delirium except:
    A. iatrogenic delirium is common
    B. involvement of the patient and relatives in the management should be encouraged
    C. more common in the elderly
    D. not associated with higher morbidity and mortality rates after discharge from the hospital
    E. reduction of risk factors can prevent further episodes

23. Wernicke's encephalopathy is characterized by all of the following except:
    A. gait ataxia
    B. ophthalmoplegia
    C. memory loss out of proportion relative to other cognitive impairments
    D. confusion

24. All of the following are true about Korsakoff's syndrome except:
    A. it can be caused by continuous vomiting
    B. chronic alcoholism is a common cause
    C. memory loss out of proportion relative to other cognitive impairments
    D. clouding of consciousness is characteristic
    E. immediate memory is preserved

25. Human immunodeficiency virus (HIV) infection can cause a variety of physical, neurological, and mental symptoms. It can manifest itself as all of the following except:
    A. hypomania
    B. Alzheimer's disease
    C. depression
    D. panic attacks
    E. schizophreniform psychosis

26. All of the following are true regarding HIV encephalopathy except:

   A. symptoms of subcortical dementia
   B. depressive symptoms
   C. movement disorders
   D. well-demarcated, asymmetrical lesions in the brain
   E. memory and psychomotor speed impairment

27. Which of the following statements is TRUE about suicide in medically ill patients?

   A. Most terminally ill patients develop a psychiatric disorder.
   B. Most terminally ill patients are at risk of suicide.
   C. Anger is an important factor in suicide.
   D. Mental illness is not common in patients who commit suicide.
   E. Suicide in medically ill patients is not preventable.

28. One of the most important questions psychiatrists ask a patient is about past history of suicide attempt. The risk of completed suicide in a person who has made a previous suicide attempt is:

   A. two times higher
   B. 25 times higher
   C. 50 times higher
   D. 100 times higher
   E. 75 times higher

29. Confidentiality is an important aspect of any doctor-patient relationship, and it is more important when it comes to mental health services. Which of the following is NOT an exception to confidentiality between a psychiatrist and the patient?

   A. Child abuse
   B. Danger to self or others
   C. Intent to commit a crime
   D. Communication with other physicians not involved in the care of the patient
   E. Competency procedures

30. The neurology team requests a psychiatric consultation for competency on a 56-year-old male with suspected depression and cognitive impairment. Which of the following statements is true regarding competency?
    A. Most depressed patients are incompetent.
    B. Cognitively impaired patients do not have the capacity to make decisions.
    C. Competency is a clinical determination.
    D. Capacity and competency are the same.
    E. Capacity to consent is issue and situation specific.

31. Which of the following is true regarding advance directives?
    A. Advance directives are a means for making future health care decisions in the event of incompetence.
    B. Power of attorney is valid even if the person becomes incompetent.
    C. Durable power of attorney does not empower an agent to make decisions even if the principal becomes incompetent.
    D. Healthcare proxy is illegal.

32. Seclusion and restraint, although undesirable, are sometimes used when absolutely necessary. Which the following is not an indication to the use of seclusion and restraint?
    A. To prevent harm to the patient or others
    B. Staff shortages
    C. To assist in treatment
    D. To prevent significant disruption to the treatment program
    E. To decrease sensory stimulation

33. All of the following are true about depression associated with medical illness except:
    A. earlier age of onset
    B. no increased rates of family history of depression
    C. no increased rates of alcoholism in family members
    D. less likely to result in suicide
    E. good response to treatment

34. Patients with strokes are thought to be at a higher risk of depression and other psychiatric problems. Depression following stroke is more likely to be associated with a lesion in which of the following regions of the brain?

    A. Left occipital
    B. Left temporal
    C. Left frontal
    D. Right parietal
    E. Right frontal

35. Dementia affects 20% to 30% of patients with AIDS. What type of dementia is typically seen in patients with AIDS?

    A. Alzheimer's dementia
    B. Subcortical dementia
    C. Lewy body dementia
    D. Infectious dementia
    E. Vascular dementia

36. What is the most common neuropsychiatric complication seen in hospitalized patients with AIDS?

    A. Depression
    B. Dementia
    C. Psychosis
    D. Mania
    E. Delirium

37. Which of the following is commonly seen in AIDS dementia complex?

    A. Psychosis
    B. Aphasia
    C. Agnosia
    D. Word-finding difficulties
    E. Steady gait

38. Substance abuse is frequently seen in individuals with HIV infection. Use of which of the following is associated with high HIV risk behaviors?

    A. Marijuana
    B. Alcohol
    C. Lysergic acid diethylamide (LSD)
    D. Crack cocaine

39. Electroconvulsive therapy (ECT) is a well-established, safe, and effective treatment for depression. Which of the following is also true about ECT?

    A. It can be administered to patients with epilepsy.
    B. It is contraindicated in patients with Parkinson's disease.
    C. Seizures are the most common cause of death in patients who undergo ECT.
    D. The use of bilateral electrodes reduces the risk of cognitive deficits.
    E. ECT is contraindicated in catatonia.

40. A 56-year-old obese male admitted to the medical unit for exacerbation of asthma is found to wake up several times at night gasping for air. He also reports daytime sleepiness and fatigue. The nurse reports that at night, the patient snored loudly, and his oxygen saturation dropped to the low 60s, and when she woke him up, the saturations went back to the low 90s. What is the most likely diagnosis in this patient?

    A. Exacerbation of asthma at night
    B. Sleep apnea
    C. Nightmare disorder
    D. Obesity hypoventilation syndrome
    E. Periodic limb movement disorder

41. A 76-year-old male admitted to the neurology inpatient unit for further assessment and stroke management is found to be screaming in the middle of the night. He could not recognize the nursing staff or the on-call resident and appears to be confused. He mistakes the resident's stethoscope to be a snake and tries to run away from his room. The resident believes that the patient is delirious and tries to calm down the patient's wife who is scared. Which of the following is affected in delirium?

    A. Attention
    B. Consciousness
    C. Perception
    D. Cognition
    E. All of the above

42. A 64-year-old male admitted to the hospital for a hip replacement procedure ends up with renal failure. He develops complications and is found to be delirious. Even after 3 weeks of intensive care by the treatment team, he continues to be confused and misperceives things. What is the percentage of patients who have delirium for more than 1 month?
    A. 5%
    B. 10%
    C. 15%
    D. 20%
    E. 50%

43. All of the following can aggravate delirium except:
    A. clock in the room
    B. hearing impairment
    C. visual impairment
    D. quiet environment
    E. similar environment regardless of the time of the day

44. Which of the following statements is true about the use of benzodiazepines in the management of delirium?
    A. It is the treatment of choice for delirium related to alcohol or benzodiazepine withdrawal.
    B. Few controlled studies have evaluated the efficacy of benzodiazepines as a monotherapy in general cases of delirium.
    C. The combination of intravenous haloperidol and benzodiazepine is more effective than either of the drugs on their own.
    D. Benzodiazepines alone can worsen delirium in some elderly patients.
    E. All of the above

45. Which of the following statements is true about delirium?
    A. ECT can cause delirium.
    B. Anticholinergic medications have been implicated as a cause of delirium.
    C. Intravenous haloperidol results in fewer extrapyramidal side effects compared to oral or intramuscular administration.
    D. Benzodiazepines are contraindicated in cases of delirium associated with hepatic insufficiency.
    E. All of the above

46. All of the following are true about delirium in the elderly except:
    A. delirium is more common in the elderly
    B. low doses of antipsychotics are recommended in the treatment of delirium in elderly
    C. medications with anticholinergic side effects often cause delirium in the elderly
    D. nursing home patients are at increased risk of delirium
    E. All of the above

ANSWERS

1. **Answer: B.** Graves' disease is the most common cause of hyperthyroidism. Hashimoto's disease causes hypothyroidism and not hyperthyroidism. A hyperthyroid state resulting from excess administration of exogenous thyroid hormone preparation is not uncommon. TSH-secreting pituitary adenoma is very rare.

2. **Answer: C.** Studies have found that depression is very common in patients who are in rehabilitation, and it is also one of the most common reasons for psychiatric consultation. Depression in rehabilitation patients is associated with longer duration of stay as well as delay in resumption of premorbid social and occupational activities.

3. **Answer: E.** The most common psychiatric manifestation in patients with Cushing's syndrome is depression. Cushing's syndrome refers to a diverse symptom complex resulting from excess steroid hormone production by the adrenal cortex or excessive administration of exogenous glucocorticoids. Depression is very common and is seen in up to 50% of patients with Cushing's syndrome. Some patients also have symptoms of mania and psychosis.

4. **Answer: B.** Hyperparathyroidism is characterized by hypercalcemia. Depression is common in patients with hypercalcemia. Symptoms become worse as the hypercalcemia levels increase. At calcium levels of more than 50 mg/dL, delirium, psychosis, and cognitive impairment are seen.

5. **Answer: B.** About 30% to 70% of patients with diabetes mellitus have psychiatric disorders including anxiety, depression, and substance use.

6. **Answer: D.** Hyperthyroidism is associated with a wide variety of psychiatric manifestations including anxiety, depression, psychosis, and cognitive impairment. The majority of patients who present with depression and anxiety secondary to hyperthyroidism will experience a resolution of symptoms once hyperthyroidism is treated. Although subjects with anxiety disorders and other psychiatric disorders often abuse opiates, opiate dependence is not known to be associated with hyperthyroidism.

7. **Answer: A.** Psychiatric disorders with steroid use are more likely to be associated with female gender, high doses of steroids, longer treatment duration, previous history of any psychiatric illness, and depressed mood.

8. **Answer: D.** Most SSRIs have been shown to be effective in the treatment of PMDD. Some SSRIs, given in the latter half of the cycle, have been found to be as effective as continuous daily dosing. Many of the SSRIs can be combined with other hormonal treatments, and the side effects of SSRIs in PMDD are not different from side effects noticed when SSRIs are used to treat depression or anxiety. SSRIs are not found to inhibit ovulation.

9. **Answer: B.** Vitamin B_{12} deficiency can cause macrocytosis, polyneuropathy, dementia, and memory impairment. Its association with depression is not established.

10. **Answer: B.** Wilson's disease is a rare autosomal recessive disorder. It is characterized by the excessive deposition of copper in the tissues, mainly in the liver and brain. The neurological features are related to basal ganglia dysfunction and include resting, postural, or kinetic tremor as well as rigidity and dystonia of the bulbar musculature with dysarthria and dysphagia. Psychiatric features include behavioral and personality changes and emotional problems. The pathognomonic sign is the golden-brown or orange Kayser-Fleischer ring in the cornea caused by copper deposition in Descemet's membrane.

11. **Answer: C.** The DSM-IV criteria for diagnosing PMDD include prospective documentation of physical and behavioral symptoms (using diaries) being present for most of the preceding year. Five or more of the following symptoms must have been present during the week prior to menses, resolving within a few days after menses starts. At least one of the five symptoms must be one of the first four on this list: (1) feeling sad, hopeless, or self-deprecating; (2) feeling tense, anxious, or "on edge"; (3) marked lability of mood interspersed with frequent tearfulness; (4) persistent irritability, anger, and increased interpersonal conflicts; (5) decreased interest in usual activities, which may be associated with withdrawal from social relationships; (6) difficulty concentrating; (7) feeling fatigued, lethargic, or lacking in energy; (8) marked changes in appetite, which may be associated with binge eating or craving certain foods; (9) hypersomnia or insomnia; (10) a subjective feeling of being overwhelmed or out of control; and (11) other physical symptoms, such as breast tenderness or swelling, headaches, joint or muscle pain, a sensation of bloating, and weight gain.

12. **Answer: D.** A number of studies have shown an association between serotonin dysfunction and PMDD. Estimates of prevalence of PMDD vary between 4% to 7%. The presence of PMDD does not indicate abnormal ovarian function, and women with PMDD show no consistent differences in basal levels of ovarian hormones. Younger age and low education levels have been associated with more severe symptoms of PMDD. Past sexual abuse is reported by a significant proportion of woman seeking treatment for PMDD.

13. **Answer: B.** intermittent porphyria is the most common form of this disorder. It is an autosomal dominant condition. Many drugs including barbiturates, carbamazepine, tricyclic antidepressants, phenytoin and valproic acid may precipitate the attacks. Patients present with abdominal pain, autonomic and peripheral neuropathy, seizures, and psychosis. Benzodiazepines are generally considered to be safe for use in porphyria, and elevated ceruloplasmin levels are associated with Wilson's disease.

14. **Answer: A.** Prion disorders, also known as subacute spongiform encephalopathies, are associated with the accumulation in the brain of abnormal partially protease-resistant glycoprotein known as prion protein. The human prion diseases can be inherited, sporadic, and acquired forms.

    CJD is a rapidly progressive dementia with myoclonus. It usually affects people 45 to 75 years of age. The clinical progression typically occurs over weeks, progressing to akinetic mutism and death within about 2 to 3 months. Patients with progressive dementia and two or more of the symptoms of myoclonus, cortical blindness, pyramidal, cerebellar, or extrapyramidal signs or akinetic mutism, in the setting of an EEG finding of pseudoperiodic sharp wave activity nearly always have CJD.

    The familial form of prion disease, called Gerstmann-Sträussler-Scheinker disease, has an onset in the third and fourth decades of life and is characterized by cerebellar ataxia with pyramidal features and dementia. It is an autosomal dominant disorder.

15. **Answer: B.** The most common psychiatric diagnoses in patients with ESRD and undergoing dialysis are adjustment disorders (30%), mood disorders (24%), and organic mental disorders. Symptoms useful in identifying major depressive disorders are low mood, reduced interest in usual activities, worthlessness, hopelessness, excess guilt, anorexia, weight-loss, and psychomotor retardation. Symptoms that are not found to be helpful in making a diagnosis of depression are lack of energy, insomnia, and reduced libido as these are very common in patients with ESRD.

16. **Answer: D.** Cognitive therapy can be used to treat psychological problems related to physical illness in hospital settings. Studies have shown that as patients perceive themselves as having no control in a situation, it is more likely they will be depressed. One of the important requirements is that the therapist should be empathetic and understand patients' perception of problems. Cognitive therapy aims to improve patients' sense of control over their physical state and educate them in techniques that can be used to deal with future problems. Cognitive therapy focuses more on "here and now" rather than exploring psychodynamic issues.

17. **Answer: D.** Depression is sometimes difficult to diagnose in patients with physical illness. Depressed mood, hopelessness, inappropriate guilt feelings, and suicidal thoughts are more suggestive of depression. Other symptoms such as sleep disturbances, anorexia, lethargy, and psychomotor retardation, although common in depression, can also be the result of physical illness.

18. **Answer: B.** Psychiatric disorders are common in patients with diabetes mellitus, and treatment of comorbid psychiatric conditions leads to better outcomes. There are reports of SSRIs sometimes causing hypoglycemia and not hyperglycemia. All the other statements are true.

19. **Answer: B.** The majority of the psychotropic medications are metabolized in the liver, and therefore, psychiatric treatment in patients with hepatic failure presents with unique challenges. Fluoxetine and paroxetine cause significant inhibition of CYP 450 2D6 enzymes and both are cleared by hepatic enzymes. The other SSRIs (citalopram, sertraline, and escitalopram) cause relatively less inhibition of hepatic CYP 450 enzymes. For drugs that are metabolized by the liver, the half-lives are increased and not decreased. Lithium is often considered as the mood stabilizer of choice in patients with hepatic failure because it is cleared almost entirely by the kidneys.

20. **Answer: D.** Delirium is characterized by waxing and waning of consciousness. Impaired attention is considered to be the core cognitive disturbance. In addition, most patients experience disturbances of memory, orientation, language, mood, thinking, perception, motor behavior, and the sleep-wake cycle. Although individual delirium symptoms are nonspecific, their pattern is highly characteristic with acute onset, fluctuant course, and transient nature. Delirium is common in general hospital settings with a point prevalence of 10% to 30%. It is more frequent in older patients and those with pre-existing cognitive impairment and medical or surgical problems.

21. **Answer: C.** Although delirium is common in patients admitted to the hospital, the diagnosis is frequently missed, causing increased morbidity and mortality. Cases of hypoactive delirium are more likely to be missed because they are not disruptive like agitated delirium patients. The prognosis of patients with hypoactive delirium is poorer than those with agitated delirium, and patients are usually arousable, although they are lethargic. Psychotic symptoms are common and respond well to antipsychotics and the treatment of the underlying condition.

22. **Answer: D.** Delirium results in longer hospital stays, reduced independence after discharge, and increased morbidity and mortality. Involvement of relatives and patients should be encouraged, as it has shown to decrease the severity of delirium. Iatrogenic causes are common in the etiology of delirium, and reducing risk factors is helpful in preventing further episodes of delirium.

23. **Answer: C.** Wernicke's encephalopathy is characterized by confusion, gait ataxia, and ophthalmoplegia. Memory loss out of proportion relative to other cognitive impairments is a feature of Korsakoff's syndrome. In 1881, Carl Wernicke described this condition that was associated with autopsy findings of punctate hemorrhages around the third and fourth ventricles and the aqueduct. It results from deficiency of vitamin B_1 (thiamine).

24. **Answer: D.** Korsakoff's syndrome is caused by thymine deficiency, which can be secondary to a variety of conditions including chronic alcohol abuse, continuous vomiting, and anorexia nervosa. The patients are not disorientated and retain a clear consciousness. Immediate memory is preserved, but learning over more prolonged periods is severely impaired. There is usually a retrograde memory loss, which characteristically extends back many years. Memory loss out of proportion relative to other cognitive impairments is a striking feature.

25. **Answer: B.** HIV infection can present as dementia, but Alzheimer's disease is a distinct type of dementia, and it is not caused by HIV infection.

26. **Answer: D.** HIV encephalopathy is characterized by symmetrical and less well-demarcated lesions in the brain. All the other features listed are seen in HIV encephalopathy.

27. **Answer: C.** The majority of terminally ill patients do not develop depressive disorder and suicidal ideation. Most of them are able to cope. Anger is an important factor in suicide. Suicides in medically ill patients are often associated with other unrecognized psychiatric conditions (mainly depression). Suicide is preventable, and its causes are treatable.

28. **Answer: E.** History of suicide attempts is an important predictor of future suicide. One of every 100 suicide-attempt survivors will die by suicide within 1 year of their index attempt. Of those who complete suicide, 25% to 50% would have attempted suicide in the past.

29. **Answer: D.** Once the doctor-patient relationship is established, the clinician assumes a duty to safeguard the patient's interests and do everything that is good for the patient. This duty is not absolute, however, and in some circumstances, breaking confidentiality is both ethical and legal.

30. **Answer: E.** The presence of mental illness or cognitive impairment does not necessarily render a person incompetent. Competency is a legal decision, whereas capacity is a clinical determination. Capacity to consent is issue and situation specific. Patients should be examined to determine whether specific functional incapacities render the person incapable of making a particular kind of decision or performing a particular type of task.

31. **Answer: A.** Advanced directives provide a method for individuals, while competent, to choose alternative health care decision makers in the event of future incompetence. An ordinary power of attorney becomes null and void if the person becomes incompetent. Durable power of attorney empowers an agent to make decisions even if the principal becomes incompetent. The health care proxy is a legal instrument akin to the durable power of attorney, but it is specifically created for the delegation of health care decisions.

32. **Answer: B.** Restraints and seclusion are appropriate when a patient presents a risk of harm to him or herself or others and when less restrictive alternatives are ineffective. They are also sometimes used to assist in treatment and to decrease sensory stimulation in an agitated patient. However, staff shortage is not a valid indication for seclusion or patient restraint.

33. **Answer: A.** Depression secondary to medical illness is more likely to begin at a later age in response to the medical illness. It is less likely to be associated with a family history of alcoholism or depression (compared to patients with endogenous depression), and individuals respond well to treatment.

34. **Answer: C.** The association between lesion location and depression following a stroke is controversial. Some studies support the contention that the risk of depression is higher the closer the lesion is to the left frontal pole, and left anterior frontal lesions are most likely associated with depression. There is also evidence that left frontal cortical and left basal ganglial strokes produce depression to a greater degree than do lesions elsewhere in the brain.

35. **Answer: B.** The dementia associated with AIDS is typically a subcortical dementia with difficulties regarding attention, concentration, and psychomotor impairment. Alzheimer's dementia is a distinct type of dementia, and Lewy body dementia is seen in Parkinson's disease.

36. **Answer: E.** Delirium is the neuropsychiatric complication that occurs most frequently in hospitalized patients with AIDS. Patients with advanced systemic disease and HIV dementia are at a higher risk for delirium. In the management of delirium, the primary goal is identification and treatment of underlying factors that can cause or exacerbate delirium.

37. **Answer: D.** AIDS dementia complex (ADC) is characterized by cognitive, affective, behavioral, and motor dysfunction. Patients describe short-term memory loss, word finding difficulties, and difficulty with sequential tasks. They also report depressed mood, social withdrawal, and reduced energy. They also have problems with movement, clumsiness, and gait disturbances. Aphasia and agnosia are rare, and psychosis is seen more often in patients with end-stage AIDS dementia complex.

38. **Answer: D.** Substance abuse-related disorders occur frequently in patients with HIV disease. The prevalence of substance abuse-related disorders in ambulatory patients with HIV referred for psychiatric evaluations may be as high as 45%. Psychoactive drugs impair judgment and may lead to risky behaviors that increase the risk of HIV infection. Crack cocaine and inhalant abuse are more commonly associated with high HIV risk behaviors.

39. **Answer: A.** Patients with concurrent psychiatric illness and epilepsy may be safely treated with ECT. Patients should continue to receive their anticonvulsant medication during ECT, and higher stimulus settings are typically necessary. ECT is effective for the mood and motor symptoms in patients with Parkinson's disease. Cardiac complications are the most common cause of death in patients who undergo ECT. The use of unilateral electrodes is associated with reduced cognitive deficits. ECT is not contraindicated in patients with catatonia, and it is in fact sometimes used as first-line treatment in these individuals.

40. **Answer: B.** The history is very typical for obstructive sleep apnea syndrome (obesity, snoring, waking up gasping for air, and oxygen desaturation while asleep). Obesity hypoventilation syndrome is not associated with snoring unless there is comorbid sleep apnea. Nightmare disorder is not associated with snoring, and patients wake up with anxiety and panic and remember the dreams. Periodic limb movement disorder is characterized by leg jerks that may or may not awaken the patient at night, and if it were to be exacerbation of asthma, the patient's oxygen levels would still be low even after he wakes up and last until the asthma is treated.

41. **Answer: E.** The essential features of delirium include disturbances of consciousness, attention, cognition, and perception. The disturbance develops over a short period of time (usually hours to days) and tends to fluctuate during the course of the day.

42. **Answer: C.** In approximately 15% of patients, delirium lasts for more than a month. Chronic delirium is more common in the elderly and in patients with multiple medical problems and polypharmacy.

43. **Answer: A.** A clock in the room helps recovery from delirium by orienting the patient to the time. A similar environment regardless of the time of day worsens delirium by promoting disorientation to day/time. Any sensory impairment can worsen delirium. Both quiet and noisy environments are known to exacerbate delirium, and a moderate degree of stimulation helps recovery.

44. **Answer: E.** Although benzodiazepines are often used in the treatment of delirium, there is a paucity of evidence for their use on their own, except in cases of benzodiazepine or alcohol withdrawal. Benzodiazepine in combination with haloperidol has been found to be more efficacious than using either of the medications alone. In the elderly and in subjects with brain injury, benzodiazepines can cause paradoxical agitation leading to worsening of delirium.

45. **Answer: E.** ECT has been used as a treatment for delirium in some cases, but ECT itself is associated with ictal and postictal delirium. Anticholinergic medications can cause delirium, especially in the elderly. Benzodiazepines are generally contraindicated in delirium from hepatic encephalopathy due to accumulation of glutamine, which is related chemically to gamma-aminobutyric acid (GABA).

46. **Answer: E.** Delirium is especially common in the elderly. Occult infections and medications are the common causes of delirium in these patients. Patients in nursing homes, possibly because of suboptimal stimulation, are more likely to develop delirium.

DSM-IV Diagnostic Criteria

QUESTIONS

1. According to the *Diagnostic and Statistical Manual of Mental Disorders*, 4th edition (DSM-IV), all of the following are the characteristic symptoms of schizophrenia except:

   A. hallucinations
   B. disorganized speech
   C. delusions
   D. disorganized behavior
   E. low mood

2. According to the DSM-IV, the duration criterion for the diagnosis of schizophrenia is:

   A. 6 months
   B. 1 month
   C. 3 months
   D. 1 week
   E. 2 months

3. All of the following are features of schizophrenia, disorganized type except:

   A. insidious onset and continuous course
   B. disorganized speech
   C. disorganized behavior
   D. flat or inappropriate affect
   E. prominent delusions and hallucinations

4. According to the DSM-IV, all of the following are recognized features of schizophrenia, catatonic type except:

   A. motor immobility
   B. excessive motor activity
   C. disorganized behavior
   D. echolalia or echopraxia
   E. extreme negativism

5. According to the DSM-IV, the duration criterion for the diagnosis of schizophreniform disorder is:

   A. at least 1 month but less than 6 months
   B. at least 6 months
   C. less than 1 month
   D. more than 12 months
   E. at least 1 week but less than 1 month

6. All of the following are considered to be good prognostic features of schizophrenia except:

   A. prominent psychotic symptoms within 4 weeks of onset of change in behavior
   B. disorganized speech
   C. confusion at the height of psychotic episode
   D. good premorbid functioning
   E. absence of blunted or flat affect

7. According to the DSM-IV, the diagnostic features of schizoaffective disorder include all of the following except:

   A. an uninterrupted period of illness during which there is an episode of mood disorder and characteristic symptoms of schizophrenia
   B. delusions or hallucinations for at least 4 weeks in the absence of prominent mood symptoms
   C. mood episode present for a substantial portion of the total duration of the illness
   D. the disturbance is not caused by substance abuse or a general medical condition
   E. can be specified as bipolar type or depressive type

8. According to the DSM-IV, all of the following are diagnostic features of delusional disorder except:
   A. nonbizarre delusions
   B. duration of at least 3 months
   C. criteria for characteristic symptoms (criterion A) of schizophrenia are never met
   D. apart from the impact of delusions, function is not markedly impaired
   E. duration of mood episodes (if present) is brief relative to the total duration of delusional beliefs

9. According to the DSM-IV, to make a diagnosis of brief psychotic disorder, at least one of the following symptoms has to be present except:
   A. delusions
   B. hallucinations
   C. disorganized speech
   D. disorganized behavior
   E. negative symptoms

10. According to the DSM-IV, which of the following symptoms has to be present to diagnose major depressive disorder?
    A. Depressed mood or loss of interest/pleasure in daily activities
    B. Lack of energy or motivation
    C. Suicide ideation or homicide ideation
    D. Hopelessness or helplessness
    E. Guilt or worthlessness

11. According to the DSM-IV, all of the following symptoms are included in the diagnostic criteria for major depressive disorder except:
    A. depressed mood
    B. suicide ideation
    C. lack of concentration
    D. fatigue
    E. decreased need to sleep

12. According to the DSM-IV, one of the criterion to diagnose major depressive disorder is either significant weight loss or weight gain. A change of more than what percentage is considered to be a significant change in weight?
    A. 10%
    B. 5%
    C. 15%
    D. 7.5%
    E. 20%

13. The symptoms of major depressive disorder and bereavement are often similar. Sometimes, even an experienced clinician might have a problem in distinguishing the two conditions. There are certain clinical features, however, that are not found in bereavement but are often found in patients with major depressive disorder. All of the following are suggestive of major depressive disorder rather than bereavement except:
    A. symptoms lasting for more than 2 months after bereavement
    B. marked functional impairment
    C. worthlessness
    D. helplessness
    E. suicide ideation

14. Major depressive disorder is a common condition with a high recurrence rate. Treatment with antidepressant medication decreases both the frequency and duration of episodes of major depressive disorder. How long does an episode of untreated depression last for?
    A. 12 months
    B. 2 years
    C. 3 months
    D. 6 months or longer
    E. Less than 6 months

15. According to the DSM-IV, the duration criterion for the diagnosis of major depressive disorder is:
    A. 4 weeks
    B. 2 weeks
    C. 8 weeks
    D. 10 weeks
    E. 1 week

16. According to the DSM-IV, the duration criterion (if the patient is not hospitalized) for the diagnosis of a manic episode is:
    A. 4 days
    B. 2 weeks
    C. 4 weeks
    D. 2 days
    E. 1 week

17. According to the DSM-IV, the duration criterion for the diagnosis of a hypomanic episode is:
    A. 10 days
    B. 2 weeks
    C. 4 weeks
    D. 3 months
    E. 4 days

18. According to the DSM-IV, the essential criterion for the diagnosis of a manic episode is:
    A. irritable mood
    B. expansive mood
    C. irritable or expansive mood
    D. grandiosity
    E. flight of ideas

19. According to the DSM-IV, the duration criterion for the diagnosis of dysthymic disorder in adults is:
    A. 2 years
    B. 2 months
    C. 1 year
    D. 2 weeks
    E. 6 months

20. The term *double depression* is often used to indicate:
    A. major depressive disorder lasting for more than 2 years
    B. dysthymic disorder with superimposed episode of major depressive disorder
    C. major depressive disorder not responding to electroconvulsive therapy (ECT)
    D. major depressive disorder with some features of hypomania
    E. major depressive disorder with psychotic features

21. According to the DSM-IV, the diagnostic criteria for bipolar disorder II include all of the following except:
    A. one or more major depressive episodes
    B. at least one hypomanic episode
    C. at least one manic episode
    D. mood symptoms not better accounted for by schizoaffective disorder
    E. course specification

22. According to the DSM-IV, all of the following are the diagnostic features of cyclothymic disorder except:
    A. numerous periods of hypomanic and depressive symptoms for at least 2 years
    B. duration criterion in children and adolescents are at least 1 year
    C. absence of symptoms for no more than 2 months during the 2-year period in adults
    D. at least one major depressive episode
    E. symptoms cause significant distress or impairment

23. According to the DSM-IV, the criterion for rapid cycling as a course specifier for bipolar I or bipolar II disorder is:
    A. at least four episodes of mood disturbance in the previous 12 months
    B. at least four episodes of mood disturbance in 1 month
    C. cycling from depression to mania every month
    D. less than 1 month between each episode of mood disturbance
    E. at least eight episodes of mood disturbance in the previous 12 months

24. According to the DSM-IV, all of the following are diagnostic criteria for the diagnosis of personality disorder except:
    A. an enduring pattern of inner experience and behavior
    B. clinically significant distress or impairment
    C. onset traced to at least adolescence or early adulthood
    D. behavior consistent with the individual's culture
    E. behavior is pervasive

25. Personality disorders are grouped into three clusters based on descriptive similarities. Cluster A includes all of the following except:
    A. schizoaffective
    B. schizoid
    C. paranoid
    D. schizotypal

26. Personality disorders are grouped into three clusters based on descriptive similarities. Cluster B includes all of the following except:
    A. antisocial
    B. borderline
    C. dependent
    D. histrionic
    E. narcissistic

27. Personality disorders are grouped into three clusters based on descriptive similarities. Cluster C includes all of the following except:
    A. avoidant
    B. dependent
    C. obsessive-compulsive
    D. antisocial

28. A 46-year-old male reports to his psychiatrist in distress and frustration. He states that all of his life he has been a victim of untrustworthy friends and feels reluctant to confide in others. He also believes that others are exploiting him, and he would never forgive his family members for the insults he suffered because of them. He also believes that his wife is cheating on him, although he has never found any evidence. A detailed mental status assessment does not reveal any evidence of schizophrenia, mood disorders with psychotic features, or any other psychotic disorders. What is this patient's most likely diagnosis?
    A. Borderline personality disorder
    B. Schizoid personality disorder
    C. Schizotypal personality disorder
    D. Paranoid personality disorder
    E. Obsessive-compulsive personality disorder

29. A 34-year-old male comes in reluctantly to see a psychiatrist because his family believes he has mental illness. The patient, however, thinks that he is fine. The family members report that as long as they remember, the patient has little interest in meeting others, pleasurable activities, or having girlfriends/sexual relationships. He often appears detached, prefers solitary activities, and does not have a desire for close relationships. A detailed mental status assessment does not reveal any evidence of schizophrenia, mood disorders with psychotic features, or any other psychotic disorders. What is this man's most likely diagnosis?

    A. Narcissistic personality disorder
    B. Schizoid personality disorder
    C. Schizotypal personality disorder
    D. Dependent personality disorder
    E. Obsessive-compulsive personality disorder

30. A 40-year-old male is referred from his workplace for a psychiatric evaluation. His colleagues noted him to be "bizarre" and "eccentric, suspicious of others." On assessment, it appears this individual has some ideas of reference and believes in telepathy. His speech was overelaborate and circumstantial. His affect was constricted and his behavior peculiar. He remained anxious and uncomfortable throughout the interview. A detailed mental status assessment did not reveal any evidence of schizophrenia, mood disorders with psychotic features, or any other psychotic disorders. What is this subject's most likely diagnosis?

    A. Narcissistic personality disorder
    B. Schizoid personality disorder
    C. Schizotypal personality disorder
    D. Paranoid personality disorder
    E. Avoidant personality disorder

31. A 28-year-old male is brought in for a psychiatric evaluation by his parents. The parents "cannot understand why he is doing this." They mention that he was doing well until the age of 10 years after which he started getting into trouble for breaking laws. He started lying and became impulsive and aggressive. He has no remorse and a complete disregard for the safety of self and others. A detailed mental status assessment does not reveal any evidence of schizophrenia, mood disorders with psychotic features, or any other psychotic disorders. What is this subject's most likely diagnosis?
    A. Narcissistic personality disorder
    B. Borderline personality disorder
    C. Schizotypal personality disorder
    D. Antisocial personality disorder
    E. Paranoid personality disorder

32. A 24-year-old female comes for a psychiatric evaluation because her husband has threatened her with "the marriage will end if there is no change in behavior." During the evaluation, it appears that she has a pattern of unstable and intense relationships, identity disturbance, and impulsivity. She has made "hundreds of suicide threats" and cut her wrist several times. She feels "empty" most of the time and has difficulty controlling her anger. A detailed mental status assessment does not reveal any evidence of schizophrenia, mood disorders with psychotic features, or any other psychotic disorders. What is the most likely diagnosis in this subject?
    A. Narcissistic personality disorder
    B. Borderline personality disorder
    C. Schizotypal personality disorder
    D. Antisocial personality disorder
    E. Histrionic personality disorder

33. A 36-year-old male comes for a psychiatric evaluation because he believes there is something wrong with him. He joined a new company a few months ago and has been having serious problems with his boss. At his previous workplace, he did not have any problems, and in fact, he was very much liked by everyone. During the evaluation, there was no evidence of any Axis I or Axis II disorder. He describes his boss, Mr. D as "always craving for attention," and others see the boss's interactions with female workers as inappropriate and seductive. Mr. D's speech is impressionistic but lacks details; he dramatizes and exaggerates emotions and is sometimes very suggestible; his emotions are shallow but shift rapidly; and he is very conscious about his physical appearance. What is the most likely diagnosis of his boss's personality?

    A. Narcissistic personality disorder
    B. Borderline personality disorder
    C. Schizotypal personality disorder
    D. Obsessive-compulsive personality disorder
    E. Histrionic personality disorder

34. A 54-year-old male is admitted to the neurology inpatient unit for unexplained weakness in his right arm. Within hours of admission to the unit, the nursing staff, residents, and fellow patients say they have had enough of this patient. The attending neurologist noticed that the patient has an exaggerated sense of self-importance and believes only the "neurology chief, not residents or fellows" should see him. He has unreasonable expectations of everyone and a sense of entitlement. The neurologist suspects an Axis I disorder but did not find any evidence of mood, anxiety, or psychotic disorders. What is the most likely diagnosis in this subject?

    A. Narcissistic personality disorder
    B. Borderline personality disorder
    C. Schizotypal personality disorder
    D. Obsessive-compulsive personality disorder
    E. Histrionic personality disorder

35. A 34-year-old male is brought in for a psychiatric evaluation by his wife because she believes that her husband is a very nice and caring individual but has a lot of social inhibitions and avoids activities that involve interpersonal contacts. He is preoccupied with being criticized by others and feels inadequate. Although he is a good-looking intelligent man, he believes he is socially inept and will not get involved with people unless he is certain of being liked. A detailed mental status assessment does not reveal any evidence of schizophrenia, mood disorders with psychotic features, or any other psychotic disorders. What is the most likely diagnosis in this subject?

A. Paranoid personality disorder
B. Avoidant personality disorder
C. Schizotypal personality disorder
D. Obsessive-compulsive personality disorder
E. Histrionic personality disorder

36. A young couple is seen for marital therapy by a psychiatrist. During the course of therapy, it becomes clear that the husband is unhappy because his wife has difficulty making trivial decisions and does not want to assume responsibilities. She almost never disagrees with him because she fears losing him. She has difficulty in doing anything on her own and is preoccupied by the fears of being left alone to take care of herself. She also goes to excessive lengths to obtain support from others and sees relationships as a source of care and support. A detailed mental status assessment does not reveal any evidence of schizophrenia, mood disorders with psychotic features, or any other psychotic disorders. What is the most likely diagnosis in this subject?

A. Paranoid personality disorder
B. Avoidant personality disorder
C. Dependent personality disorder
D. Obsessive-compulsive personality disorder
E. Histrionic personality disorder

37. A young couple is seen for marital therapy by a psychiatrist. The wife states that it is becoming increasingly difficult for her to stay in the marriage because of her husband's behavior. She states her husband is preoccupied with orderliness and perfectionism to the point it makes her crazy. He is very devoted to his work and is not involved in any leisure activities. He is inflexible about morality, ethics, and is reluctant to delegate tasks to others. He is very rigid and constantly thinks about rules, tasks, and lists. A detailed mental status assessment does not reveal any evidence of schizophrenia, mood disorders with psychotic features, or any other psychotic disorders. What is the most likely diagnosis in this subject?
    A. Schizoid personality disorder
    B. Avoidant personality disorder
    C. Dependent personality disorder
    D. Obsessive-compulsive personality disorder
    E. Schizotypal personality disorder

38. A 20-year-old male is referred for further assessment and management for suspected intellectual impairment. An IQ test reveals an overall score of 65. This puts him in which of the following categories?
    A. Normal
    B. Mild mental retardation
    C. Moderate mental retardation
    D. Severe mental retardation
    E. Profound mental retardation

39. According to the DSM-IV, all of the following are included in the diagnostic features of Asperger's syndrome except:
    A. impairment in social interaction
    B. restricted repetitive and stereotyped patterns of behavior
    C. significant delay in language
    D. normal age-appropriate self-help skills
    E. absence of other specific pervasive developmental disorders

40. According to the DSM-IV, to diagnose autistic disorder, the abnormalities in at least one of the three areas of social interaction, language, or symbolic play must be present prior to the age of:
    A. 3 years
    B. 6 years
    C. 7 years
    D. 6 months
    E. 1 year

41. According to the DSM-IV, to diagnose attention-deficit hyperactivity disorder (ADHD), some hyperactive-impulsive or inattentive symptoms that cause impairment must have been present before the age of:
    A. 3 years
    B. 12 years
    C. 7 years
    D. 5 years
    E. 1 year

42. The DSM-IV specifies three subtypes of ADHD, based on the predominant symptom pattern in the past 6 months. These include all of the following except:
    A. ADHD, combined type
    B. ADHD, disruptive type
    C. ADHD, predominantly inattentive type
    D. ADHD, predominantly hyperactive-impulsive type

43. According to the DSM-IV, conduct disorder is characterized by behaviors in which basic rights of others or rules are violated. These patterns of behaviors fall into the following categories except:
    A. aggression to people and animals
    B. destruction of property
    C. deceitfulness or theft
    D. serious violations of rules
    E. hyperactivity-impulsivity

44. According to the DSM-IV, all of the following are diagnostic features of oppositional defiant disorder except:
    A. hostile and defiant behavior
    B. lasts at least 12 months
    C. behavior results in significant impairment in social, academic, or occupational functioning
    D. criteria for conduct disorder are not met
    E. if 18 years or older, criteria for antisocial personality disorder are not met

45. According to the DSM-IV, all of the following are included in the criteria for substance dependence except:

    A. tolerance
    B. withdrawal
    C. unsuccessful efforts to cut down
    D. cessation of use on obtaining information on the harmful effects of the substances
    E. cessation of important social, occupational activities in preference to using the substance

46. According to the DSM-IV, all of the following are characteristic features of anorexia nervosa except:

    A. body mass index (BMI) of less than 19
    B. intense fear of gaining weight
    C. body image disturbance
    D. amenorrhea

47. According to the DSM-IV, all of the following are characteristic features of bulimia nervosa except:

    A. recurrent episodes of binge eating
    B. recurrent inappropriate compensatory behavior to prevent weight gain
    C. binge eating and compensatory behaviors occur at least twice a week for 6 months
    D. self-evaluation unduly influenced by body weight and shape
    E. the disturbance does not occur exclusively during episodes of anorexia nervosa

ANSWERS

1. **Answer: E.** According to the DSM-IV, there are five characteristic symptoms of schizophrenia including delusions, hallucinations, disorganized speech, disorganized or catatonic behavior, and negative symptoms (affective flattening, alogia, or avolition).

2. **Answer: A.** According to the DSM-IV, there should be continuous signs of disturbance persisting for at least 6 months. This 6-month period must include at least 1 month of characteristic symptoms (or less if successfully treated) and may include periods of prodromal or residual symptoms.

3. **Answer: E.** Schizophrenia, disorganized type, is not characterized by prominent delusions or hallucinations. Delusions and hallucinations, if present, are fragmentary and are not organized into a coherent theme. This type of schizophrenia has a continuous course with no significant remissions.

4. **Answer: C.** According to the DSM-IV, all of the choices are recognized features of schizophrenia, catatonic type, except disorganized behavior (which is a feature of Schizophrenia, disorganized type). The other feature of schizophrenia, catatonic type is peculiar voluntary movements such as posturing stereotyped movements, prominent mannerisms, or grimacing.

5. **Answer: A.** According to the DSM-IV, the duration criterion for the diagnosis of schizophreniform disorder is at least 1 month but less than 6 months (including prodromal, active, and residual phases). Brief psychotic disorder has a duration criterion of less than 1 month, and schizophrenia requires a duration criterion of at least 6 months.

6. **Answer: B.** Disorganized speech or behavior is a bad prognostic feature of schizophrenia.

7. **Answer: B.** According to the DSM-IV, to diagnose schizoaffective disorder, delusions or hallucinations must be present for at least 2 weeks (not 4 weeks) in the absence of prominent mood symptoms.

8. **Answer: B.** According to the DSM-IV, to diagnose delusional disorder, non-bizarre delusions must be present for at least 1 month (not 3 months). Delusional disorder has various subtypes including erotomanic type, grandiose type, jealous type, persecutory type, somatic type, mixed type, and unspecified type.

9. **Answer: E.** According to the DSM-IV, negative symptoms are not included in the diagnostic criteria for brief psychotic disorder. The duration criteria specify that one of the above four symptoms should last for at least 1 day but less than 1 month, with eventual full return to premorbid function. It is further specified as with marked stressor, without marked stressor, and with postpartum onset.

10. **Answer: A.** According to the DSM-IV, to diagnose major depressive disorder, the subject should have at least five of the nine symptoms of depression over a 2-week period. At least one of the symptoms should be either depressed mood or loss of interest or pleasure in usual activities.

11. **Answer: E.** According to the DSM-IV, to diagnose major depressive disorder, the subject should have at least five of the nine symptoms of depression over a 2-week period. At least one of the symptoms should be either depressed mood or loss of interest or pleasure in usual activities. The other seven symptoms are significant weight loss or weight gain, insomnia or hypersomnia, psychomotor agitation or retardation, fatigue/loss of energy, worthlessness, diminished concentration, and suicide ideation. Decreased need to sleep is a symptom of hypomania or mania.

12. **Answer: B.** According to the DSM-IV, to diagnose major depressive disorder, the subject should have at least five of the nine symptoms of depression over a 2-week period. At least one of the symptoms should be either depressed mood or loss of interest or pleasure in usual activities. Significant change in weight is also one of the criteria. The DSM-IV specifies a change of more than 5% of body weight in a month (either weight gain or weight loss) as significant.

13. **Answer: D.** The symptoms of major depressive disorder and bereavement are very similar, and the fact that some of the subjects with bereavement develop major depressive disorder makes it even harder to distinguish the two conditions. In subjects with bereavement, however, the symptoms last for less than 2 months, and they do not experience marked functional impairment, worthlessness, suicide ideation, psychotic symptoms, or psychomotor retardation. Helplessness is a common symptom in bereavement.

14. **Answer: D.** An untreated episode of major depressive disorder typically lasts for 6 months or longer. In about 5% to 10% of individuals, the full criteria for a major depressive disorder continue to be met for 2 or more years, in which case it is considered as chronic. Subjects with untreated or partially treated episodes of depression are more likely to relapse.

15. **Answer: B.** According to the DSM-IV, to diagnose major depressive disorder, the subject should have at least five of the nine symptoms of depression over a 2-week period. At least one of the symptoms should be either depressed mood or loss of interest or pleasure in usual activities.

16. **Answer: E.** According to the DSM-IV, to diagnose a manic episode, the subject should have the symptoms for at least 1 week or for any duration if hospitalization is necessary.

17. **Answer: E.** According to the DSM-IV, to diagnose a hypomanic episode, the subject should have the symptoms for at least 4 days.

18. **Answer: C.** According to the DSM-IV, to diagnose a manic episode, the subject should have abnormally and persistently elevated, expansive, or irritable mood lasting for at least 1 week or for any duration if hospitalization is necessary.

19. **Answer: A.** According to the DSM-IV, to diagnose dysthymic disorder, the subject must have depressed mood for most of the day, for more days than not, as indicated by subjective account or observation by others, for at least 2 years. Of note, in children and adolescents, mood can be irritable, and the duration must be at least 1 year.

20. **Answer: B.** When subjects with dysthymic disorder have superimposed major depressive disorder, it is often referred as *double depression.*

21. **Answer: C.** According to the DSM-IV, to diagnose bipolar II disorder, it is necessary to have one or more major depressive episodes and at least one hypomanic episode. These mood symptoms should not be accounted for by other disorders such as schizoaffective, schizophrenia, etc. Manic episode is a characteristic feature of bipolar I disorder.

22. **Answer: D.** According to the DSM-IV, to diagnose cyclothymic disorder, there should be no major depressive episode, manic episode, or mixed episode during the first 2 years of the disturbance. After the initial 2 years of cyclothymic disorder, however, there may be superimposed manic or mixed or major depressive episodes.

23. **Answer: A.** According to the DSM-IV, the criteria for rapid cycling specifier is at least four episodes of mood disturbance in the previous 12 months that meet the criteria for a major depressive, manic, mixed, or hypomanic episode. These episodes are demarcated by partial or full remission for at least 2 months or a switch to an episode of opposite polarity (e.g., major depressive episode to manic episode).

24. **Answer: D.** According to the DSM-IV, a personality disorder is an enduring pattern of inner experience and behavior that deviates markedly from the expectations of the individual's culture, is pervasive and inflexible, has an onset in adolescence or early adulthood, is stable over time, and leads to distress or impairment.

25. **Answer: A.** The common characteristics of cluster A personality disorders are that these individuals often appear odd or eccentric. Cluster A includes three personality disorders, and they are schizoid, paranoid, and schizotypal. Schizoaffective is not a personality disorder. Of note, the clustering system of personality disorders is not consistently validated.

26. **Answer: C.** The common characteristics of cluster B personality disorders are that these individuals often appear dramatic, emotional, or erratic. Cluster B includes four personality disorders: antisocial, borderline, histrionic, and narcissistic. Of note, the clustering system of personality disorders is not consistently validated.

27. **Answer: D.** The common characteristics of cluster C personality disorders are that these individuals often appear anxious or fearful. Cluster C includes three personality disorders: avoidant, dependent, and obsessive-compulsive. Of note, the clustering system of personality disorders is not consistently validated.

28. **Answer: D.** Paranoid personality disorder is characterized by pervasive suspiciousness of others such that their motives are interpreted as malevolent, beginning by early childhood. Individuals are suspicious of others, preoccupied about loyalty of friends/relatives, reluctant to confide in others, feel threatened by benign remarks, bear grudges, perceive attacks on their character or reputation that are not apparent to others, and they are also suspicious of their spouse or sexual partner.

29. **Answer: B.** Schizoid personality disorder is characterized by a pervasive pattern of detachment from social relationships and a restricted range of expressions of emotions in social settings, beginning by early adulthood. Affected individuals do not have any desire to have close relationships, choose solitary activities, have little interest in sexual experiences, lack close friends, are indifferent to praise or criticisms and show emotional coldness, detachment, or flattened affect.

30. **Answer: C.** Schizotypal personality disorder is characterized by a pervasive pattern of social and interpersonal deficits marked by acute discomfort with, and reduced capacity for, close relationships as well as by cognitive or perceptual distortions and eccentricities of behavior, beginning by early adulthood. These individuals have ideas of reference but not delusions, magical thinking, unusual perceptual experiences, odd thinking and speech, paranoid ideation, inappropriate or constricted affect, peculiar/odd/eccentric behavior, lack of close friends, and excessive social anxiety that does not diminish with familiarity.

31. **Answer: D.** Antisocial personality disorder is characterized by a pervasive pattern of disregard and violation of the rights of others occurring since the age of 15 years. They fail to conform to the social norms and involve in law-breaking behavior. They are deceitful, impulsive, and aggressive. They also exhibit complete disregard for the safety of self or others and lack remorse. To make this diagnosis, the individual should be at least 18 years of age and there should be evidence of conduct disorder with onset before the age of 15 years.

32. **Answer: B.** Borderline personality disorder is characterized by a pervasive pattern of instability in interpersonal relationships, self-image, and affect and marked impulsivity beginning by early adulthood and present in a variety of contexts. Affected individuals make frantic efforts to avoid real or imagined abandonment, have a pattern of unstable and intense personal relationships, identity disturbance, impulsivity that is potentially self-damaging, recurrent suicidal behavior, marked mood reactivity, difficulty controlling anger, and transient stress-related paranoid ideation or severe dissociative symptoms.

33. **Answer: E.** Histrionic personality disorder is characterized by a pervasive pattern of excessive emotionality and attention seeking, beginning by early adulthood and present in a variety of contexts. Affected individuals are uncomfortable in situations in which they are not the center of attention, often exhibit inappropriate sexually seductive behavior, have rapidly shifting and shallow emotions, use physical appearance to draw attention, and their speech is impressionistic but lacks details. Those with histrionic personality disorder are also known for dramatization, theatricality, suggestibility, and consider relationships to be more intimate than they actually are.

34. **Answer: A.** Narcissistic personality disorder is characterized by a pervasive pattern of grandiosity, need for admiration, and lack of empathy, which begins by early adulthood and present in a variety of contexts. Affected individuals have a grandiose sense of self-importance, are preoccupied with fantasies of unlimited success and power, tend to associate with high-status people, have a sense of entitlement, lack empathy, and are exploitative. They are often envious of others and show arrogant, haughty behaviors or attitudes.

35. **Answer: B.** Avoidant personality disorder is characterized by a pervasive pattern of social inhibition, feelings of inadequacy, and hypersensitivity to negative evaluation, beginning by early adulthood and present in a variety of contexts. Affected individuals avoid occupational activities that involve significant interpersonal contacts because of fears of criticism, show restraint with intimate relationships, are preoccupied with being criticized in social situations, are viewed as socially inept and personally unappealing, and they are usually reluctant to take any personal risks or engage in any new activities because such endeavors may prove embarrassing.

36. **Answer: C.** Dependent personality disorder is characterized by a pervasive pattern of excessive need to be taken care of that leads to submissive and clinging behavior and fears of separation, beginning by early adulthood and present in a variety of contexts. Affected individuals have difficulty making everyday decisions and need others to assume responsibility for major areas of their life. They have difficulty expressing disagreement for fear of losing support and go to great lengths to obtain support and nurturance. They feel helpless when they are on their own and are unrealistically preoccupied with fears of being left alone to take care of themselves.

37. **Answer: D.** Obsessive-compulsive personality disorder is characterized by a pervasive pattern of preoccupation with orderliness, perfectionism, and mental/interpersonal control, at the expense of flexibility, openness and efficiency, beginning in early adulthood and present in a variety of contexts. Affected individuals are preoccupied with rules, order, and show perfectionism that interferes with task completion. They are excessively devoted to work to the exclusion of leisure activities and are overconscientious, scrupulous, and inflexible about morality, ethics, and values. They often cannot discard worthless objects even when they are not associated with any sentimental values. They are reluctant to delegate tasks to others and adopt miserly spending habits. They are very rigid and stubborn.

38. **Answer: B.** According to the DSM-IV, the four degrees of severity of mental retardation are specified, reflecting the individual's level of intellectual impairment: mild mental retardation (IQ level 50–55 to 70); moderate mental retardation (35–40 to 50–55); severe mental retardation (20–25 to 35–40); and profound mental retardation (IQ level below 20 or 25).

39. **Answer: C.** According to the DSM-IV, the essential features of Asperger's disorder are severe and sustained impairment in social interaction and the development of restricted, repetitive patterns of behavior, interests, and activities. In contrast to autistic disorder, there are no clinically significant delays in language. Also, there are no clinically significant delays in cognitive development or age-appropriate self-help skills.

40. **Answer: A.** According to the DSM-IV, to diagnose autistic disorder, the abnormalities in at least one of the three areas of social interaction, language, or symbolic play must be present prior to the age of 3 years. The essential features of autistic disorder are the presence of markedly abnormal or impaired development in social interaction and communication and a markedly restricted repertoire of activity and interests.

41. **Answer: C.** According to the DSM-IV, to diagnose ADHD, some hyperactive-impulsive or inattentive symptoms that cause impairment must have been present before the age of 7 years. The essential features of ADHD are a persistent pattern of inattention and/or hyperactivity-impulsivity that is more frequent and severe than is typically observed in individuals at a comparable level of development.

42. **Answer: B.** According to the DSM-IV, there are three subtypes of ADHD, based on the predominant symptom pattern in the past 6 months. These include ADHD, combined type; ADHD, predominantly inattentive type; and ADHD, predominantly hyperactive-impulsive type.

43. **Answer: E.** According to the DSM-IV, conduct disorder is characterized by a repetitive and persistent pattern of behavior in which the basic rights of others or major age-appropriate societal norms or rules are violated. These behaviors fall into the four main groups of aggression to people or animals, destruction of property, deceitfulness, or theft and serious violations of rules. Conduct disorder may be diagnosed in individuals who are older than 18 years but only if the criteria for antisocial personality disorder are not met.

44. **Answer: E.** According to the DSM-IV, oppositional defiant disorder is characterized by recurrent pattern of negativistic, defiant, disobedient, and hostile behavior toward authority figures and persists for at least 6 months. This diagnosis is not made if the behavior occurs exclusively during the course of a psychotic or mood disorder or if criteria are met for conduct disorder or antisocial personality disorder (in an individual over the age of 18 years).

45. **Answer: D.** According to the DSM-IV, substance dependence is defined as a maladaptive pattern of substance use, leading to clinically significant distress or impairment for 12 months or more. During this period, tolerance, withdrawal, unsuccessful attempts to cut down, spending an extended period of time obtaining/using substance, and giving up important activities is noted. Also, in substance dependence, the individual uses the substance despite knowing that its use can cause significant psychological or physical problems.

46. **Answer: A.** The essential features of anorexia nervosa are that the affected individual refuses to maintain a minimal body weight, is intensely afraid of gaining weight, and exhibits a significant disturbance in the perception of the shape or size of his or her body. Amenorrhea is noted in postmenarcheal females. BMI of less than 17.5 (or less than 85% of weight for the height) is considered as one of the features of anorexia nervosa.

47. **Answer: C.** The essential features of bulimia nervosa are binge eating and inappropriate compensatory methods to prevent weight gain. Individuals' self-evaluation is excessively influenced by body shape and weight. The binge eating and compensatory behaviors must occur, on average, at least twice a week for 3 months.

Psychopharmacology

QUESTIONS

1. A 20-year-old Caucasian female diagnosed with paranoid schizophrenia was started on an atypical antipsychotic. She is concerned that the antipsychotic medication will cause weight gain. Which of the following is the most accurate statement regarding weight gain and antipsychotics?

   A. No significant weight gain is observed with atypical antipsychotics.
   B. Weight gain occurs mainly in the first 2 weeks.
   C. Weight gain is related to the pretreatment body mass index (BMI).
   D. All antipsychotics cause the same amount of weight gain.
   E. Weight gain is associated with clinical improvement.

2. Benzodiazepine withdrawal symptoms include all of the following except:

   A. depersonalization and derealization
   B. perceptual disturbances
   C. anxiety
   D. constipation
   E. rhinorrhea

3. Which of the following antipsychotics also has an antidepressant effect?

   A. Flupentixol
   B. Chlorpromazine
   C. Haloperidol
   D. Trifluoperazine
   E. Fluphenazine

4. A 46-year-old male is referred to a neurologist for tingling and burning sensations in his feet. He also has a history of depression and has been on many antidepressant medications. The neurologist diagnoses him to have peripheral neuropathy after a detailed history and physical examination. Which of the following classes of antidepressants can cause peripheral neuropathy?

   A. Selective serotonin reuptake inhibitors (SSRIs)
   B. Tricyclic antidepressants
   C. Serotonin and norepinephrine reuptake inhibitors
   D. Monoamine oxidase inhibitors (MAOIs)
   E. Norepinephrine reuptake inhibitors

5. A 48-year-old male patient with treatment-resistant depression has tried all the antidepressants except for MAOIs. He is currently on an SSRI. You would like to get the patient off the SSRI before starting MAOIs because of the risk of serotonin syndrome. Which of the following SSRIs needs the longest washout period before switching over to MAOIs?

   A. Paroxetine
   B. Fluoxetine
   C. Citalopram
   D. Sertraline
   E. Escitalopram

6. A neurologist is consulted by a psychiatrist to assess a 42-year-old depressed female with recent onset of "muscle twitches." She was taking citalopram 80 mg, and duloxetine 40 mg was recently added because of suboptimal response to citalopram alone; she denies any alcohol or substance abuse. On examination, the neurologist notes that the patient is slightly disoriented and also has mild tremors and hyperreflexia. What is the most likely cause of the "muscle twitches" in this patient?

   A. Serotonin syndrome
   B. Alcohol withdrawal syndrome
   C. Neuroleptic malignant syndrome
   D. Malingering
   E. Encephalitis

7. Serotonin syndrome is characterized by a spectrum of signs and symptoms. According to Hunter criteria for serotonin syndrome, the patient must have taken a serotonergic agent and should have at least one symptom. All of the following are listed in Hunter criteria except:

   A. tremor and hyperreflexia
   B. spontaneous clonus
   C. inducible clonus plus agitation or diaphoresis
   D. ocular clonus plus agitation or diaphoresis
   E. temperature above 32°C plus ocular clonus or inducible clonus
   F. hypertonia

8. Which of the following tricyclic antidepressants has a strong serotonin reuptake inhibition effect?

   A. Amitriptyline
   B. Nortriptyline
   C. Imipramine
   D. Clomipramine
   E. Doxepin

9. Which of the following antidepressants blocks reuptake of dopamine?

   A. Venlafaxine
   B. Bupropion
   C. Buspirone
   D. Mirtazapine
   E. Fluoxetine

10. Which of the following medications is associated with depression?

    A. Methyldopa
    B. Procyclidine
    C. Tryptophan
    D. Flupentixol
    E. Testosterone

11. Which of the following is used as an augmenting agent in the treatment of depression?

    A. Propranolol
    B. Pindolol
    C. Metoprolol
    D. Sotalol
    E. Labetalol

12. The advancement in central nervous system (CNS) pharmacology is attributed to the better understanding of neurotransmitters and neuro-receptors. Which of the following is TRUE about neuroreceptors?

    A. $5\text{-}HT_{2A}$ antagonists enhance rapid eye movement (REM) sleep.
    B. $5\text{-}HT_{1A}$ antagonists are anxiolytic.
    C. Most typical antipsychotics are D_2 agonists.
    D. D_2 receptors are found in the limbic system.
    E. Alpha-2 adrenergic agonists cause increased norepinephrine release.

13. A majority of psychotropic drugs are considered to be lipophilic. All of the following are true about lipophilic drugs except:

    A. they are rapidly absorbed
    B. they have a large volume of distribution
    C. they have a high first-pass aspect
    D. they cross the blood-brain barrier slowly
    E. they are completely absorbed

14. The hepatic cytochrome P450 system is important in drug metabolism. All of the following induce hepatic cytochrome P450 enzymes except:

    A. alcohol
    B. smoking
    C. carbamazepine
    D. paroxetine
    E. isoniazid

15. Serotonin is considered as one of the most important neurotransmitters in the regulation of various psychophysiological functions. Serotonin is thought to be involved in all of the following except:

    A. aggressive behavior
    B. sleep and wakefulness
    C. muscle tone
    D. weight gain
    E. sexual behavior

16. A 46-year-old male with alcohol-induced cirrhosis is admitted to the neurology in-patient unit for seizure disorder. He becomes agitated following an argument with the nurse and requests "some benzodiazepines" as they have helped him in the past "to relax." Which of the following benzodiazepines is safe in patients with hepatic insufficiency i.e., the elimination of which of the following benzodiazepines is NOT influenced by liver disease?

    A. Midazolam
    B. Lorazepam
    C. Chlordiazepoxide
    D. Alprazolam
    E. Diazepam

17. Benzodiazepines act by:

    A. increasing K^+ channel opening
    B. decreasing the frequency of opening of Na^+ channels
    C. increasing the frequency of opening of Na^+ channels
    D. increasing the duration of opening of Cl^- channels
    E. increasing the frequency of opening of Cl^- channels

18. A 34-year-old female who is breast-feeding her 2-month-old infant would like to know if she can restart diazepam as needed, that her family physician had prescribed her many years ago. She states that it helps her control acute stress-related anxiety. All of the following are true about diazepam except:

    A. peak plasma concentrations are reached in 30 to 90 minutes
    B. intramuscular absorption is faster than oral
    C. it is highly lipid soluble
    D. it is about 90% to 95% protein bound
    E. it is secreted in breast milk

19. Which of the following is NOT a side effect of benzodiazepines?

    A. Ataxia
    B. Postural hypotension
    C. Drowsiness
    D. Amnesia
    E. Nightmares

20. The following are recognized to be associated with benzodiazepine use except:
    A. induction of hepatic microsomal enzymes
    B. leucopenia
    C. eosinophilia
    D. change in plasma cortisol
    E. respiratory depression

21. Benzodiazepines are often used in combination with SSRIs in the treatment of panic disorder until the full effects of SSRIs are realized. Among other variables, the choice of benzodiazepines depends on the drug's half-life. Which of the following has the longest half-life?
    A. Alprazolam
    B. Oxazepam
    C. Temazepam
    D. Flurazepam
    E. Lorazepam

22. Which of the following benzodiazepines have the US Food and Drug Administration (FDA) approval as hypnotic medications for insomnia?
    A. Triazolam
    B. Temazepam
    C. Estazolam
    D. All of the above
    E. None of the above

23. All of the following are common symptoms associated with benzodiazepine withdrawal except:
    A. paranoia
    B. tremors
    C. derealization
    D. tinnitus
    E. depersonalization

24. A 56-year-old male with a history of chronic benzodiazepine use for insomnia is brought to the emergency department (ED) by his daughter with complaints of sedation, incoherence, and problems with coordination. His daughter states that he had been using diazepam 10 to 20 mg every night for many, many years. She also recalls that a few days ago her father saw his family physician and got a new medication for some other problem. The ED physician checks the current medication list and believes the patient has benzodiazepine overdose. Which of the following can increase the levels of benzodiazepines?

    A. Topiramate
    B. Cimetidine
    C. Phenytoin
    D. Carbamazepine
    E. Rifampicin

25. The use of benzodiazepines during pregnancy especially during the first trimester is associated with several complications in the fetus. All of the following are known to occur following benzodiazepine use during pregnancy except:

    A. cleft lip
    B. cleft palate
    C. respiratory depression
    D. absent arms and legs
    E. neonatal withdrawal symptoms

26. All of the following changes in sleep and sleep architecture are associated with benzodiazepine use except:

    A. decrease in sleep latency
    B. increase in total sleep time
    C. decrease in REM sleep
    D. decrease in stage II sleep
    E. increase in sleep spindles

27. A 38-year-old business executive from Japan comes to the United States for a meeting. He is worried, however, that he will not be able to do a good presentation because he is not able to sleep at night. He sees a physician who prescribes a short-acting hypnotic for 3 days to help him sleep, but the patient is worried that he might develop "addiction." How long does it usually take to develop tolerance to benzodiazepines?

    A. Two days of daily use
    B. Two to 3 weeks of daily use
    C. One to 2 months of intermittent use
    D. Four to 6 months of daily use
    E. One year of daily use

28. A person taking benzodiazepines can have cross-tolerance to which of the following?

    A. Antipsychotics
    B. SSRIs
    C. MAOIs
    D. Alcohol
    E. Noradrenergic reuptake inhibitors

29. All of the following are true about benzodiazepine dependence except:

    A. it is more common with rapidly acting drugs
    B. it is more common in patients with history of other substance abuse
    C. it is less likely in patients with passive and dependent personality traits
    D. withdrawal symptoms begin from 24 to 48 hr after last use to 3 weeks after last use depending on the half-life of the drug
    E. withdrawal symptoms can sometimes be fatal

30. A 26-year-old female with bipolar disorder, stable on lithium would like to know the effects of lithium on the fetus if she becomes pregnant. Lithium administration during pregnancy is associated with which of the following?

    A. Epstein's anomaly
    B. Depression in the infant
    C. Neural tube defects
    E. Hyperglycemia in the newborn
    F. Phacomelia

31. A 28-year-old male with a complicated psychiatric history is on multiple psychotropic medications. His psychiatrist requests a neurology consultation for ataxia. A review of the patient's current medication list shows that he is on the following medications. Which of these drugs can produce ataxia at therapeutic doses?
    A. Imipramine
    B. Carbamazepine
    C. Quetiapine
    D. Chlorpromazine
    G. Fluoxetine

32. A 38-year-old male presents with multiple symptoms. A detailed history and physical examination leads to a suspicion of benzodiazepine withdrawal. The physician is not sure, however, if the symptoms are because of benzodiazepine withdrawal or anxiety disorder. All of the following are more likely to be secondary to benzodiazepine withdrawal rather than anxiety except:
    A. sensory hyperawareness
    B. tremors
    C. dysphoria
    D. difficulty to stop worrying
    E. tongue fasciculations

33. All of the following are recognized side effects of benzodiazepines except:
    A. ataxia
    B. confusional state
    C. acute dystonia
    D. aggression
    E. drowsiness

34. All of the following are true about benzodiazepines except:
    A. they potentiate Gamma-aminobutyric acid (GABA)
    B. they may have hangover effects
    C. they modulate chloride channel flow
    D. they are used to abort seizures
    E. their effects are antagonized by naloxone

35. All of the following drugs can cause tremors except:

    A. amitriptyline
    B. diazepam
    C. lithium
    D. haloperidol
    E. phenelzine

36. A 75-year-old female with headaches is prescribed a low dose of amitriptyline, which was gradually increased. Although she reports feeling better, she complains about dry mouth and difficulty in swallowing. All of the following are side effects of tricyclic antidepressants except:

    A. blurred vision
    B. tachycardia
    C. tremors
    D. impotence
    E. diarrhea

37. Tricyclic antidepressants can result in severe toxicity at high doses. Which of the following tricyclics has a therapeutic window?

    A. Amitriptyline
    B. Nortriptyline
    C. Protriptyline
    D. Imipramine
    E. Clomipramine

38. A 72-year-old female with chronic major depressive disorder is brought to the ED by ambulance for confusion and disorientation. She has been taking amitriptyline for the past 36 years for depression. The ED physician suspects possibility of accidental tricyclic antidepressant overdose. All of the following are true about tricyclic antidepressant overdose except:

    A. gastric aspiration is helpful
    B. intravenous sodium bicarbonate is often used
    C. cardiac monitoring is important
    D. convulsions can occur
    E. tricyclics have a high therapeutic index

39. Which of the following tricyclics is a secondary amine?
    A. Clomipramine
    B. Desipramine
    C. Amitriptyline
    D. Imipramine
    E. Doxepin

40. A 37-year-old male with headaches, insomnia, and depression is pre-scribed a tricyclic antidepressant with the hope of treating all of these problems with one medication. Two days after starting treatment, he calls the physician with complaints of dry mouth and blurred vision. Which of the following tricyclics has the most anticholinergic effects?
    A. Clomipramine
    B. Amitriptyline
    C. Nortriptyline
    D. Desipramine
    E. Amoxapine

41. A 56-year-old female with postural hypotension and chronic migraine headaches is prescribed amitriptyline. The patient reports improvement in headaches but mentions an increase in dizziness symptoms, especially when she gets out of bed in the morning. Which of the following drugs has the least effect on blood pressure?
    A. Amitriptyline
    B. Clomipramine
    C. Nortriptyline
    D. Imipramine
    E. Desipramine

42. Nortriptyline is one of the very few psychotropic medications that is known to have a therapeutic window. The most effective therapeutic plasma concentrations for nortriptyline are in the range of:
    A. 150 to 200 ng/mL
    B. 200 to 250 ng/mL
    C. 50 to 150 ng/mL
    D. 115 to 150 ng/mL
    E. 25 to 50 ng/mL

43. A 52-year-old female presents with depressed mood and diminished interests for the past 2 months. Her appetite has increased and so has her weight. She reports sleeping up to 15 hours per day but continues to feel tired. She mentions that typically her mood gets worse during the winter and she feels better during summer months. What would be the most appropriate antidepressant to prescribe for this patient?

   A. Fluoxetine
   B. Paroxetine
   C. Mirtazapine
   D. Bupropion
   E. Trazodone

44. A 56-year-old male with recurrent depression resistant to standard antidepressant medications is started on phenelzine and advised dietary and other restrictions. The patient has a hard time understanding why he would develop hypertensive crisis if he eats cheese. The hypertensive crisis seen with MAOIs are caused by the patient's inability to deaminate:

   A. tryptophan
   B. leucine
   C. tyramine
   D. tyrosine
   E. tranylcypromine

45. All of the following foods are contraindicated in individuals taking MAOIs except:

   A. cheese
   B. bananas
   C. red wine
   D. yeast extracts
   E. aged meats

46. A 54-year-old male on phenelzine for depression presents with confusion and agitation. On examination, he is diaphoretic, and his reflexes are brisk. His partner reports that the physician had recently started taking a new medication, sumatriptan, for migraine headaches. The patient is most likely having:

   A. rhabdomyolysis
   B. neuroleptic malignant syndrome
   C. respiratory infection
   D. cheese reaction
   E. serotonin syndrome

47. When switching from an SSRI to an MAOI, a washout period of at least 2 weeks is recommended for all of the following, except:
    A. citalopram
    B. paroxetine
    C. venlafaxine
    D. fluoxetine
    E. sertraline

48. All of the following are true about mirtazapine except:
    A. it has antihistamine effects
    B. it is a central presynaptic alpha-2 adrenergic receptor antagonist
    C. sedation is a common side effect
    D. it decreases appetite
    E. It rarely causes agranulocytosis

49. Which of the following antidepressants has the shortest half-life?
    A. Fluoxetine
    B. Paroxetine
    C. Sertraline
    D. Fluvoxamine
    E. Citalopram

50. All of the following are known side effects of SSRIs except:
    A. diarrhea
    B. stomach upset
    C. change in appetite
    D. cardiac arrhythmias
    E. headaches

51. Which of the following is a common side effect of SSRIs?
    A. Anorgasmia
    B. Hypertension
    C. Urinary hesitancy
    D. Alopecia
    E. Itching

52. All of the following can be caused by SSRIs except:

   A. nausea
   B. diarrhea
   C. agitation
   D. akathisia
   E. premature ejaculation

53. A 46-year-old male is very unhappy that when he missed two doses of paroxetine, he felt nauseous, anxious, irritable, and agitated. He requests his physician to prescribe a medication that is unlikely to cause these symptoms if he accidentally misses any dose of medication. Discontinuation syndrome is least likely to be associated with:

   A. fluoxetine
   B. citalopram
   C. venlafaxine
   D. sertraline
   E. fluvoxamine

54. An 86-year-old female with coronary artery disease and congestive heart failure is admitted to the neurology department after a stroke. She is on multiple medications, and the neurologist attending to her diagnosed her to have clinical depression. He decides to start her on an SSRI. One of the important considerations in choosing an appropriate SSRI in this patient includes:

   A. affinity for opiate receptors
   B. potency in inhibiting 5-HT reuptake
   C. selectivity in inhibiting 5-HT reuptake
   D. inhibition of dopamine reuptake
   E. inhibition of hepatic cytochrome P450 isoenzymes

55. What is the most common adverse effect reported with SSRIs use?

   A. Constipation
   B. Nausea
   C. Diarrhea
   D. Tremor
   E. Headaches

56. Priapism is most commonly associated with which of the following anti-depressant medications?
    A. Trazodone
    B. Paroxetine
    C. Effexor
    D. Wellbutrin
    E. Amitriptyline

57. The antidepressant effect of trazodone is because of its action at which of the following receptors?
    A. Histamine receptors
    B. Muscarinic receptors
    C. 5-HT$_{2A}$ receptors
    D. Dopamine receptors
    E. Norepinephrine receptors

58. Which of the following is NOT a side effect of trazodone?
    A. Priapism
    B. Orthostatic hypotension
    C. Drowsiness
    D. Seizures
    E. Headaches

59. Lithium is primarily excreted through which of the following organ systems?
    A. Lungs
    B. Kidneys
    C. Sweat
    D. Feces
    E. Liver

60. A 54-year-old male with chronic recurrent depression is admitted to the hospital for confusion and disorientation. A review of his medications shows that he is on lithium. Further collateral history from his psychiatrist reveals that he was getting depressed again recently, and he had in fact decreased his food intake due to lack of appetite but continued to take lithium as prescribed. What is the most likely cause for this patient's confusion?

    A. Lithium toxicity
    B. Worsening of depression
    C. Dementia
    D. Psychosis
    E. Postictal confusion

61. All of the following drugs are lipophilic except:

    A. lithium
    B. haloperidol
    C. nortriptyline
    D. propranolol
    E. diazepam

62. Clozapine is indicated for treatment-resistant schizophrenia. All of the following are dose-limiting side effects of clozapine except:

    A. agranulocytosis
    B. sedation
    C. seizures
    D. hypotension
    E. all of the above

63. Although agranulocytosis associated with clozapine is considered to be largely an idiosyncratic reaction, certain risk factors have been identified. All of the following are considered to increase the risk of agranulocytosis except:

    A. female gender
    B. older age
    C. low baseline white cell count
    D. first few months of treatment
    E. African American race

64. Which of the following medications is generally not administered with clozapine?

   A. escitalopram
   B. clonazepam
   C. sertraline
   D. risperdal
   E. propranolol

65. A 52-year-old female with schizophrenia who was in remission with olanzapine decided to stop taking olanzapine because of a 30-pound weight gain in the past 3 months since she started taking olanzapine. She is now back in the inpatient unit with paranoia and auditory hallucination but refuses to take olanzapine because of weight gain. Which of the following antipsychotics is least likely to cause weight gain?

   A. Risperidone
   B. Molindone
   C. Haloperidol
   D. Chlorpromazine
   E. Clozapine

66. Which of the following medications, in combination with neuroleptics, can increase the risk of neuroleptic malignant syndrome (NMS)?

   A. Lithium
   B. Valproic acid
   C. Lamotrigine
   D. Clonazepam
   E. Benzatropine

67. Although NMS is typically associated with neuroleptics, other drugs can cause symptoms that are very similar to NMS. Which of the following drugs are known to cause symptoms similar to NMS?

   A. Reserpine
   B. Metoclopramide
   C. Methylphenidate
   D. Lithium
   E. All of the above

68. All of the neuroleptics are known to decrease the seizure threshold to some extent. Which of the following neuroleptics causes the largest decrease in seizure threshold?
    A. Olanzapine
    B. Risperidone
    C. Molindone
    D. Clozapine
    E. Aripiprazole

69. A 24-year-old female with rapid-cycling bipolar disorder is in remission with carbamazepine. She has a new boyfriend and would like to start taking birth control pills. What is the effect of carbamazepine on birth control pill levels in the blood?
    A. Decreases the levels of birth control pills
    B. Increases the levels of birth control pills
    C. No effect on the levels of birth control pills
    D. None of the above
    E. All of the above

70. Which of the following medications can increase serum lithium levels?
    A. Ibuprofen
    B. Diclofenac sodium
    C. Spironolactone
    D. Tetracycline
    E. All of the above

71. Which of the following are noted in electrocardiogram (EKG) with lithium?
    A. T-wave flattening
    B. T-wave inversion
    C. Prolongation of atrioventricular conduction
    D. All of the above

72. Which of the following antidepressant medications is available in the parenteral form?
    A. Citalopram
    B. Amitriptyline
    C. Fluoxetine
    D. Doxepin
    E. Sertraline

73. Which of the following antidepressant medications should be avoided in patients with Parkinson's disease?

A. Amoxapine
B. Amitriptyline
C. Bupropion
D. Fluoxetine
E. Venlafaxine

74. Which of the following SSRIs has the most anticholinergic effects?

A. Paroxetine
B. Fluoxetine
C. Sertraline
D. Fluvoxamine
E. Citalopram

75. A 65-year-old male with narrow-angle glaucoma is diagnosed to have major depressive disorder and is considered for antidepressant medications. All of the following antidepressants are considered to be relatively safe except:

A. Paroxetine
B. Venlafaxine
C. Bupropion
D. Trazodone
E. Nefazodone

76. A 28-year-old female is diagnosed to have seasonal affective disorder. She is not keen to try antidepressants but is willing to try bright light therapy. She would like to know how quickly she can expect a response. What is the average length of time for patients to show response to bright light therapy in seasonal affective disorder?

A. 8 weeks
B. 4 weeks
C. 2 months
D. 2 to 4 days
E. 30 days

77. A 36-year-old male with a history of drug abuse is admitted to the hospital for disorientation and possible psychosis. Over the next 2 days, he is noticed to be doing well on the unit. The night before planned discharge, however, he is noted to be hallucinating again and becomes extremely agitated. Intermittent psychotic episodes are noticed in the next 2 to 3 weeks. The resident decides to take another look at this patient's medical records and checks for his urine toxicology on admission. Given the above presentation, what is it most likely to show?

    A. Amphetamines
    B. Benzodiazepines
    C. Cocaine
    D. Marijuana
    E. Phencyclidine (PCP)

78. Which of the following benzodiazepines is metabolized in the gastrointestinal tract prior to its absorption?

    A. Clonazepam
    B. Diazepam
    C. Clorazepate
    D. Alprazolam
    E. Temazepam

79. Bupropion is known to decrease the seizure threshold. What is the incidence of seizures in patients taking bupropion in doses greater than 450 mg per day?

    A. 0.4%
    B. 4%
    C. 2%
    D. 0.2%
    E. 10%

80. The incidence of aplastic anemia with carbamazepine is:

    A. one in 1,000
    B. one in 10,000
    C. one in 100,000
    D. one in 20,000
    E. one in 5,000

81. All of the following are side effects associated with use of the clozapine except:

    A. hyperprolactinemia
    B. weight gain
    C. sedation
    D. seizures
    E. hypotension

82. Aripiprazole has all of the following FDA approvals except for the treatment of:

    A. schizophrenia
    B. acute agitation in schizophrenia
    C. mixed bipolar disorder
    D. manic bipolar disorder
    E. acute agitation in depression

83. All of the following are true regarding aripiprazole except:

    A. half-life of 75 hours
    B. partial agonist at D_2 and 5-HT_{1A}
    C. it is a substrate of CYP2D6 and 3A4
    D. indicated for dementia-related psychosis
    E. can lower seizure threshold

84. A 72-year-old female with panic disorder was prescribed paroxetine and clonazepam. Her past medical history is significant for seizure disorder, which is treated with phenytoin. During the follow-up appointment, the patient complains of unsteady gait. On examination, except for unsteady gait, no focal neurological abnormalities are noted. What is the most likely cause for unsteady gait in this patient?

    A. Paroxetine
    B. Clonazepam
    C. Phenytoin
    D. Phenytoin toxicity
    E. All of the above

85. A 26-year-old Asian American male with mental retardation is evaluated for aggressive behavior. The patient was tried on several antipsychotic and mood stabilizers with no benefit. His mother mentions to you that she tried carbamazepine 500 mg, which she got from one of her colleagues at work. It has worked well for her colleague's son who also has similar problems. Before prescribing carbamazepine for this patient, which of the following blood tests should you perform?

    A. Thyroid-stimulating hormone (TSH) levels
    B. HLA-B*1502
    C. HLA-DQB106
    D. Cortisol levels
    E. Prolactin levels

86. All of the following are true about carbamazepine except:

    A. can cause syndrome of inappropriate antidiuretic hormone secretion (SIADH)
    B. it induces its own metabolism
    C. eliminated by extrahepatic metabolism
    D. reduces levels of valproic acid
    E. plasma levels are not an accurate indicator of toxicity

87. A 62-year-old male with bipolar disorder presents with complaints of double vision. On reviewing his medications, he was noted to be on lithium. His psychiatrist has been prescribing lithium for more than 20 years, and the patient's most recent lithium levels done 4 weeks ago were within normal range. The patient would like to know more about lithium side effects. The following are the recognized side effects of lithium at a therapeutic dose except:

    A. thirst
    B. fine tremors
    C. polydipsia
    D. diplopia
    E. erection problems

88. An 18-year-old male has been taking paroxetine for the past 8 weeks for anxiety disorder. He forgets to pick up the refill and does not take paroxetine for more than 48 hours. He calls the physician's office and complains of anxiety, irritability, and feeling uncomfortable. He is worried that he has become "hooked on the medicine." All of the following are true regarding antidepressant discontinuation syndromes except:

    A. more common with short half-life drugs
    B. most of them can cause discontinuation syndrome
    C. abrupt discontinuation is a risk factor
    D. indicate that the patient is dependent on these medicines
    E. cause irritability, insomnia, and restlessness

89. A 36-year-old anxious executive complains of difficulty falling and staying asleep because of the "stress" associated with several deadlines at his workplace. He believes that lack of sleep at night is affecting his performance during the day and makes him more worried at night. He was prescribed a short course of eszopiclone and referred for relaxation therapy. After a week, he calls, however, and mentions that his insomnia is getting worse. The patient has not tried eszopiclone because he is now "worried about getting dependent on sleeping medicines." All of the following are true about eszopiclone except:

    A. potential for tolerance exists
    B. it is thought to bind preferentially to the alpha subunit of the GABA-BDZ receptor complex
    C. it is a benzodiazepine derivative
    D. dose to be reduced in the elderly
    E. The FDA has approved this drug for "long-term" use

90. A 54-year-old male with generalized anxiety disorder (GAD) was prescribed buspirone. He calls the doctor's office after 2 weeks and complains of persistent anxiety. One of the features of treatment with buspirone the patient should be aware is:

    A. it can cause dependence
    B. it takes 4 to 6 weeks for symptomatic relief
    C. causes sedation
    D. sexual dysfunction is not common
    E. low doses are effective

91. A 32-year-old female with panic disorder is terrified by panic attacks and requests immediate symptomatic relief. The panic attacks are debilitating, and she is not able to function. She is otherwise fit and healthy and has no history of any substance abuse or dependence. A reasonable approach would be:
    A. intensive psychodynamic psychotherapy
    B. combination of bupropion and clonazepam
    C. start the patient on any SSRI
    D. start the patient on an SSRI and refer to cognitive behavioral therapy (CBT)
    E. start the patient on a combination of an SSRI for the long term and low-dose clonazepam for a short duration

92. A 26-year-old schizophrenic African American male is administered 10 mg of haloperidol following an episode of acute agitation and aggressive behavior in the emergency department (ED). After a few hours, he is noticed to have sustained contraction of the neck muscles and complains of severe pain. All of the following are true about dystonia except:
    A. more common in men than in women
    B. more common in younger than older individuals
    C. is more common than akathisia in patients treated with neuroleptics
    D. treated with lorazepam or diphenhydramine hydrochloride
    E. can cause trismus

93. A 52-year-old male admitted to an acute psychiatric unit for psychosis and agitation is given 10 mg intramuscular (IM) haloperidol. Later in the evening, the resident on call is called by the nursing staff, as the patient was noticed to be having muscle rigidity and fever. He suspects neuroleptic malignant syndrome (NMS). All of the following are features of NMS except:
    A. clear consciousness
    B. muscle rigidity
    C. elevated temperature
    D. leukocytosis
    E. elevated creatine kinase levels

94. A 42-year-old male with bipolar disorder is admitted to the hospital for acute mania. He is pacing up and down the hallway and agitating other patients. He believes he has divine powers and offers to "cure everyone." All of the following drugs are effective in the treatment of the acute phase of mania except:

    A. lithium
    B. lamotrigine
    C. olanzapine
    D. valproic acid
    E. haloperidol

95. What is the mechanism of action of venlafaxine?

    A. Inhibition of reuptake of dopamine
    B. 5-HT$_1$ receptor agonist
    C. Inhibition of reuptake of serotonin and noradrenaline
    D. Stimulation of glutamate receptors
    E. Inhibition of gamma-aminobutyric acid (GABA) receptors

96. A 48-year-old male with profound mental retardation is noted to be sexually aggressive and inappropriate. He has sexually assaulted several patients and staff members in the nursing home. The physicians decide to administer cyproterone acetate after getting permission from the family members and the legal guardian. All of the following are true about cyproterone acetate except:

    A. used in the treatment of sexually disinhibited behavior in the context of mental illness
    B. decreases the erectile response to stimulation
    C. can be given orally or IM
    D. more effective in older men with low testosterone levels
    E. has been used in to control sexual disinhibition in mentally retarded people

97. A 48-year-old female with bipolar disorder is considered for treatment with lithium. After discussing the risks, benefits, and alternatives, the patient agrees to take lithium. All of the following tests are relevant in this patient except:

    A. pregnancy test
    B. TSH
    C. urea and creatinine
    D. electrocardiogram (EKG)
    E. liver function tests

98. A 48-year-old male with treatment-resistant schizophrenia has been relatively stable for the past 6 months on clozapine. On a routine follow-up visit, the patient is noticed to be depressed with lack of appetite, difficulty staying asleep, problems with concentration, energy, and motivation. He also complains of feeling helpless and worthless. The treating physician decides to start antidepressant medication. Which of the following antidepressants would mandate particular caution in this patient?

    A. Mirtazapine
    B. Fluoxetine
    C. Sertraline
    D. Citalopram
    E. Trazodone

99. A 38-year-old male with a history of coronary artery disease was diagnosed with psychosis not otherwise specified following an episode of paranoia associated with third-person auditory hallucinations. The patient was started on an atypical antipsychotic (ziprasidone 20 mg twice per day). The pharmacy requests an EKG before they could dispense ziprasidone. What is the most important feature to look for on the EKG in this patient?

    A. QT$_c$ interval
    B. Heart rate
    C. Signs of ischemia
    D. Signs of old infarction
    E. Signs of hypokalemia

100. Serotonin discontinuation syndrome is caused by abrupt discontinuation of an SSRI. However, different SSRIs cause varying severities of symptoms. Which of the following SSRIs is least likely to cause discontinuation syndrome?

    A. Sertraline
    B. Citalopram
    C. Escitalopram
    D. Paroxetine
    E. Fluoxetine

101. A 46-year-old female with GAD admits to using alcohol to "control anxiety." She requests her physician to prescribe diazepam because it helped one of her friends. Her physician refuses to prescribe any benzodiazepines, however, because of her substance abuse history. Instead, he prescribes her buspirone. Buspirone acts by:

    A. $5\text{-}HT_{2C}$ agonist
    B. $5\text{-}HT_{1A}$ agonist
    C. $5\text{-}HT_{1A}$ antagonist
    D. GABA agonist
    E. serotonin reuptake inhibition

102. A 57-year-old male was treated for depression with an SSRI. He made a less-than-full recovery despite taking the highest recommended dose. The treating physician thinks about using an augmenting agent. All of the following can be used except:

    A. thyroxine
    B. lithium
    C. tryptophan
    D. propranolol
    E. pindolol

103. Serotonin deficiency is thought to be one of the most important causes of depression. All of the following facts support the serotonin deficiency hypothesis for depression except:

    A. decreased 5-HT platelet uptake
    B. decreased plasma tryptophan levels
    C. decreased 5-hydroxy-indoloacetic acid (5-HIAA) levels in cerebrospinal fluid
    D. decreased 5-HIAA levels in brain
    E. blunted $5\text{-}HT_1$-mediated prolactin release in response to L-tryptophan

104. A 36-year-old obese female with a history of bulimia characterized by binge eating and induced vomiting is admitted to a psychiatry inpatient unit following an overdose of an acetaminophen (Tylenol). She is diagnosed to have major depressive disorder. Which of the following is the least appropriate choice of antidepressant in this patient?
    A. Fluoxetine
    B. Bupropion
    C. Venlafaxine
    D. Citalopram
    E. Sertraline

105. Clozapine, a potent atypical antipsychotic is associated with the adverse effect of agranulocytosis. What is the incidence of agranulocytosis in patients taking clozapine?
    A. 5%
    B. 10%
    C. 3% to 5%
    D. 1% to 2%
    E. 10% to 15%

106. Which of the following statements are true about the pharmacological treatment of generalized anxiety disorder (GAD)?
    A. SSRIs can cause temporary worsening of some of the symptoms.
    B. It usually takes about 4 to 6 weeks to notice any significant improvement.
    C. Beta-blockers are helpful mainly because of their peripheral effect.
    D. If benzodiazepines are used at all, a relatively longer half-life drugs are preferred.
    E. All of the above

107. A 56-year-old male with panic disorder takes almost 60 mg of clonazepam to "get rid of bad panic attack." His wife calls 911 because he is not responding now, and he is breathing very shallow. Which of the following statements regarding benzodiazepine intoxication is true?
    A. Flumazenil is the treatment of choice.
    B. A single dose of flumazenil reverses all the symptoms of benzodiazepine intoxication permanently.
    C. Benzodiazepine intoxication is never fatal.
    D. Short half-life benzodiazepines are less likely to cause intoxication.
    E. CYP450-1A2 is very important in the metabolism of benzodiazepines.

108. All of the following statements regarding lamotrigine are true except:

  A. rapid increase in dose is more likely to cause rash
  B. has been found to be effective in bipolar depression
  C. promotes glutamate release
  D. it is thought to stabilize sodium channels
  E. the usual starting dose in patients with bipolar depression in 25 mg once per day

109. Which of the following statements regarding lithium are true?

  A. It is a monovalent cation.
  B. Dialysis is one of the treatments in overdose.
  C. It is thought to affect second messenger systems.
  D. Can cause leucocytosis.
  E. All of the above

110. Which of following statements about acamprosate are true?

  A. It is a taurine derivative.
  B. It is an N-methyl-D-aspartate (NMDA) antagonist.
  C. It is contraindicated in severe hepatic damage.
  D. It helps with abstinence in alcohol dependence.
  E. All of the above

111. A 45-year-old registered nurse would like to quit smoking because her new workplace has a no-smoking policy. Although she never bothered to learn how nicotine affects her health despite smoking for more than 20 years, she is now interested in knowing more about nicotine and believes that this knowledge will help her to quit smoking. Which of the following statements about nicotine are true?

  A. It increases dopamine release in the nucleus accumbens.
  B. It is a stimulant.
  C. Bupropion has been found to be effective in smoking cessation.
  D. Nicotine primarily acts at nicotinic acetyl receptors.
  E. All of the above

ANSWERS

1. **Answer: C.** Weight gain with antipsychotic medications seems to be associated with pre-treatment BMI such that the greatest weight gain is seen in individuals with low baseline BMI. Although all antipsychotics cause a certain amount of weight gain, some of them cause more than others, and it is likely to plateau only after 6 months.

2. **Answer: E.** Benzodiazepine withdrawal symptoms are very uncomfortable and sometimes serious. Symptoms of benzodiazepine withdrawal include anxiety, delirium, increase in breathing rate, tachycardia, high blood pressure, hyperreflexes, depression, depersonalization and derealization, perceptual disturbances, and seizures. Both constipation and diarrhea are recognized features of benzodiazepine withdrawal. Rhinorrhea is a feature of opiate withdrawal.

3. **Answer: A.** Flupentixol, which is a typical antipsychotic, also has an antidepressant effect. Similarly, amoxapine has both an antipsychotic and an antidepressant effect.

4. **Answer: D.** MAOIs can cause pyridoxine deficiency. Pyridoxine deficiency is associated with peripheral neuropathy.

5. **Answer: B.** Norfluoxetine, the active metabolite of fluoxetine has a half-life of up to 5 to 7 days, and therefore, a washout period of at least 5 weeks is recommended before switching over to MAOIs. The other SSRIs' half-life is less than 24 hours.

6. **Answer: A.** Serotonin syndrome is a potentially life-threatening condition associated with increased serotonergic activity in the CNS. It is seen in patients with an excess of serotonin either due to high doses of serotonergic medications, drug interactions, and sometimes drug overdoses. The diagnosis of serotonin syndrome is made on clinical grounds. Mental status changes include anxiety, delirium, and disorientation. Autonomic manifestations can include diaphoresis, tachycardia, hyperthermia, hypertension, vomiting, and diarrhea. Neuromuscular hyperactivity presents as tremors, muscle rigidity, myoclonus, hyperreflexia, and bilateral Babinski sign. NMS is associated with neuroleptics and not serotonergic medications. There is no history of alcohol abuse in this patient, and therefore, alcohol withdrawal syndrome is not the correct choice.

7. **Answer: E.** Serotonin syndrome can be a difficult condition to diagnose and is easily overlooked due to the high prevalence of use of SSRIs. Several criteria for the diagnosis of serotonin syndrome have been used. The Hunter criteria are 84% sensitive and 97% specific when compared with the gold standard (diagnosis by blood serotonin levels). One of the criteria is "temperature above 38°C plus ocular clonus or inducible clonus," not 32°C.

8. **Answer: D.** Clomipramine, although classified as a tricyclic antidepressant, has a strong serotonin reuptake inhibition effect. It is indicated for the treatment of depression and obsessive-compulsive disorder (OCD). The serotonin reuptake inhibition is thought to be responsible for its anti-OCD properties.

9. **Answer: B.** Bupropion blocks reuptake of both noradrenaline and dopamine. This mechanism of action is particularly useful in patients with depression associated with psychomotor retardation. Buspirone is a 5-HT$_{1A}$ agonist and is effective in treating anxiety. Fluoxetine is an SSRI, and venlafaxine is a serotonin-norepinephrine reuptake inhibitor.

10. **Answer: A.** Methyldopa is an antihypertensive drug that is converted to alpha-methylnoradrenaline in the central presynaptic neurons. This acts as a false neurotransmitter and reduces the overall noradrenergic neurotransmission to the postsynaptic neurons, resulting in depression.

11. **Answer: B.** Pindolol is a nonselective beta-blocker in terms of cardioselectivity but possesses intrinsic sympathomimetic activity. It acts on serotonin (5-HT$_{1A}$) receptors in the brain resulting in increased postsynaptic serotonin concentrations. Pindolol is sometimes added to SSRIs (particularly fluoxetine), if the patient fails to respond to standard therapy alone.

12. **Answer: D.** D$_2$ receptors are found in the mesolimbic, mesocortical, and nigrostriatal systems. There are five subtypes of dopamine receptors: D$_1$, D$_2$, D$_3$, D$_4$, and D$_5$. The D$_1$ and D$_5$ receptors are members of the D$_1$-like family of dopamine receptors, whereas the D$_2$, D$_3$ and D$_4$ receptors are members of the D$_2$-like family. There is some evidence to suggest that 5-HT$_{2A}$ antagonists improve slow-wave sleep and no evidence to suggest they enhance REM sleep. 5-HT$_{1A}$ agonists such as buspirone have anxiolytic properties. Most typical antipsychotics are D$_2$ antagonists rather than agonists. Alpha-2 adrenergic agonists decrease the release of norepinephrine and cause hypotension.

13. **Answer: D.** Lipophilic drugs are rapidly and completely absorbed from the gastrointestinal tract. They have a large volume of distribution and a high first-pass effect. They rapidly cross the blood-brain barrier.

14. **Answer: D.** All of the drugs mentioned except paroxetine induce hepatic cytochrome P450 enzymes. Knowledge of the cytochrome P450 enzyme system helps in choosing appropriate medicines and prevents untoward drug interactions in patients taking multiple medicines.

15. **Answer: C.** Serotonin is now considered to be an important neurotransmitter that is responsible for the regulation of various brain functions. Serotonin is implicated in alertness, activation, aggression, sleep and wakefulness regulation, weight gain, and sexual behavior. However, serotonin has no known role in the maintenance of muscle tone.

16. **Answer: B.** Most of the benzodiazepines are metabolized in the liver, except lorazepam, oxazepam, and temazepam.

17. **Answer: E.** Benzodiazepines act by increasing the frequency of Cl^+ channel opening, and barbiturates increase the duration of Cl^+ channel opening.

18. **Answer: B.** Diazepam is highly lipid soluble and diffuses rapidly into the CNS. It is 90% to 95% protein bound, stored in body fat and brain tissue, is found in breast milk, and crosses the placenta. Peak plasma levels are reached in 30 to 90 minutes. The elimination half-life is between 30 to 100 hours. Oral absorption is faster than IM absorption.

19. **Answer: E.** Ataxia is common in the elderly. Sedation, drowsiness, anterograde amnesia, and postural hypotension are side effects of most of the benzodiazepines. Paradoxical restlessness and behavioral disinhibition is also seen in some patients. Nightmares are a withdrawal symptom and not a side effect of benzodiazepines.

20. **Answer: A.** Leucopenia, eosinophilia, and changes in plasma cortisol are associated with benzodiazepine use. Respiratory depression is mainly seen with intravenous use. Benzodiazepines do not cause induction of hepatic microsomal enzymes, whereas barbiturates and alcohol do induce hepatic enzymes.

21. **Answer: D.** Flurazepam has a half-life that ranges between 40 to 250 hours. The half-lives of the other drugs are as follows: lorazepam, 10 to 12 hours; alprazolam, 6 to 10 hours; oxazepam, 4 to 15 hours; and temazepam, 8 to 22 hours.

22. **Answer: D.** The five benzodiazepines that have received FDA approval for the treatment of insomnia are temazepam, triazolam, estazolam, flurazepam, and quazepam.

23. **Answer: A.** Tremors, depression, tinnitus, depersonalization, derealization, insomnia, fatigue, sweating, concentration difficulties, restlessness, labile blood pressure, and heart rate are all features of benzodiazepine withdrawal. Psychotic symptoms are not common.

24. **Answer: B.** Cimetidine inhibits hepatic enzymes and hence raises levels of many drugs including benzodiazepines. The other drugs listed are hepatic enzyme inducers, which increase metabolism and decrease the levels of drugs metabolized by the hepatic enzymes.

25. **Answer: D.** Cleft lip, cleft palate, respiratory depression, and withdrawal symptoms have been reported in children born to mothers taking benzodiazepines. Absent arms and legs is a teratogenic effect of thalidomide, which was banned many years ago but is now found to have some chemotherapeutic activity.

26. **Answer: D.** Benzodiazepines increase stage II sleep and sleep spindles seen in this stage. A relative decrease in REM and stage III sleep is noted. Sleep latency, total sleep time, and sleep efficiency all improve depending on the half-life of the benzodiazepine used.

27. **Answer: B.** The risk of tolerance or dependence depends on several factors associated with the patient and the drug used. In general, tolerance to the sedative effects of benzodiazepines is seen after 2 to 3 weeks of daily use.

28. **Answer: D.** Cross-tolerance in patients taking benzodiazepines can occur with other benzodiazepines, barbiturates, and alcohol. This is presumed to be due to their proximity of sites of action.

29. **Answer: C.** Personality profiles of patients with benzodiazepine abuse and dependence have shown that it is relatively more common in individuals with passive and dependent personality traits.

30. **Answer: A.** Epstein's anomaly is the downward displacement of the tricuspid valve in the right ventricle. It is relatively rare in the general population with an incidence of one in 20,000. Lithium during pregnancy is associated with a 400 times increased incidence of Epstein's anomaly. Neural tube defects are associated with certain drugs such as sodium valproate that cause vitamin B_{12} deficiency; and phacomelia (congenital absence of limbs) is caused by thalidomide.

31. **Answer: B.** Carbamazepine can produce ataxia at therapeutic doses. Imipramine, quetiapine, chlorpromazine, and fluoxetine do not typically produce ataxia.

32. **Answer: D.** Hyperawareness of senses, dysphoria, tremors, and tongue fasciculations are more suggestive of benzodiazepine withdrawal. Difficulty to stop worrying and the inability to relax are more commonly seen in patients with anxiety disorder.

33. **Answer: C.** Acute dystonia is associated with dopamine receptor antagonists, and benzodiazepines are one of the classes of drugs used to treat acute dystonia. Ataxia, confusion, drowsiness, and aggression (especially in individuals with traumatic brain injury) are recognized side effects of benzodiazepines.

34. **Answer: E.** Benzodiazepines act at the GABA-BDZ receptor complex and potentiate the effects of GABA. They increase the frequency of opening of chloride ion channels and cause hyperpolarization of the cells. Flumazenil, a benzodiazepine receptor antagonist is used to reverse the effects of benzodiazepines. Naloxone is used in patients with opiate toxicity.

35. **Answer: B.** Amitriptyline, lithium, haloperidol, and phenelzine are all associated with tremors. Diazepam is not associated with tremors.

36. **Answer: E.** Tricyclic antidepressants have anticholinergic effects that result in blurred vision, dry mouth, urinary hesitancy, delirium, and constipation. Paralytic ileus may occasionally occur. Desipramine and nortriptyline have a lower incidence of anticholinergic effects compared with other tricyclics.

37. **Answer: B.** Nortriptyline is the only tricyclic antidepressant that has good evidence for an effective therapeutic window. Blood levels in the range of 50 to 150 ng/mL are considered to be therapeutic, whereas levels >500 ng/mL are considered toxic.

38. **Answer: E.** Tricyclics have a low therapeutic index, that is, the therapeutic dose is close to the toxic dose. Tricyclic overdose (deliberate or accidental) can be lethal. Intravenous sodium bicarbonate is often used as an antidote to neutralize metabolic acidosis.

39. **Answer: B.** Tricyclics are sometimes classified as tertiary amines and secondary amines. In general, the tertiary amines inhibit reuptake of serotonin as well as norepinephrine and produce more sedation, anticholinergic effects, and orthostatic hypertension. The secondary amines act primarily on norepinephrine and tend to have a lower side effect profile. Secondary amine tricyclics include nortriptyline, desipramine, and protriptyline.

40. **Answer: B.** Of all the tricyclics, amitriptyline has the most anticholinergic effects, and desipramine has the least anticholinergic effects.

41. **Answer: C.** Nortriptyline, a secondary amine tricyclic, which predominantly inhibits the reuptake of norepinephrine, is least likely to cause postural hypotension.

42. **Answer: C.** Nortriptyline is the only tricyclic antidepressant that has good evidence for an effective therapeutic window. Blood levels in the range of 50 to 150 ng/mL are considered to be therapeutic, whereas levels >500 ng/mL are considered toxic.

43. **Answer: D.** The symptoms suggest seasonal affective disorder. Bupropion has been found to be more effective in these patients. SSRIs are also useful but lack the activating effects of bupropion. Mirtazapine is not a good choice, as it is likely to worsen hypersomnia and enhance appetite further.

44. **Answer: C.** Tyramine, a substrate of MAO enzymes is present in certain fermented foodstuffs such as red wine, cheese, yeast extracts, and pickled fish. Patients taking MAOIs are unable to deaminate tyramine, normally broken down by MAO-A in the gut. This results in the displacement of intracellular stores of norepinephrine and can cause a pressor response resulting in hypertensive crisis.

45. **Answer: B.** Tyramine, a substrate of MAO enzymes is present in high concentrations in certain foods such as cheese, red wine, and yeast extracts. Ingestion of these foods results in hypertensive crisis. Bananas do not cause a hypertensive crisis with MAOIs, although the skin of banana can.

46. **Answer: E.** The symptoms described are typical of serotonin syndrome. The combination of sumatriptan and MAOIs can result in serotonin syndrome. This reaction is commonly seen when MAOIs are combined with SSRIs or other tricyclic antidepressants. For this reason, when switching from MAOIs to SSRIs or tricyclics or vice versa, a minimum of a 2-week washout period is required.

47. **Answer: D.** When switching from an SSRI to a MAOI, a washout period of 2 weeks is recommended for all SSRIs, except for fluoxetine, which requires a washout period of 5 weeks because of its relatively long half-life.

48. **Answer: D.** Mirtazapine is a novel antidepressant that acts by blocking presynaptic alpha-2 adrenergic receptors. It is also a potent antagonist of H1 receptors, which explains its somnolent effects. There are reports of agranulocytosis with mirtazapine. Mirtazapine increases appetite, and weight gain is a common side effect.

49. **Answer: D.** The half-life of fluvoxamine is about 15 hours. The half-lives of the other drugs are as follows: fluoxetine, 4 to 6 days; paroxetine, 21 hours; sertraline, 26 hours; and citalopram, 35 hours.

50. **Answer: D.** SSRIs are one of the safest groups of antidepressants and do not cause arrhythmias. They can cause diarrhea or constipation and have variable effects on the appetite. They can cause tremors and headaches.

51. **Answer: A.** SSRIs commonly cause sexual side effects. The range of problems includes anorgasmia, delayed ejaculation, and impotence. Sometimes, SSRIs are used to treat premature ejaculation. SSRIs do not have significant effects on blood pressure and cause clinically insignificant slowing of the heart rate. They do not cause alopecia, urinary hesitancy, or itching.

52. **Answer: E.** SSRIs do not cause premature ejaculation. They cause delay in ejaculation and are sometimes used in the treatment of premature ejaculation. SSRIs are associated with nausea, vomiting, diarrhea, agitation, and akathisia.

53. **Answer: A.** Fluoxetine is least likely to cause discontinuation syndrome because of its long half-life of 4 to 6 days.

54. **Answer: E.** The main consideration in choosing an appropriate SSRI in this patient would be their action on the P450 isoenzymes. Because this patient is on multiple medications, it is important to make sure that there are no significant interactions with other medications via inhibition of hepatic cytochrome P450 isoenzymes. The other considerations listed are not very important, as all of the SSRIs are comparable in their efficacy, and they do not have any significant actions at either opiate or dopamine receptors.

55. **Answer: B.** The most common adverse effects reported with SSRIs use are gastrointestinal, and nausea is the most common side effect reported.

56. **Answer: A.** Priapism is a known side effect of trazodone. The incidence varies from one in 6,000 to 10,000 individuals. There are case reports of priapism in association with various other medications including other antidepressants and antipsychotic medications. It is not as common as it is seen with trazodone.

57. **Answer: C.** Trazodone has significant antagonistic activity at 5-HT_{2A} receptors. Chronic administration of trazodone causes down-regulation of 5-HT_{2A} receptors, which is thought to have an antidepressant effect. Trazodone has very little affinity for muscarinic, histamine, dopamine, and norepinephrine receptors.

58. **Answer: D.** Trazodone is not associated with seizures or lowering of the seizure threshold. Priapism, orthostatic hypotension, drowsiness, and headaches are all recognized side effects of trazodone.

59. **Answer: B.** Lithium is an elemental drug that is not bound to plasma protein, is not metabolized, and is excreted unchanged by the kidneys.

60. **Answer: A.** Renal lithium clearance is relatively constant for each individual, but it is proportional to glomerular filtration as measured by creatinine clearance. If creatinine clearance decreases, lithium excretion will be reduced, and serum lithium levels will rise. Sodium is required for renal lithium excretion. When sodium is depleted as in decreased food intake, excessive sweating, diarrhea, lithium renal clearance etc; is reduced leading to lithium toxicity.

61. **Answer: A.** Lithium is an element that is not lipophilic. It is rapidly and completely absorbed. It has low-protein binding properties and no metabolites. All of the other drugs mentioned are lipophilic.

62. **Answer: A.** Agranulocytosis is an idiosyncratic reaction to clozapine and is not related to the dose. The other three side effects mentioned are dose related and worsen with increasing dose.

63. **Answer: E.** A higher risk for agranulocytosis in patients treated with clozapine is noted in the Jewish population and not in African Americans. The risk among women is two times higher than men.

64. **Answer: B.** Benzodiazepines are generally not administered with clozapine because of the reports of circulatory collapse and respiratory arrest.

65. **Answer: B.** Molindone has an appetite suppressant effect and is least likely to cause weight gain. Other antipsychotics, which cause relatively less weight gain, are ziprasidone and aripiprazole.

66. **Answer: A.** Lithium is known to increase the risk of NMS when used in combination with antipsychotics.

67. **Answer: E.** Although NMS is typically associated with neuroleptics, other drugs can cause symptoms that are very similar to NMS. These include reserpine, metoclopramide, methylphenidate, dextroamphetamines, lithium, MAOIs, and tricyclic antidepressants.

68. **Answer: D.** Of all the antipsychotics, clozapine causes the largest decrease in seizure threshold. It is not uncommon to start seizure prophylaxis above the dose of clozapine 600 mg per day.

69. **Answer: A.** Carbamazepine induces CYP 450 3A4 enzymes, which is also the enzyme system that metabolizes carbamazepine. Therefore, it not only accelerates its own metabolism, but it also lowers the levels of other drugs that are metabolized by CYP 450 3A4 enzymes including birth control pills.

70. **Answer: E.** Several medications can increase the lithium levels including diuretics, non-steroidal anti-inflammatory drugs, and tetracycline.

71. **Answer: D.** Apart from the changes mentioned, lithium is also known to affect the sinus node, and therefore, it is contraindicated in patients with sick sinus syndrome.

72. **Answer: B.** Amitriptyline and imipramine are the only two antidepressants that are available in the parenteral form.

73. **Answer: A.** Amoxapine should be avoided in patients with Parkinson's disease. Amoxapine has dopamine-blocking effects that can make Parkinson's disease symptoms worse. Bupropion is the preferred antidepressant in treating patients with Parkinson's disease because of its dopamine reuptake blocking properties.

74. **Answer: A.** Compared to all other SSRIs, paroxetine has the most anticholinergic effects.

75. **Answer: A.** Of all the antidepressant medications, venlafaxine, bupropion, trazodone, and nefazodone are considered to have the least anticholinergic effects and are therefore relatively safe to use in narrow-angle glaucoma.

76. **Answer: D.** Patients with seasonal affective disorder who use bright light therapy usually respond within 2 to 4 days, but full response is noticed only after 1 to 2 weeks.

77. **Answer: E.** PCP abuse is characterized by recurring psychotic episodes and aggression over a period of time, and sometimes, it can last up to 2 to 3 months. This is because of its high lipid solubility, and it is released intermittently in the blood stream. Patients taking amphetamines and cocaine can present with a similar clinical picture, but the effects usually do not last for more than 72 hours. Marijuana and benzodiazepines rarely produce acute psychosis with aggression.

78. **Answer: C.** Clorazepate is metabolized in the gastrointestinal tract to desmethyl diazepam prior to its absorption.

79. **Answer: C.** The incidence of seizures in patients taking bupropion less than 450 mg per day is 0.4%. The risk of seizures increases to 2%, however, if the dose range is between 450 to 600 mg per day.

80. **Answer: D.** The incidence of aplastic anemia associated with carbamazepine is one in 20,000. Therefore, a complete blood count is done before starting carbamazepine.

81. **Answer: A.** Hyperprolactinemia is not associated with clozapine because unlike typical and some atypical antipsychotics (particularly risperidone), clozapine does not cause D_2 receptor blockade in the tuberoinfundibular pathways.

82. **Answer: E.** Aripiprazole is an atypical antipsychotic that has FDA approval for treating schizophrenia, bipolar disorder (both mania and mixed), and acute agitation in schizophrenia and mania (not depression).

83. **Answer: D.** Aripiprazole is an atypical antipsychotic that acts as a partial agonist at D_2 and 5-HT_{1A} receptors, and it is a $5H\text{-T}_{2A}$ receptor antagonist. Like all other atypical antipsychotics, it can lower the seizure threshold and is not indicated for dementia-related psychosis in the elderly population. In fact, atypical antipsychotics are associated with an increased incidence of cerebrovascular events when used in the elderly for dementia-related psychosis.

84. **Answer: B.** Benzodiazepines commonly cause ataxia at therapeutic doses, especially in the elderly. Phenytoin toxicity can cause ataxia, which is a possibility in this patient, as paroxetine increase the levels of phenytoin. Phenytoin toxicity is associated with other signs and symptoms, however, including nystagmus, blurred vision, diplopia, slurred speech, drowsiness, lethargy, confusion, and mood changes.

85. **Answer: B.** Carbamazepine is associated with rare but serious skin reactions that include toxic epidermal necrolysis and Stevens-Johnson syndrome. The risk of these reactions is estimated to be about one to six per 10,000 new users of the drug in countries with mainly white populations. However, the risk is estimated to be about 10 times higher in some Asian countries. Studies have found a strong association between serious skin reactions and an inherited variant of a gene, HLA-B*1502, an immune system gene, found almost exclusively in people of Asian ancestry. Patients testing positive for this gene should not be treated with carbamazepine unless the benefit clearly outweighs the increased risk of these serious skin reactions.

86. **Answer: C.** Carbamazepine is a potent inducer of hepatic enzymes and promotes the metabolism of many other drugs including its own. It is metabolized mainly by CYP3A4 and other oxidative mechanisms in the liver. Plasma levels of carbamazepine are not very useful in determining the seriousness of carbamazepine toxicity. Therapeutic levels are thought to range between 4 to 12 mcg/mL, and side effects including CNS effects occur commonly at higher dosage levels. Symptoms of carbamazepine toxicity include dizziness, ataxia, drowsiness, nausea, vomiting, tremor, agitation, nystagmus, urinary retention, coma, seizures, respiratory depression, and neuromuscular disturbances.

87. **Answer: D.** Thirst, polyuria, and polydipsia are some of the early side effects related to Na-K pump changes in the renal tubule. Fine tremors are associated with therapeutic levels of lithium, and toxic levels cause coarse tremors. About 7% of patients report problems with erection on therapeutic doses of lithium. Lithium causes blurred vision but not diplopia.

88. **Answer: D.** Discontinuation syndrome following abrupt stopping of antidepressants does not indicate dependence on antidepressant medications. Patients on antidepressants do not show evidence of tolerance, a compulsive desire to take the drug, or drug-seeking behavior.

89. **Answer: C.** Eszopiclone is a cyclopyrrolone and not a benzodiazepine derivative. It belongs to a newer class of hypnotics, commonly known as benzodiazepine receptor agonists. Although the potential for tolerance and dependence exists, these medicines are thought to be relatively safer.

90. **Answer: B.** Buspirone, an azaspirodecanedione is a non-benzodiazepine anxiolytic and does not cause sedation or dependence. It acts as a 5-HT_{1A} presynaptic receptor partial agonist. It takes up to 4 to 6 weeks before symptomatic relief is noted. It is usually started at 10 to 20 mg in two divided doses and can be titrated up to a maximum of 60 mg per day in three divided doses.

91. **Answer: E.** Although SSRIs are effective in treating anxiety disorders, it usually takes 4 to 6 weeks before they can be effective, and therefore, clonazepam is often used for symptomatic relief until SSRIs are effective. Bupropion is activating and can make the patient's anxiety worse. CBT is effective treating in anxiety disorders but does not provide immediate relief.

92. **Answer: C.** Acute dystonia, characterized by sustained muscle contraction, is usually seen in the first few days after starting neuroleptics, although it can occur anytime. Akathisia, a subjective sense of psychomotor restlessness is more common than acute dystonia.

93. **Answer: A.** Clear consciousness is not a feature of NMS. Patients with NMS have altered sensorium. NMS is a medical emergency and needs aggressive treatment including immediate discontinuation of neuroleptics. The mortality rate is high, if untreated.

94. **Answer: B.** Lamotrigine is not effective for treating acute mania. It is approved by the FDA for the maintenance treatment of bipolar I disorder to delay the recurrence of mania, hypomania, mixed and depression episodes in patients treated with standard therapy for acute mood episodes. Lamotrigine is started at a small dose and titrated gradually over the next few weeks.

95. **Answer: C.** Venlafaxine inhibits the reuptake of serotonin and noradrenaline, which is dose dependent. Venlafaxine inhibits reuptake of serotonin only up to a dose of 150 mg, and inhibition of norepinephrine reuptake starts at a dose larger than 150 mg.

96. **Answer: D.** Cyproterone acetate is an antiandrogen that acts by blocking androgen receptors. It is indicated in the treatment of prostate cancer, benign prostate hyperplasia, and hirsutism. It is particularly effective in young individuals with high testosterone levels.

97. **Answer: E.** Lithium is eliminated almost entirely by the kidneys and does not undergo any hepatic metabolism. Therefore, there is no need for liver function tests. Baseline TSH, EKG, urea, and creatinine level tests are recommended. All women of child-bearing age should also take a pregnancy test because of the risk of cardiac defects to the fetus.

98. **Answer: A.** Clozapine is associated with the risk of agranulocytosis. Mirtazapine is also associated with rare but serious side effects of agranulocytosis in less than 1% of the patients. Therefore, patients who are on a combination of clozapine and mirtazapine should be monitored carefully.

99. **Answer: A.** Although all atypical antipsychotics can cause QT prolongation to some extent, ziprasidone is known to cause the maximum prolongation of QT interval. A prolonged QT interval predisposes to cardiac arrhythmias. Although all of the choices mentioned are important observations to make in an EKG, corrected QT interval (QT_c) is the most important feature.

100. **Answer: E.** Although all of the SSRIs can cause discontinuation syndrome, fluoxetine is least likely to cause symptoms of discontinuation because of its long half-life. Norfluoxetine, the active metabolite of fluoxetine, has a half-life of 5 to 7 days and "tapers off" on its own.

101. **Answer: B.** Buspirone decreases the symptoms of anxiety by 5-HT_{1A} agonistic action. However, it takes 4 to 6 weeks before symptomatic relief is noted. Buspirone is usually started at 10 to 20 mg twice per day, and the dose may have to be titrated up to a maximum of 60 mg given in three divided doses.

102. **Answer: D.** Propranolol is a beta-blocker, which can, in fact, worsen the patient's depression. Pindolol, another beta-blocker acts at 5-HT_{1A} receptors and is sometimes used as an adjunctive agent along with an SSRI in the treatment of depression.

103. **Answer: D.** Serotonin deficiency hypothesis for depression has considerable evidence including the effectiveness of SSRIs in depression. There is no demonstrable decrease in the brain levels of 5-HIAA, however, which is a metabolite of 5-HT.

104. **Answer: B.** Bupropion is contraindicated in individuals with anorexia and/or bulimia nervosa because of the increased risk of seizures.

105. **Answer: D.** The incidence of agranulocytosis with clozapine is around 1% to 2%. Therefore, all patients who start clozapine should be registered with the clozapine patient monitoring service.

106. **Answer: E.** In GAD, SSRIs can sometimes cause temporary worsening of some symptoms such as irritability and nervousness. It usually takes 4 to 6 weeks before there is any significant improvement. Sometimes, symptomatic treatment is recommended until SSRIs are effective. In these situations, a benzodiazepine with a relatively long half-life (8 to 10 hours) is preferred to prevent breakthrough anxiety. Beta-blockers are helpful mainly because of their peripheral effect, and they do not have any central effects.

107. **Answer: A.** Flumazenil is the treatment of choice in benzodiazepine intoxication. Intravenous flumazenil may have to be used repeatedly to treat benzodiazepine intoxication because of the short half-life of flumazenil. Benzodiazepine intoxication can be fatal, if not promptly treated. The half-life of a benzodiazepine is not a significant factor as far its potential to cause intoxication is concerned, and CYP450-2D6 is the most important enzyme in the metabolism of benzodiazepines.

108. **Answer: C.** Lamotrigine inhibits glutamate release. A rapid increase in dose is more likely to cause a rash and serious allergic reactions such as Stevens-Johnson syndrome. It has been found to be effective in treating patients with bipolar depression, and the usual starting dose is 25 mg once a day. The dose is slowly increased every 2 weeks to about 100 mg by week 5.

109. **Answer: E.** Lithium is a monovalent cation that is cleared almost entirely by the kidneys; for this reason, dialysis is one of the interventions used in overdose. Although lithium's exact mechanism of action is not known, it is thought to affect second messenger systems in cells. Lithium is also known to induce mild leucocytosis.

110. **Answer: E.** Acamprosate has been found to be effective in increasing the abstinence rates in alcohol dependence. It is a taurine derivative and acts by NMDA antagonism. It is also thought to enhance GABA function and is contraindicated in severe hepatic damage.

111. **Answer: E.** Nicotine is a stimulant, and it primarily acts at the nicotinic acetyl receptors. It increases dopamine release in the nucleus accumbens, and nicotine tolerance is associated with receptor desensitization and a compensatory up-regulation of nicotinic receptors. Although nicotine's primary site of action is at nicotinic acetyl receptors, bupropion has been found to be effective in smoking cessation

Psychotherapy

QUESTIONS

1. Defense mechanism in psychotherapy refers to:
   A. fending off an argument by not talking
   B. conscious effort to block unpleasant emotions
   C. unconscious, intrapsychic process
   D. psychological turmoil
   E. all of the above

2. Ego ideal in psychotherapy refers to:
   A. id
   B. ego
   C. defense mechanism
   D. part of superego that aspires to have higher morals and values
   E. based on pleasure principle

3. Oedipus complex refers to:
   A. internalization of maternal figure
   B. develops at the age of 10 years
   C. occurs in boys
   D. internalization of father figure
   E. proposed by Sigmund Freud

4. The three stages of development proposed by Margaret Mahler include all of the following except:
   A. separation-individuation phase
   B. autistic phase
   C. symbiotic phase
   D. all of above
   E. none of the above

5. Alexithymia refers to:

   A. difficulty reading
   B. total inability to read
   C. difficulty with writing
   D. difficulty understanding spoken language
   E. inability to verbalize feelings

6. Aaron Beck's cognitive triad in depression includes:

   A. negative cognitions about self
   B. negative cognitions about the world
   C. negative cognitions about the future
   D. all of the above
   E. none of the above

7. All of these features are characteristic of obsessions except:

   A. urge to perform a behavior
   B. persistent intrusive thoughts
   C. insight that the thoughts belong to self
   D. not amenable to logic
   E. persistent intrusive impulse or idea

8. All of these features are characteristic of compulsions except:

   A. urge to perform a behavior
   B. difficulty in resisting the behavior
   C. worsening of anxiety on resisting the urge
   D. worsening of anxiety on performing the behavior
   E. relief of anxiety on performing the behavior

9. Cognitive behavioral therapy (CBT) is effective in treating which of the following conditions?

   A. Major depressive disorder
   B. Generalized anxiety disorder (GAD)
   C. Panic disorder
   D. Social phobia
   E. All of the above

10. The theory of learned helplessness was proposed to explain which of the following disorders?
    A. Alcohol abuse
    B. Depression
    C. Phobia
    D. GAD
    E. Posttraumatic stress disorder

11. *Flooding* in the behavioral component of CBT refers to:
    A. sudden exposure to the most anxiety-provoking stimulus
    B. relaxation in water
    C. exposure to painful stimulus until the undesired behavior is terminated
    D. gradual exposure to the most anxiety-provoking stimulus
    E. challenge dysfunctional beliefs

12. The use of disulfiram in the treatment of alcoholism is an example of:
    A. punishment
    B. CBT
    C. aversion therapy
    D. systematic desensitization
    E. flooding

13. One of the symptoms that differentiates depression from bereavement is:
    A. appetite disturbance
    B. sleep disturbance
    C. lack of concentration
    D. crying spells
    E. worthlessness

14. Systematic desensitization refers to:
    A. gradual exposure to anxiety-provoking stimulus
    B. sudden exposure to anxiety-provoking stimulus
    C. application of electric shocks until the undesired behavior is extinguished
    D. modification of dysfunctional beliefs and attitudes
    E. group therapy

15. Which of the following statements are true about dialectical behavior therapy (DBT)?
    A. Designed by Marsha Linehan
    B. Goal is to reduce self-harm and hospitalizations
    C. Manual-driven therapy
    D. Helpful in borderline personality disorder patients
    E. All of the above

16. All of the following are features of CBT except:
    A. focus on dysfunctional beliefs and attitudes
    B. based on principles of learning and cognitive theory
    C. homework is often part of the treatment plan
    D. considers childhood experiences, abuse
    E. goal setting is an important part of the treatment

17. Which of the following conditions respond to CBT?
    A. Obsessive-compulsive disorder (OCD)
    B. Panic disorder
    C. Depression
    D. GAD
    E. All of the above

18. All of the following are characteristics of group therapy except:
    A. the participants have a similar problem
    B. goal is to establish premorbid function
    C. no prescreening is necessary
    D. acceptance is an important therapeutic factor
    E. therapist acts as a guide

19. Which of the following statements is true about hypnosis?
    A. Paranoia is a contraindication
    B. Effective in pain disorders
    C. Subject's ability to dissociate is important
    D. Trust between the therapist and subject is important
    E. All of the above

20. All of the following are true about Freud's psychosexual model of development except:
    A. it deals from birth to 18 years of age
    B. there are six stages of development
    C. the goal of each stage is to derive pleasure and relieve pain
    D. the phallic stage is also known as the genital stage
    E. the latency stage lasts from 6 to 11 years of age

ANSWERS

1. **Answer: C.** Defense mechanism is an unconscious, intrapsychic process that maintains psychological homeostasis and relieves emotional conflicts and anxiety.

2. **Answer: D.** Id, ego, and superego refer to the three aspects of Freud's structural theory of psyche. Superego is a symbolic internalization of the father figure and cultural regulations. It acts as conscience.

3. **Answer: D.** The Oedipus complex, proposed by Freud is formed by the identification and internalization of the father figure after a little boy cannot successfully hold his mother as a love object out of fear of castration.

4. **Answer: D.** The three stages of development proposed by Margaret Mahler include autistic phase (0 to 4 weeks), symbiotic phase (4 weeks to 5 months), and separation-individuation phase (5 months to 3 years).

5. **Answer: E.** Alexithymia refers to the inability to verbalize or become aware of one's mood or feelings.

6. **Answer: D.** Aaron Beck, who proposed CBT, described the negative cognitive triad of depression and included negative thoughts about self, others, and the future.

7. **Answer: A.** Obsessions are persistent intrusive thoughts, ideas, or impulses that cannot be eliminated by logic or reasoning and are part of the individual's thought process. An urge to perform a behavior that is irresistible is defined as a compulsion.

8. **Answer: D.** A compulsion is an irresistible urge to perform a behavior in response to an obsession, worsening of anxiety on resisting the behavior, and relief of anxiety on performing the behavior.

9. **Answer: E.** CBT has been found to be effective in a variety of mood and anxiety disorders including OCDs.

10. **Answer: B.** Martin Seligman proposed an animal model of human depression known as *learned helplessness*.

11. **Answer: A.** Flooding is a behavioral technique in which a subject is exposed to his or her most anxiety-provoking stimulus until it no longer produces any anxiety.

12. **Answer: C.** The use of disulfiram in the treatment of alcoholism is an example of aversion therapy. Here, the undesired behavior (alcohol abuse) is paired with an unpleasant stimulus (nausea, vomiting) to terminate the undesired behavior.

13. **Answer: E.** Depression and bereavement often cause similar symptoms, and sometimes depression follows a bereavement reaction. A sense of worthlessness is more suggestive of depression, which is typically absent in bereavement reaction.

14. **Answer: A.** Systematic desensitization refers to gradual exposure to increasingly more anxiety-provoking stimuli associated with relaxation techniques.

15. **Answer: E.** DBT was originally designed specifically for patients with borderline personality disorder to reduce self-harm and recurrent hospitalizations. It is manual-driven therapy that can last for more than 1 year.

16. **Answer: D.** CBT is based on principles of learning, cognitive theory, and focuses on dysfunctional beliefs and attitudes. It is goal oriented and uses a collaborative approach. Patients are expected to practice relaxation techniques and other coping techniques taught in the sessions. CBT does not involve dwelling into childhood experiences and deals with the "here and now" approach.

17. **Answer: E.** CBT has been found to be effective in treating a wide variety of anxiety disorders (GAD, panic disorder, phobias, social anxiety disorder), mood disorders (depression, bipolar disorders), eating disorders, substance abuse, as well as some of the psychotic and personality disorders.

18. **Answer: C.** Group therapy is a form of psychotherapy that is very effective in certain conditions. Alcoholics Anonymous is one example of group therapy. Group therapies have been found to be effective in treating other conditions such as mood disorders, eating disorders, anxiety disorders, and substance abuse problems. Prescreening is important to ensure the patient's values and goals match the group's objectives and that the patient does not disrupt the group.

19. **Answer: E.** Hypnosis is characterized by the therapeutic use of suggestion to bring about a change in the subject. The subject's ability to trust the therapist, ability to dissociate, and the relationship between the therapist and the subject are important factors in hypnosis. It has been used effectively in various conditions including pain, smoking cessation, and weight reduction. Some studies have confirmed the efficacy of hypnosis, but many physicians have not received it enthusiastically.

20. **Answer: B.** Freud's psychosexual model of development has five stages: (1) oral phase (0 to 1 year); (2) anal phase (1 to 3 years); (3) phallic or genital stage (3 to 5 years); (4) latency (6 to 11 years); and (5) adolescence (12 to 18 years). The goal of each stage is to derive pleasure and relieve pain.

Miscellaneous

QUESTIONS

1. The prevalence of personality disorders in the general population is:

   A. 20%
   B. 1%
   C. 5% to 10%
   D. 20% to 40%
   E. 30 % to 60%

2. What is the most common defense mechanism in patients with paranoid personality disorders?

   A. Regression
   B. Suppression
   C. Denial
   D. Projection
   E. Reaction formation

3. According to the *Diagnostic and Statistical Manual of Mental Disorders*, 4th edition (DSM-IV), violent behavior is a characteristic feature of all of the following disorders except:

   A. paranoid personality disorder
   B. borderline personality disorder
   C. antisocial personality disorder
   D. intermittent explosive disorder
   E. conduct disorder

4. All of the following are known to increase the risk of antisocial behavior except:
   A. substance abuse
   B. family history of alcoholism
   C. adoption
   D. childhood abuse
   E. easy access to guns

5. A 26-year-old female presents to the emergency department (ED) with superficial scratches on her left forearm. While in the ED, she gets into an argument with the nurse and swears at her. When the doctor comes to see her, however, she becomes very pleasant and tells him that he is the best doctor she has ever seen. The ED physician feels very good about this but suspects the patient has borderline personality traits. All of the following defense mechanisms are commonly seen in patients with borderline personality disorder except:
   A. idealization and devaluation
   B. projection
   C. projective identification
   D. acting out
   E. reaction formation

6. All of the following defense mechanisms are commonly seen in individuals with obsessive-compulsive personality disorders except:
   A. reaction formation
   B. undoing
   C. isolation of affect
   D. projection
   E. rationalization

7. Which of the following conditions can cause catatonia?
   A. Viral encephalitis
   B. Head injury
   C. Cerebrovascular disorders
   D. Brain tumors
   E. All of the above

8. All of the following are features of Huntington's disease except:

   A. autosomal recessive
   B. abnormality on chromosome 4
   C. dementia
   D. chorea
   E. anticipation

9. What is the trinucleotide repeat sequence characteristic of Huntington's disease?

   A. CAG
   B. AAG
   C. CCG
   D. GCC
   E. ACC

10. Which of the following psychiatric disorders is very common in patients with cardiovascular disorders?

    A. Mania
    B. Hypomania
    C. Psychosis
    D. Depression
    E. Phobia

11. Which of the following conditions can cause dementia?

    A. Hypercalcemia
    B. Vitamin B_{12} deficiency
    C. Hypothyroidism
    D. Normal pressure hydrocephalus
    E. All of the above

12. All of the following are features of pellagra except:

    A. thiamine deficiency
    B. psychiatric disturbances
    C. dermatitis
    D. diarrhea
    E. dementia

13. Rapid eye movement (REM) sleep behavior disorder (RBD) is associated with a higher incidence of which of the following disorders?
    A. Strokes
    B. Seizures
    C. Synucleinopathies
    D. Depression
    E. Psychosis

14. A 72-year-old male is consulted for grimacing, tongue protrusion, and lip-smacking movements. He was diagnosed with schizoaffective disorder when he was 40 years old and has been taking trifluoperazine since then. The neurologist diagnoses him to have tardive dyskinesia. All of the following are risk factors for tardive dyskinesia except:
    A. old age
    B. diffuse brain damage
    C. duration of antipsychotic treatment
    D. affective psychosis
    E. substance abuse

15. All of the following are associated with a higher risk of mental illness in children except:
    A. living in inner cities
    B. learning disability
    C. physical disability
    D. adoption
    E. chronic physical illness

16. Untreated attention-deficit hyperactivity disorder (ADHD) in children is associated with an increased risk of:
    A. conduct disorder
    B. substance abuse
    C. poor academic performance
    D. increase in motor vehicle accidents
    E. all of the above

17. A 56-year-old female with a history of depression characterized by psychomotor retardation is treated with venlafaxine. Although she responds well to the medication, she complains of "uncomfortable sensations" in her legs during the evening. These symptoms worsen gradually to the point that she finds it hard to fall asleep because she has to walk or shake her legs to get rid of these sensations. The treating psychiatrist diagnosed her to have restless legs syndrome (RLS) precipitated by venlafaxine and considers changing the antidepressant. Which of the following antidepressant medications is not associated with RLS?
    A. Escitalopram
    B. Bupropion
    C. Mirtazapine
    D. Fluvoxamine
    E. Paroxetine

18. A 32-year-old male is diagnosed to have attention-deficit disorder (ADD) after neuropsychological testing. He states that he is happy because "finally, there is some explanation" to all the problems he has had with concentration and memory all his life. He also states that as a child, he was not just having attention problems but he was also "very hyperactive." However, the symptoms of hyperactivity have subsided over the past decade. He states that he was "self-medicating" with stimulants including methylphenidate that he got off the streets and sometimes drank large quantities of alcohol to "calm" himself. He was admitted twice to an alcohol rehabilitation center. Which of the following will be the first choice to treat ADD in this patient?
    A. Methylphenidate
    D. Amphetamines
    C. Provigil
    D. Atomoxetine
    E. All of the above

19. Freud's psychosexual model of development includes all the following stages except:
    A. adolescence
    B. anal phase
    C. oral phase
    D. Oedipus complex
    E. genital phase

20. Which of the following statements about separation anxiety disorder is true?
    A. Found in 1% of adolescents
    B. Equally common in both boys and girls
    C. Found in 4% of school-age children
    D. CBT is effective
    E. All of the above

ANSWERS

1. **Answer: C.** The prevalence of personality disorders in the general population is 5% to 10%. It is higher in psychiatric outpatients (20% to 40%) and very common in psychiatric inpatients (30% to 60%).

2. **Answer: D.** Projection is the most common defense mechanism associated with paranoid personality disorder.

3. **Answer: A.** Violent behavior is not a characteristic feature of paranoid personality disorder.

4. **Answer: C.** There is no increased prevalence of antisocial behavior in adopted children. Apart from the risk factors mentioned, poverty, lack of education, and absence of family contributes to antisocial behavior.

5. **Answer: E.** Reaction formation is often seen in individuals with obsessive-compulsive personality rather than borderline personality. Acting out, splitting, and denial are other defense mechanisms seen in patients with borderline personality disorder.

6. **Answer: D.** Projection and projective identification are often seen in patients with borderline personality disorder. Other typical defense mechanisms seen in individuals with obsessive-compulsive personality disorders are intellectualization and displacement.

7. **Answer: E.** All of these conditions can cause catatonia.

8. **Answer: A.** Huntington's disease is an autosomal dominant disorder with trinucleotide repeat abnormality on chromosome 4. It is characterized by dementia and chorea. Anticipation is a genetic concept wherein the disorder appears at a younger age, and the symptoms become more severe in successive generations.

9. **Answer: A.** The genetic defect responsible for Huntington's disease is a small sequence of DNA on chromosome 4 in which the trinucleotide sequence CAG repeats many times.

10. **Answer: D.** Depression is very common in patients with cardiovascular disorders and is often associated with increased morbidity.

11. **Answer: E.** Many other medical conditions such as encephalitis, strokes, brain tumors, and metabolic problems can cause dementia.

12. **Answer: A.** Pellagra results from a deficiency of vitamin B_3 (niacin). The psychiatric disturbances include aggression, delirium, depression, and dementia.

13. **Answer: C.** Longitudinal follow-up of patients with RBD have shown a higher incidence of synucleinopathies (particularly Parkinson's disease).

14. **Answer: D.** Increasing age is a strong risk factor and is thought to be a much stronger risk factor for men than women. Having an affective psychosis lowers the risk of tardive dyskinesia. The risk of tardive dyskinesia increases with the duration of antipsychotics and not the dose. Comorbid substance abuse increases the risk of tardive dyskinesia.

15. **Answer: D.** Adoption is not associated with increased incidence of mental illness in children. In fact, adoption into a stable and caring family will decrease the risk of mental illness.

16. **Answer: E.** Untreated, ADHD is associated with a higher incidence of a number of problems that can significantly affect various aspects of life.

17. **Answer: B.** Bupropion is not associated with RLS. Although the exact mechanism that causes RLS with antidepressants is not known, it is thought to be caused by the serotonergic effects.

18. **Answer: D.** In patients with a history of substance abuse, it is always wise not to use as a first choice, any medications that have a potential for tolerance and abuse. Atomoxetine is a norepinephrine reuptake inhibitor that is approved by the FDA for the treatment of ADD. Methylphenidate and amphetamines are helpful with ADD but have a potential for tolerance and abuse. Some of the newer preparations of these drugs are thought to be safer as far as abuse potential is concerned. Provigil is not approved for the treatment of ADD.

19. **Answer: D.** Freud's psychosexual model of development includes five stages: (1) oral phase; (2) anal phase; (3) phallic or genital phase; (4) latency; and (5) adolescence. The Oedipus complex is part of the genital phase.

20. **Answer: E.** Separation anxiety disorder is the only childhood-onset anxiety disorder recognized by the DSM-IV. It occurs when a child is separated from home or from a significant attachment figure. It is found in 4% of school-age children and 1% of adolescents. The symptoms should last for at least 4 months, and the onset should be prior to the age of 18 years. It is equally common in both boys and girls, and both CBT and selective serotonin reuptake inhibitors have been found to be effective treatment.

Psychiatry High-Yields

DEPRESSION

1. According to the *Diagnostic and Statistical Manual of Mental Disorders*, 4th edition (DSM-IV), the time criterion to diagnose depression is if the patient has symptoms lasting for at least 2 weeks.

2. The mechanism of action of mirtazapine is central, presynaptic, alpha-2 receptor antagonism.

3. Priapism is one of the rare but serious side effects of trazodone.

4. A patient is said to have recurrent depression when he or she has two or more episodes of depression.

5. Of all the antidepressants, bupropion and paroxetine are less likely to precipitate a hypomanic or manic episode in patients with bipolar affective disorder.

6. Mirtazapine, although a sedating antidepressant, can be activated at doses higher than 30 mg.

7. The medications approved by the Food and Drug Administration (FDA) for the treatment of bipolar depression are lithium and lamotrigine.

8. Lithium and clozapine are known to specifically decrease suicidal ideation.

9. All patients presenting with depression should be screened for bipolar disorder.

10. Depression is twice as common in women compared to men.

11. Atypical depression is characterized by hypersomnia, hyperphagia, fatigue, and rejection sensitivity.

12. The risk of recurrence of depression after one episode is 50%. After two episodes, the recurrence risk increases to 70% to 90%.

13. The most important factor in predicting suicide is a past history of suicide attempt.

14. Of all the selective serotonin reuptake inhibitors (SSRIs), paroxetine is more likely to cause serotonin discontinuation symptoms because of the way it is metabolized.

15. Venlafaxine is a serotonin and norepinephrine reuptake inhibitor (SNRI).

16. Venlafaxine acts as an SSRI until the dose of 150 mg. A higher dose will inhibit the reuptake of norepinephrine.

17. All patients with depression should be screened for suicide risk.

18. The highest risk for suicide is associated with bipolar depression (20%), followed by major depressive disorder (15%) and schizophrenia (10%).

19. Cognitive behavioral therapy (CBT) has been found to be effective for patients with mild-to-moderate depressive disorders.

20. Dialectical behavioral therapy (DBT) has been found to be effective with patients who repeatedly harm themselves (especially patients who have borderline personality traits).

21. The risk of suicide increases with certain factors such as male gender, age (elderly individuals), physical health problems, chronic pain, lack of social support, access to firearms, and past history of suicide attempt.

22. Women attempt suicide more often than men, but men are more likely to complete suicide.

23. Comorbid alcohol and substance abuse greatly increases the risk of suicide.

24. Electroconvulsive therapy (ECT) is indicated for treatment-resistant depression. The most important predictor of response to ECT is a past history of response to ECT.

25. Vagus nerve stimulation (VNS) was recently approved by the FDA for depression. It is indicated for patients with chronic or recurrent depression who are at least 18 years old, who have a current episode of major depression that has not responded to an adequate trial of at least four different antidepressant treatments.

BRAIN LOBE SYNDROMES

1. In a right-handed person, the left hemisphere is dominant in 90%, and the right hemisphere is dominant in 10%.

2. In a left-handed person, the left hemisphere is dominant in 64%, and the right hemisphere is dominant in 20%. In 16% of individuals, both hemispheres are dominant.

3. Frontal lobe damage results in changes in personality, perseveration; pallilalia, psychomotor retardation, and urinary incontinence.

4. Pallilalia is repetition of phrases and sentences.

5. Lesions in Broca's area result in problems with verbal expression characterized by poor articulation and sparse speech.

6. Lesions in the dominant temporal lobe result in sensory or receptive aphasia.

7. Lesions within Wernicke's area result in problems with decreased verbal comprehension and reading and writing abilities. Speech remains fluent but it is semantically inappropriate.

8. Lesions in the nondominant temporal lobe result in hemisomatognosia, prosognosia, and visuospatial problems.

9. Bilateral medial temporal lobe lesions cause amnesia.

10. Hippocampal lesions result in impaired memory of verbal information.

11. Gerstmann's syndrome is a neurological disorder characterized by a lesion in the dominant parietal lobe, dyscalculia, agraphia, finger agnosia, and right-left disorientation.

12. Features of lesions in the dominant parietal lobe are motor aphasia, sensory aphasia, agraphia, alexia, apraxia, bilateral tactile agnosia, visual agnosia, and Gerstmann's syndrome.

13. Features of lesions in the nondominant parietal lobe are anosognosia, hemisomatognosia, dressing apraxia, and prosopagnosia.

14. Anosognosia is failure to recognize a disabled limb.

15. Prosopagnosia is an inability to recognize faces.

16. Lesions in the dominant occipital lobe result in alexia without agraphia, color agnosia, and visual object agnosia.

17. Lesions in the nondominant occipital lobe result in visuospatial agnosia, prosopagnosia, metamorphosia, and complex visual hallucinations.

18. Metamorphosia is image distortion.

19. Klüver-Bucy syndrome results from bilateral ablation of temporal lobes including the uncus, amygdala, and hippocampus. It is characterized by oral tendencies, placidity, visual agnosia (and sometimes prosopagnosia), altered sexual activity, and hypermetamorphosis.

20. Apraxia is the inability to carry out purposeful voluntary movements, which cannot be accounted for by paresis, incoordination, sensory loss, or involuntary movements.

21. Ideomotor apraxia: lesion in parietotemporal lesions.

22. Ideational apraxia: lesion in temporoparietal.

23. Dressing apraxia: lesion in parietooccipital.

24. Constructional apraxia: lesion in parietooccipital.

25. Agnosia is an impaired recognition of an object despite an intact sensory system.

PSYCHOTHERAPY

1. Sigmund Freud is the author of *Mourning and Melancholia*, *Cocaine Papers*, and *The Psychopathology of Everyday Life*.

2. According to Freud's dream analysis, primary process thinking includes condensation, displacement, and symbolization.

3. Freud proposed three models: affect trauma, topographical, and structural.

4. The structural model is composed of id, ego, and superego.

5. Superego refers to conscience and ideals.

6. Defense mechanisms are functions of ego.

7. The basic defense mechanism is repression.

8. The defense mechanism of projection is associated with paranoia.

9. Homework is typically a part of treatment in cognitive behavioral therapy (CBT).

10. Analysis of transference is important in psychoanalytic psychotherapy.

11. Transference refers to the process whereby a patient displaces onto the analyst his or her feelings and ideas that derive from previous figures in life.

12. Countertransference refers to the therapist's emotional attitude toward the patient, including his or her response to specific forms of the patient's behavior.

13. Winnicott introduced the term, *transitional objects* and has argued, "There is no such thing as a baby."

14. Melanie Klein, a pioneer in child psychoanalysis, coined the term *projective identification.*

15. Brief dynamic therapy has been shown to be effective in treating irritable bowel syndrome.

16. In chronic fatigue syndrome, CBT and graded exercise has been found to be helpful.

17. Ainsworth devised the Strange Situation Test to study the effects of separating primary school-aged children from their parents.

18. John Bowlby contributed extensively to the understanding of attachment behavior.

19. Konrad Lorenz proposed the theory of "imprinting."

20. Joseph Wolpe was the original proponent of systemic desensitization.

21. Alcoholics Anonymous is an example of group therapy.

22. High expressed emotion (EE) in families of patients with schizophrenia is associated with poor prognosis.

23. EE in family members of patients with schizophrenia include criticism, hostility, and emotional overinvolvement.

24. A paradoxical injunction is a technique in psychotherapy in which the presenting symptom is prescribed as the treatment.

25. The ability to become hypnotized depends on the subject's dissociative ability.

PSYCHOPHARMACOLOGY

1. The most annoying side effect associated with clozapine is hypersalivation. The exact cause is not known but is probably related to an impaired swallowing mechanism rather than excessive saliva secretion.

2. Clozapine is sometimes helpful in reversing tardive dyskinesia caused by chronic administration of typical antipsychotics.

3. Pimozide has been found to be most effective in the treatment of delusional disorders.

4. The use of prophylactic anticholinergic drugs to prevent extrapyramidal side effects of neuroleptics is a relative contraindication in the elderly due to the risk of memory problems and delirium.

5. "Rabbit syndrome" is a focal, perioral tremor seen in patients on typical antipsychotics.

6. Thirty percent of patients with major depressive disorder do not respond to the first trial of antidepressant medication.

7. The antidepressants that are known to decrease seizure threshold are bupropion, amoxapine, maprotiline, and trimipramine.

8. SSRIs can cause recurrent flashbacks in post—d-lysergic acid diethylamide (LSD) depression.

9. Drugs are metabolized mainly by oxidation, reduction, hydrolysis, and conjugation.

10. Therapeutic index is the ratio of median toxic dose to the median effective dose.

11. Approximately 7% of Caucasians are considered poor 2D6 metabolizers.

12. Lithium and carbamazepine both can cause hypothyroidism.

13. Carbamazepine is contraindicated in patients taking clozapine because of the additive risk of agranulocytosis.

14. The incidence of clinical hypothyroidism associated with lithium is about 5%.

15. Methadone is a mu opioid receptor agonist.

16. The most serious side effect associated with mirtazapine is agranulocytosis. Therefore, it is contraindicated in patients taking clozapine.

17. Use of lithium during pregnancy is associated with Epstein's anomaly.

18. Age less than 10 years is considered as one of the important risk factors for valproate-induced hepatotoxicity.

19. Citalopram is the most effective SSRI.

20. Low-potency neuroleptics can cause significant orthostatic hypotension. Therefore, these drugs are started at a low dose and are titrated up slowly.

21. All tricyclic antidepressants and many of the antipsychotics can cause prolongation of the QT_c interval.

22. Lithium can cause sinus node dysfunction, especially in the elderly.

23. Disulfiram acts by inhibiting acetaldehyde dehydrogenase enzyme in the liver.

24. Modafinil can decrease the levels of birth control pills and increase the risk of accidental pregnancy.

25. All atypical antipsychotics have been associated with an increased incidence of type II diabetes mellitus.

PERSONALITY DISORDERS

1. Nature and nurture are both thought to be important factors in personality development.

2. There is an increased incidence of schizophrenia in individuals and relatives of people with schizotypal personality disorders.

3. Paranoid ideation is often associated with violent behavior.

4. Antisocial behavior is more common in men, whereas borderline personality traits are more common in women.

5. Common defense mechanisms seen in individuals with borderline personality disorder are splitting, denial, projection, projective identification, and acting out.

FORENSIC PSYCHIATRY

1. *Mens rea* implies capacity to form intent to do harm.

2. A physician who treats a patient without obtaining informed consent may be charged with battery.

3. Under certain circumstances, breach of confidentiality is allowed by law (e.g., duty to warn).

4. The most common reason for malpractice lawsuits against psychiatrists is related to suicide/suicide attempts.

5. Pathological jealously is often associated with homicide followed by suicide.

6. Although a majority of individuals who commit crimes do not have mental illness, those with mental retardation are often involved in arson.

7. Command hallucinations in schizophrenia are associated with an increased risk of violence.

8. A past history of violence is the most important predictor of future violence.

9. Testamentary capacity is the capacity to make a legal will.

10. Autonomy is a patient's right to self-determination.

11. Beneficence is the physician's duty to act in the best interests of his or her patients.

12. Medical malpractice cases fall into two categories: intentional torts and unintentional torts.

13. The American Psychiatry Association rules that, "once a patient, always a patient." It is unethical to have a sexual relationship with a current or a former patient.

14. The Health Insurance Portability and Accountability Act (HIPPA) is a federal law that deals with privacy protection in clinical care and research.

15. The Health Care Quality Improvement Act (HCQIA) of 1986 makes it mandatory to report any actions taken by any state board on medical licensure, any payments made in malpractice claims, and any adverse actions taken by health care entities.

PSYCHIATRIC EMERGENCIES

1. Women attempt suicide twice as often as men.

2. Men complete suicide at a rate four times that of women.

3. History of suicide attempt is more common in women than in men, with a gender ratio of 2:1.

4. Firearms are now the leading method of suicide in women, as well as men.

5. The suicide rates for men rise with age, most significantly after age 65.

6. The rate of suicide in men 65+ years old is seven times that of women in the same age group.

7. Women often attempt suicide after interpersonal loss or crises in significant social or family relationships.

8. Two thirds of those who die by suicide suffer from a depressive illness.

9. Thirty percent of all depressed inpatients attempt suicide.

10. Ninety percent of all people who die by suicide have a diagnosable psychiatric disorder at the time of their death.

11. Suicide is the fifth leading cause of death among those 5 to 14 years old.

12. Suicide is the third leading cause of death among those 15 to 24 years old.

13. Most people who are violent are not mentally ill, and most people who are mentally ill are not violent.

14. Alcohol abuse/dependence is associated with up to 12 times increased risk of violence compared to the general population.

15. Past history of violence is the most reliable predictor of future violence.

PARAPHILIAS

1. Exhibitionism is the recurrent urge or behavior to expose one's genitals to an unsuspecting person.

2. Fetishism is the use of inanimate objects to gain sexual excitement.

3. Frotteurism is the recurrent urges or behavior of touching or rubbing against a nonconsenting person.

4. Pedophilia is sexual attraction toward prepubescent or peripubescent children.

5. Sexual masochism is the recurrent urge or behavior of wanting to be humiliated, beaten, bound, or otherwise made to suffer for sexual pleasure.

6. Sexual sadism is the recurrent urge or behavior involving acts in which the pain or humiliation of a person is sexually exciting.

7. A transvestite is the sexual attraction, usually of a man toward the clothing and behavior of the opposite gender.

8. Voyeurism is the recurrent urge or behavior to observe an unsuspecting person who is naked, disrobing, or engaging in sexual activities.

9. Zoophilia (or bestiality) is the recurrent urge or behavior of sex with animals.

10. Coprophilia is deriving sexual pleasure from feces.

11. Klismaphilia is deriving sexual pleasure from enemas.

12. Urophilia is sexual pleasure from urine or urinating on others.

13. Emetophilia is deriving sexual pleasure by vomiting or observing others vomiting.

14. Paraphilias almost always occur in males.

15. There is a strong association between paraphilias and substance abuse, depression, and phobic disorders.

ANTIDOTES

1. Benzodiazepines: flumazenil

2. Tricyclic antidepressants: sodium bicarbonate

3. Anticholinergic overdose: physostigmine

4. Beta-blocker overdose: glucagon

5. Carbon monoxide poisoning : oxygen

6. Heparin overdose: protamine

7. Iron poisoning: deferoxamine

8. Isoniazid overdose: pyridoxine

9. Methanol poisoning: ethanol

10. Methemoglobinemia: methylene blue

11. Opiate overdose: naloxone

12. Acetaminophen overdose: N-acetylcysteine

13. Thallium poisoning: Prussian blue

14. Warfarin overdose: vitamin K and fresh frozen plasma

15. Calcium channel blockers overdose: calcium

16. Cholinergics overdose: atropine, pralidoxime

17. Digoxin overdose: digoxin Fab antibodies

TIME CRITERIA FOR DSM-IV DIAGNOSIS

1. Adjustment disorder occurs within 3 months of stressor and lasts less than 6 months.

2. Major depressive disorder: 2 weeks

3. Manic episode: 1 week

4. Bipolar I: one or more manic or mixed episodes

5. Bipolar II: at least one hypomanic episode and one or more major depressive episodes

6. Hypomania: 4 days

7. Recurrent brief depressive disorder: at least 2 days but less than 2 weeks. At least once a month for 12 months, unrelated to menses

8. Minor depressive disorder: At least 2 weeks, but there are two to five symptoms

9. Cyclothymia: greater than 2 years of alternating hypomania and depression

10. Dysthymia: depressed mood for at least 2 years with no major depressive disorder episode at onset and no hypomania/mania. In children, at least 1 year. Early onset if <21 years of age; late onset if >21 years of age.

11. Mixed episode: mania and major depression for more than 1 week

12. Generalized anxiety disorder: at least 6 months

13. Acute stress disorder: 2 days to 4 weeks and within 1 month of event

14. Tourette's syndrome vocal and motor tics >1 year, < age 18

15. Transient tic disorder—vocal and/or motor tics <1 year, < age 18, >4 weeks

16. Chronic tic disorder—vocal or motor tics >1year, < age 18

17. Tic disorder not otherwise specified <4 weeks or onset > age 18

18. Conduct disorder: three criteria in past 12 months and age <18 years

19. Oppositional defiance disorder (ODD): 6 months and age <18 years.

20. Schizophrenia: at least 6 months with 1 month of symptoms

21. Schizophreniform disorder: 1 to 6 months

22. Schizoaffective disorder: delusions or hallucinations in the absence of mood symptoms for at least 2 weeks

23. Delusional disorder: nonbizarre delusions for greater than 1 month

24. Brief psychotic disorder: minimum of 1 day but less than 1month

25. Paraphilias: at least 6 months

PHOBIAS

1. Amaxophobia: fear of riding in a car

2. Cynophobia: fear of dogs

3. Ailurophobia: fear of cats

4. Xenophobia: fear of strangers or foreign people

5. Mysophobia: fear of dirt or germs

6. Agoraphobia: fear of open spaces or of being in crowded, public places

7. Acrophobia: fear of heights

8. Necrophobia: fear of death or dead things

9. Mnemophobia: fear of memories

10. Nosophobia: fear of becoming ill

11. Oneirophobia: fear of dreams

12. Ornithophobia: fear of birds

13. Paraphobia: fear of sexual perversion

14. Pteromerhanophobia: fear of flying

15. Pyrophobia: fear of fire

16. Rupophobia: fear of dirt

17. Thanatophobia: fear of death or dying

18. Zelophobia: fear of jealousy

19. Zoophobia: fear of animals

20. Dystychiphobia: fear of accidents

21. Algophobia: fear of pain

22. Agliophobia: fear of pain

23. Carnophobia: fear of meat

24. Hominophobia: fear of men

25. Isolophobia: fear of solitude

26. Pedophobia: fear of children

27. Scoleciphobia: fear of worms

SYNDROMES ASSOCIATED WITH SPECIFIC CULTURES

1. Koro: Intense anxiety about retraction of one's genitalia leading to attachment of devices to prevent imagined retraction. Often seen in China and Malaysia.

2. Latah: Characterized by echo phenomenon (e.g., echolalia, echopraxia) following a sudden stimulus that causes a startle response. Seen in Indonesia and Malaysia.

3. Amok: Sudden, unprovoked rage leading to the bizarre attacking or killing of people or animals until the person is overpowered by authorities or commits suicide. Seen in Malaysia and Indonesia.

4. Piblokto: Episodes of screaming associated with bizarre behavior including tearing clothes off, running, and rolling over on ice. Seen in Eskimos.

5. Bouffée délirante: Sudden episodes of agitation, aggression, and confusion seen in West Africa and Haiti.

6. Susto: Loss of soul following a frightening event. Seen in Latinos.

7. Taijin kyofusho: Phobic belief that one's body parts embarrass or displease others. Seen in Japan.

8. Dhat: Anxiety associated with the belief that semen is being passed in urine. Seen in Indian subcontinent.

9. Mal de ojo: Crying without a reason, vomiting, and diarrhea. The symptoms are thought to be due to the "evil eye." Seen in Mediterranean cultures.

10. Shenjing shuairuo: Physical and mental fatigue, headaches, problems with concentration, memory, and sleep. Seen in China.

MISCELLANEOUS

1. Capgras' syndrome: Delusion that imposters have replaced familiar people

2. Fregoli's syndrome: Delusion that a persecutor is taking on a variety of faces

3. Cotard's syndrome: Delusion of negation (i.e., belief of losing everything)

4. De Clerambault's syndrome: Erotomania

5. Othello syndrome: Pathological jealousy

6. Medications are one of the most common causes of delirium in the elderly.

7. Left frontal lesions are most commonly associated with depression.

8. Right temporal lesions are most commonly associated with mania.

9. Women are six times more likely than men to be victims of domestic violence by their partners.

10. Violence in homosexual couples is as common as in heterosexual couples.

11. Perpetrators of domestic violence often tend to have low self-esteem.

12. The hypothalamus, limbic system, and prefrontal cortex have all been implicated in the neurobiology of aggression.

13. Pregnancy is a high-risk period for battering.

14. Conversion disorder is the most common form of somatoform disorder.

15. Binge eating disorder is more common than anorexia nervosa.

16. Sleep paralysis is seen not only in patients with narcolepsy but also in sleep deprivation and in people without any sleep problems.

17. Cataplexy is specific to narcolepsy and it is not seen in any other conditions.

18. Rapid eye movement sleep behavior disorder is when a person acts out dream content.

19. Restless legs syndrome (RLS) is a clinical diagnosis, which usually does not require an overnight polysomnogram.

20. About one third of patients with RLS have periodic limb movement disorder, whereas more than two thirds of patients with periodic limb movement disorder have RLS.

Psychiatry Factoids

SUBSTANCE ABUSE

1. Opiates

   SYMPTOMS OF INTOXICATION

   Miosis

   Pruritus

   Bradycardia

   Constipation

   Anorexia

   Decreased libido

   Slurred speech

   Impaired attention/concentration

   Impaired memory

   SYMPTOMS OF WITHDRAWAL

   Pupillary dilation

   Piloerection

   Sweating

   Diarrhea

   Yawning

   Lacrimation

   Rhinorrhea

   Insomnia

2. Amphetamines and Cocaine

   SYMPTOMS OF INTOXICATION

   Mydriasis

   Halitosis

Impotence

Delirium

Seizures

SYMPTOMS OF WITHDRAWAL

Dysphoria

Fatigue

Insomnia

Agitation

Craving

3. Benzodiazepines

SYMPTOMS OF INTOXICATION

Sedation

Slurred speech

Incoordination

Unsteady gait

Impaired memory or attention

Central nervous system depression

Respiratory depression

SYMPTOMS OF WITHDRAWAL

Nausea and vomiting

Autonomic hyperactivity

Anxiety

Tremor

Hyperreflexes

Insomnia

Seizures

4. Phencyclidine (PCP)

SYMPTOMS OF INTOXICATION

Mydriasis

Ataxia

Downbeating nystagmus

Hyperacusis

Seizures

Agitation

Aggression

5. Hydrocarbons

SYMPTOMS OF INTOXICATION

Odor on breath

Tachycardia

Ventricular tachycardia

6. Belladonna Alkaloids

SYMPTOMS OF INTOXICATION

Mydriasis

Hypertension

Dry mouth

Urinary retention

7. Gamma hydroxybutyrate (GHB)

SYMPTOMS OF INTOXICATION

Bradycardia

Hypothermia

Coma (resolves rapidly with prompt return to alertness)

Amnesia of recent events

8. Hallucinogens

SYMPTOMS OF INTOXICATION

Mydriasis

Ataxia

Table 30.1.   Typical Antipsychotics

Agent	Potency	Sedative Properties	Anticholinergic Properties	Extrapyramidal Side Effects
Chlorpromazine	Low	High	Medium	Low
Thioridazine	Low	High	High	Low
Fluphenazine	High	Medium	Low	High
Haloperidol	High	Low	Low	High
Pimozide	High	Low	Low	High

Table 30.2.   Atypical Antipsychotics

Agent	5-HT Receptor Antagonism	Dopamine Receptor Antagonism	Important Side Effects	Weight Gain
Clozapine	$5\text{-}HT_{2A}$	D_1, D_3, D_4	Agranulocytosis	High
Risperidone	$5\text{-}HT_{2A}$	D_2	Prolactin, Extrapyramidal symptoms (EPS)	Moderate
Olanzapine	$5\text{-}HT_{2A}$	D_1, D_2, D_4	Weight gain	High
Quetiapine	$5\text{-}HT_2$, $5\text{-}HT_6$	D_1, D_2	Somnolence	Moderate
Ziprasidone	$5\text{-}HT_{2A}$, $5\text{-}HT_{1D}$, $5\text{-}HT_{2C}$	D_2, D_3, D_4	Insomnia	Minimal or no weight gain
Aripiprazole	$5\text{-}HT_{2A}$ partial agonist at the $5\text{-}HT_{1A}$	Partial agonist at D_2 receptors	Nausea, vomiting	Minimal or no weight gain

Agent	Sedation	Weight Gain
Imipramine	Moderate	Moderate
Desipramine	Mild	Mild
Amitriptyline	High	High
Nortriptyline	Moderate	Mild
Protriptyline	Moderate	Mild
Trimipramine	High	High
Doxepin	High	High
Maprotiline	High	Moderate
Amoxapine	Moderate	Mild
Trazodone	Moderate	Mild
Fluoxetine	Mild	None/Mild
Bupropion-SR	Mild	None/Mild
Bupropion	Mild	None/Mild
Sertraline	Mild	None/Mild
Paroxetine	Mild	None/Mild
Venlafaxine-XR	Mild	None/Mild
Venlafaxine	Mild	None/Mild
Nefazodone	Moderate	None/Mild
Fluvoxamine	Mild	None/Mild
Mirtazapine	Moderate	High
Phenelzine	Mild	Moderate
Tranylcypromine	Mild	Mild

Table 30.3. Antidepressants: Sedation and Weight Gain

Table 30.4.	Antidepressants and CYP 450 Enzymes
Agent	**CYP 450 Enzymes Inhibited**
Fluoxetine	2C9 (moderate)
	2C19 (minimal)
	2D6 (significant)
	3A4 (moderate)
Sertraline	2C9 (significant)
	2D6 (moderate)
	3A4 (moderate)
Paroxetine	2D6 (significant)
	3A4 (minimal)
Nefazodone	3A4 (significant)
Citalopram	Minimal inhibition of CYP enzymes
Escitalopram	Minimal inhibition of CYP enzymes

Index

In this index, *italic* page numbers designate figures; page numbers followed by the letter "t" designate tables; *(see also)* cross-references designate related topics or more detailed subtopic breakdowns.